Immunohistochemical Expression

Immunohistochemical Expression

Editors

Rosario Caltabiano
Carla Loreto

MDPI • Basel • Beijing • Wuhan • Barcelona • Belgrade • Manchester • Tokyo • Cluj • Tianjin

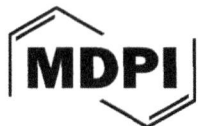

Editors
Rosario Caltabiano
University of Catania
Italy

Carla Loreto
University of Catania
Italy

Editorial Office
MDPI
St. Alban-Anlage 66
4052 Basel, Switzerland

This is a reprint of articles from the Special Issue published online in the open access journal *Applied Sciences* (ISSN 2076-3417) (available at: https://www.mdpi.com/journal/applsci/special_issues/Immunohistochemical_Expression).

For citation purposes, cite each article independently as indicated on the article page online and as indicated below:

LastName, A.A.; LastName, B.B.; LastName, C.C. Article Title. *Journal Name* **Year**, *Volume Number*, Page Range.

ISBN 978-3-0365-0400-1 (Hbk)
ISBN 978-3-0365-0401-8 (PDF)

© 2021 by the authors. Articles in this book are Open Access and distributed under the Creative Commons Attribution (CC BY) license, which allows users to download, copy and build upon published articles, as long as the author and publisher are properly credited, which ensures maximum dissemination and a wider impact of our publications.

The book as a whole is distributed by MDPI under the terms and conditions of the Creative Commons license CC BY-NC-ND.

Contents

About the Editors vii

Carla Loreto and Rosario Caltabiano
Immunohistochemical Expression
Reprinted from: *Appl. Sci.* **2021**, *11*, 360, doi:10.3390/app11010360 1

Lidia Puzzo, Giuliana Giunta, Rosario Caltabiano, Antonio Cianci and Lucia Salvatorelli
Fetal Megacystis: A New Morphologic, Immunohistological and Embriogenetic Approach
Reprinted from: *Appl. Sci.* **2019**, *9*, 5155, doi:10.3390/app9235155 5

**Rosario Caltabiano, Paola Castrogiovanni, Ignazio Barbagallo, Silvia Ravalli,
Marta Anna Szychlinska, Vincenzo Favilla, Luigi Schiavo, Rosa Imbesi,
Giuseppe Musumeci and Michelino Di Rosa**
Identification of Novel Markers of Prostate Cancer Progression, Potentially Modulated by
Vitamin D
Reprinted from: *Appl. Sci.* **2019**, *9*, 4923, doi:10.3390/app9224923 15

**Saleh A. Almatroodi, Mohammed A. Alsahli, Hanan Marzoq Alharbi, Amjad Ali Khan and
Arshad Husain Rahmani**
Epigallocatechin-3-Gallate (EGCG), An Active Constituent of Green Tea: Implications in the
Prevention of Liver Injury Induced by Diethylnitrosamine (DEN) in Rats
Reprinted from: *Appl. Sci.* **2019**, *9*, 4821, doi:10.3390/app9224821 33

**Alessandro Pitruzzella, Letizia Paladino, Alessandra Maria Vitale, Stefania Martorana,
Calogero Cipolla, Giuseppa Graceffa, Daniela Cabibi, Sabrina David, Alberto Fucarino,
Fabio Bucchieri, Francesco Cappello, Everly Conway de Macario, Alberto JL Macario and
Francesca Rappa**
Quantitative Immunomorphological Analysis of Heat Shock Proteins in Thyroid Follicular
Adenoma and Carcinoma Tissues Reveals Their Potential for Differential Diagnosis and Points
to a Role in Carcinogenesis
Reprinted from: *Appl. Sci.* **2019**, *9*, 4324, doi:10.3390/app9204324 49

**Blanka Stiburkova, Jana Bohata, Iveta Minarikova, Andrea Mancikova, Jiri Vavra,
Vladimír Krylov and Zdenek Doležel**
Clinical and Functional Characterization of a Novel URAT1 Dysfunctional Variant in a Pediatric
Patient with Renal Hypouricemia
Reprinted from: *Appl. Sci.* **2019**, *9*, 3479, doi:10.3390/app9173479 61

**Lucia Salvatorelli, Lidia Puzzo, Giovanni Bartoloni, Stefano Palmucci, Antonio Longo,
Andrea Russo, Michele Reibaldi, Manlio Vinciguerra, Giovanni Li Volti and
Rosario Caltabiano**
Immunoexpression of Macroh2a in Uveal Melanoma
Reprinted from: *Appl. Sci.* **2019**, *9*, 3244, doi:10.3390/app9163244 69

**Giuseppe Broggi, Giuseppe Musumeci, Lidia Puzzo, Andrea Russo, Michele Reibaldi,
Marco Ragusa, Antonio Longo and Rosario Caltabiano**
Immunohistochemical Expression of ABCB5 as a Potential Prognostic Factor in
Uveal Melanoma
Reprinted from: *Appl. Sci.* **2019**, *9*, 1316, doi:10.3390/app9071316 79

Michelino Di Rosa, Paola Castrogiovanni, Francesca Maria Trovato, Lorenzo Malatino, Silvia Ravalli, Rosa Imbesi, Marta Anna Szychlinska and Giuseppe Musumeci
Adapted Moderate Training Exercise Decreases the Expression of Ngal in the Rat Kidney: An Immunohistochemical Study
Reprinted from: *Appl. Sci.* **2019**, *9*, 1041, doi:10.3390/app9061041 . . . . **91**

Lucia Salvatorelli, Giovanna Calabrese, Rosalba Parenti, Giada Maria Vecchio, Lidia Puzzo, Rosario Caltabiano, Giuseppe Musumeci and Gaetano Magro
Immunohistochemical Expression of Wilms' Tumor 1 Protein in Human Tissues: From Ontogenesis to Neoplastic Tissues
Reprinted from: *Appl. Sci.* **2020**, *10*, 40, doi:10.3390/app10010040 . . . . **105**

Logan Herm, Ardit Haxhia, Flavio de Alcantara Camejo, Lobat Tayebi and Luis Eduardo Almeida
Matrix Metalloproteinases and Temporomandibular Joint Disorder: A Review of the Literature
Reprinted from: *Appl. Sci.* **2019**, *9*, 4508, doi:10.3390/app9214508 . . . . **133**

Cristian Bogdan Iancu, Mugurel Constantin Rusu, Laurenţiu Mogoantă, Sorin Hostiuc and Oana Daniela Toader
The Telocytes in the Subepicardial Niche
Reprinted from: *Appl. Sci.* **2019**, *9*, 1615, doi:10.3390/app9081615 . . . . **143**

About the Editors

Rosario Caltabiano is an Associate Professor in the Department G.F. Ingrassia Section of Anatomic Pathology at the University of Catania. He is responsible for dermatopathological diagnostics and is a lecturer in the medical and dentistry courses at the University of Catania. His total scientific production includes more than 180 scientific publications (citation number greater than 2400). He has an h-index of 27. He has carried out his research activity in the scientific disciplinary sector MED/08 continuously since 1996. In 1998, he graduated in Medicine and Surgery; in 2002, he specialized in Dermatology; and in 2007, he specialized in Surgical Pathology. The research activity was mainly oriented to dermatopathology and neuropathology.

Carla Loreto is group leader of the "Organ Functional Anatomy" laboratory in the Anatomy and Histology Section of the Department of Biomedical and Biotechnological Sciences at the University of Catania. She was also responsible in her own laboratory for the practical training activities in microscopic anatomy of the students of the first year of the degree course Biomedical Laboratory Techniques of the same university, from 2012 to 2015. Her total scientific production includes more than 170 scientific publications related to the insolvency sector (citation number greater than 3100). She has an h-index of 24. She has carried out her research activity in the scientific disciplinary sector BIO/16 continuously since 1996 when she was already an internal student at the Institute of Human Anatomy, University of Catania. In 1998, she graduated in Medicine and Surgery and in 2002, she specialized in Occupational Medicine, always with the highest marks and honors; these medical studies have left a significant imprint on her scientific career. The research activity was mainly oriented to the functional anatomy of organs, also paying attention to the microscopic and biomolecular aspects.

Editorial

Immunohistochemical Expression

Carla Loreto [1] and Rosario Caltabiano [2],*

[1] Department of Biomedical and Biotechnological Sciences Section of Anatomy and Histology, University of Catania, Santa Sofia street 87, 95123 Catania, Italy; carla.loreto@unict.it
[2] Department G.F. Ingrassia–Section of Anatomic Pathology, University of Catania, Santa Sofia street 87, 95123 Catania, Italy
* Correspondence: rosario.caltabiano@unict.it; Tel.: +39-095-378-2003

Received: 17 December 2020; Accepted: 30 December 2020; Published: 1 January 2021

1. Introduction

Immunohistochemistry (IHC) is an ancillary method, widely used in pathologist practice, that allows to identify diagnostic and prognostic/predictive therapeutic response protein markers on tissue samples by the use of specific monoclonal antibodies and chromogenic substances that guarantee the visualization of the antibody–antigen binding complex under the light microscope [1]. Coon et al. in 1941 [2] first introduced the use of fluorochrome-conjugated antibodies in clinical practice. Since then, IHC has gone from being a useful tool for identifying the differentiation line of otherwise undifferentiated cells, to a technique capable of providing not only diagnostic but also prognostic and predictive indications of response to specific therapeutic options [1,3]. The aforementioned peculiarities have made IHC one of the most used ancillary methods in the histopathological approach to human neoplastic and non-neoplastic diseases [3–5].

This Special Issue contains 11 accepted papers that provide readers with a comprehensive update on the current and future applications of IHC in medical practice.

2. Diagnostic Applications of Immunohistochemistry

The detection on tissue specimens of protein markers capable of identifying the differentiation line (melanocytic, epithelial, neural, mesenchymal or lymphoproliferative) of poorly differentiated tumors is undoubtedly one of the major advantages of IHC [3]; since its introduction, it has represented a valid diagnostic tool that, combined to the "evergreen" morphology, allowed pathologists to formulate a more accurate diagnosis of neoplasms, previously labeled as "undifferentiated" [3]. Furthermore, the increasing knowledge about the genetic landscape of human neoplasms has allowed the identification of specific genes, deriving from molecular alterations and encoding proteins, whose expression was restricted to a specific cancer type [3]; such proteins could be easily targeted by IHC, greatly improving the diagnostic accuracy of neoplasms that harbored specific molecular alterations, such as solitary fibrous tumor (SFT) [6] or glioblastoma multiforme (GBM) [7].

3. Prognostic and Predictive Value of Immunohistochemistry

However, the major clinical impact of IHC is not in the diagnostic field but that of providing the oncologist with essential prognostic and predictive information of therapeutic response [3]. The aforementioned application field of IHC was born with the introduction in clinical practice of the immunohistochemical detection of Hormone Receptors (estrogen and progesterone receptors) and HER-2/neu in the diagnostic approach to breast cancer [8,9]; in this regard, the "molecular" classification of breast cancer (Luminal A vs. Luminal B vs. HER-2/neu vs. Basal-like), based on the different combinations of Hormone Receptor and HER-2/neu immunoexpression has almost replaced the morphological one, since the former was able to select specific patient subgroups with a similar outcome and potential candidates to "personalized" treatments [8,9].

The search for new prognostic factors, promptly identifiable by IHC, has been and still is particularly intense in the field of rare malignancies with poor prognosis. In recent years, our research group reported some immunohistochemical markers with prognostic significance in terms of overall survival, disease-free survival and risk of distant metastasis in rare and prognostically poor tumors, such as uveal melanoma (UM) [10–15] and malignant mesothelioma (MM) [16–19].

4. Future Perspectives

The introduction of new molecular tests, including fluorescence in situ hybridization (FISH), real-time polymerase chain reaction (rt-PCR) or next generation sequencing (NGS) has not replaced IHC, that, due to its low costs and its immediate applicability, remains the most used first level test [3]. The 11 published papers included within this Special Issue provide the scientific community with new potential application fields of IHC in human neoplastic and non-neoplastic diseases, emphasizing the concept that the identification of new factors capable of predicting the biological behavior of diseases must represent a direction to follow in medical scientific research.

Author Contributions: C.L. and R.C. made a substantial, direct and intellectual contribution to the work, and approved it for publication. Both authors have read and agreed to the published version of the manuscript.

Funding: This research received no external funding.

Conflicts of Interest: The authors declare no conflict of interest.

References

1. Sukswai, N.; Khoury, J.D. Immunohistochemistry Innovations for Diagnosis and Tissue-Based Biomarker Detection. *Curr. Hematol. Malig. Rep.* **2019**, *14*, 368–375. [CrossRef] [PubMed]
2. Coons, A.H.; Creech, H.J.; Jones, R.N. Immunological properties of an antibody containing a fluorescent group. *Proc. Soc. Exp. Biol. Med.* **1941**, *47*, 200–202. [CrossRef]
3. Broggi, G.; Salvatorelli, L. Bio-Pathological Markers in the Diagnosis and Therapy of Cancer. *Cancers* **2020**, *12*, 3113. [CrossRef] [PubMed]
4. Castorina, S.; Lombardo, C.; Castrogiovanni, P.; Musumeci, G.; Barbato, E.; Almeida, L.E.; Leonardi, R. P53 and VEGF expression in human temporomandibular joint discs with internal derangement correlate with degeneration. *J. Biol. Regul. Homeost. Agents* **2019**, *33*, 1657–1662. [CrossRef] [PubMed]
5. Loreto, C.; Lombardo, C.; Caltabiano, R.; Filetti, V.; Vitale, E.; Seminara, D.; Castorina, S.; Fenga, C.; Ledda, C.; Rapisarda, V. Immunohistochemical expression and localization of MMP-9, MMP-13, E-Cadherin and Ki-67 in road pavers' skin chronically exposed to bitumen products. *Histol. Histopathol.* **2019**, *34*, 1141–1150. [CrossRef] [PubMed]
6. Magro, G.; Salvatorelli, L.; Puzzo, L.; Piombino, E.; Bartoloni, G.; Broggi, G.; Vecchio, G.M. Practical approach to diagnosis of bland-looking spindle cell lesions of the breast. *Pathologica* **2019**, *111*, 344–360. [CrossRef] [PubMed]
7. Certo, F.; Altieri, R.; Maione, M.; Schonauer, C.; Sortino, G.; Fiumanò, G.; Tirrò, E.; Massimino, M.; Broggi, G.; Vigneri, P.; et al. FLAIRectomy in Supramarginal Resection of Glioblastoma Correlates with Clinical Outcome and Survival Analysis: A Prospective, Single Institution, Case Series. *Oper. Neurosurg.* **2020**, opaa293. [CrossRef] [PubMed]
8. Cammarata, F.P.; Forte, G.I.; Broggi, G.; Bravatà, V.; Minafra, L.; Pisciotta, P.; Calvaruso, M.; Tringali, R.; Tomasello, B.; Torrisi, F.; et al. Molecular Investigation on a Triple Negative Breast Cancer Xenograft Model Exposed to Proton Beams. *Int. J. Mol. Sci.* **2020**, *21*, 6337. [CrossRef] [PubMed]
9. Broggi, G.; Filetti, V.; Ieni, A.; Rapisarda, V.; Ledda, C.; Vitale, E.; Varricchio, S.; Russo, D.; Lombardo, C.; Tuccari, G.; et al. MacroH2A1 Immunoexpression in Breast Cancer. *Front. Oncol.* **2020**, *10*, 1519. [CrossRef] [PubMed]
10. Caltabiano, R.; Puzzo, L.; Barresi, V.; Ieni, A.; Loreto, C.; Musumeci, G.; Castrogiovanni, P.; Ragusa, M.; Foti, P.; Russo, A.; et al. ADAM 10 expression in primary uveal melanoma as prognostic factor for risk of metastasis. *Pathol. Res. Pract.* **2016**, *212*, 980–987. [CrossRef] [PubMed]

11. Salvatorelli, L.; Puzzo, L.; Bartoloni, G.; Palmucci, S.; Longo, A.; Russo, A.; Reibaldi, M.; Vinciguerra, M.; Li Volti, G.; Caltabiano, R. Immunoexpression of Macroh2a in Uveal Melanoma. *Appl. Sci.* **2019**, *9*, 3244. [CrossRef]
12. Broggi, G.; Musumeci, G.; Puzzo, L.; Russo, A.; Reibaldi, M.; Ragusa, M.; Longo, A.; Caltabiano, R. Immunohistochemical Expression of ABCB5 as a Potential Prognostic Factor in Uveal Melanoma. *Appl. Sci.* **2019**, *9*, 1316. [CrossRef]
13. Russo, D.; Di Crescenzo, R.M.; Broggi, G.; Merolla, F.; Martino, F.; Varricchio, S.; Ilardi, G.; Borzillo, A.; Carandente, R.; Pignatiello, S.; et al. Expression of P16INK4a in Uveal Melanoma: New Perspectives. *Front. Oncol.* **2020**, *10*, 562074. [CrossRef]
14. Broggi, G.; Russo, A.; Reibaldi, M.; Russo, D.; Varricchio, S.; Bonfiglio, V.; Spatola, C.; Barbagallo, C.; Foti, P.V.; Avitabile, T.; et al. Histopathology and Genetic Biomarkers of Choroidal Melanoma. *Appl. Sci.* **2020**, *10*, 8081. [CrossRef]
15. Broggi, G.; Ieni, A.; Russo, D.; Varricchio, S.; Puzzo, L.; Russo, A.; Reibaldi, M.; Longo, A.; Tuccari, G.; Staibano, S.; et al. The Macro-Autophagy-Related Protein Beclin-1 Immunohistochemical Expression Correlates with Tumor Cell Type and Clinical Behavior of Uveal Melanoma. *Front. Oncol.* **2020**, *10*, 589849. [CrossRef] [PubMed]
16. Loreto, C.; Ledda, C.; Tumino, R.; Lombardo, C.; Vitale, E.; Filetti, V.; Caltabiano, R.; Rapisarda, V. Activation of caspase-3 in malignant mesothelioma induced by asbestiform fiber: An in vivo study. *J. Biol. Regul. Homeost. Agents.* **2020**, *34*, 1163–1166. [CrossRef] [PubMed]
17. Filetti, V.; Vitale, E.; Broggi, G.; Hagnäs, M.P.; Candido, S.; Spina, A.; Lombardo, C. Update of in vitro, in vivo and ex vivo fluoro-edenite effects on malignant mesothelioma: A systematic review (Review). *Biomed. Rep.* **2020**, *13*, 60. [CrossRef] [PubMed]
18. Loreto, C.; Caltabiano, R.; Graziano, A.C.E.; Castorina, S.; Lombardo, C.; Filetti, V.; Vitale, E.; Rapisarda, G.; Cardile, V.; Ledda, C.; et al. Defense and protection mechanisms in lung exposed to asbestiform fiber: The role of macrophage migration inhibitory factor and heme oxygenase-1. *Eur. J. Histochem.* **2020**, *64*, 3073. [CrossRef] [PubMed]
19. Loreto, C.; Lombardo, C.; Caltabiano, R.; Ledda, C.; Hagnas, M.; Filetti, V.; Rapisarda, V. An in vivo immunohistochemical study on MacroH2A.1 in lung and lymph-node tissues exposed to an asbestiform fiber. *Curr. Mol. Med.* **2020**, *20*. [CrossRef] [PubMed]

Publisher's Note: MDPI stays neutral with regard to jurisdictional claims in published maps and institutional affiliations.

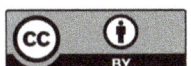

© 2021 by the authors. Licensee MDPI, Basel, Switzerland. This article is an open access article distributed under the terms and conditions of the Creative Commons Attribution (CC BY) license (http://creativecommons.org/licenses/by/4.0/).

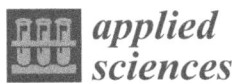

Article

Fetal Megacystis: A New Morphologic, Immunohistological and Embriogenetic Approach

Lidia Puzzo [1,*], Giuliana Giunta [2], Rosario Caltabiano [1], Antonio Cianci [2] and Lucia Salvatorelli [1]

[1] Department of Medical and Surgical Sciences and Advanced Technologies, G.F. Ingrassia, Azienda Ospedaliero-Universitaria "Policlinico-Vittorio Emanuele", Anatomic Pathology Section, School of Medicine, University of Catania, 95123 Catania, Italy; rosario.caltabiano@unict.it (R.C.); lucia.salvatorelli@unict.it (L.S.)

[2] Department of General Surgery and Medical Surgical Specialties, Department of Obstetrics and Gynecology-Policlinico Universitario G. Rodolico, University of Catania, 95123 Catania, Italy; giuntagiuliana.ct@gmail.com (G.G.); acianci@unict.it (A.C.)

* Correspondence: lipuzzo@unict.it; Tel.: +39-095-3782026; Fax: +39-095-3782023

Received: 23 September 2019; Accepted: 26 October 2019; Published: 28 November 2019

Abstract: Congenital anomalies of the kidney and urinary tract (CAKUT) include isolated kidney malformations and urinary tract malformations. They have also been reported in Prune-Belly syndrome (PBS) and associated genetic syndromes, mainly 13, 18 and 21 trisomy. The AA focuses on bladder and urethral malformations, evaluating the structural and histological differences between two different cases of megacystis. Both bladders were examined by routine prenatal ultrasound screening and immunohistochemistry, comparing the different expression of smooth muscular actin (SMA), S100 protein and WT1c in megacystis and bladders of normal control from fetuses of XXI gestational age. Considering the relationship between the enteric nervous system and urinary tract development, the AA evaluated S100 and WT1c expression both in bladder and bowel muscular layers. Both markers were not expressed in the bladder and bowel of PBS associated with anencephaly. In conclusion, megacystis could be considered only a macroscopic definition, concerning the size of the fetal bladder rather than the embryologic origin; it may be a single or multiple malformation; the possible association with the bowel and/or encephalic malformations will decide the outcome and prognosis in fetal megacystis.

Keywords: immunohistochemistry; urinary tract malformations; megacystis; enteric nervous system; outcome and prognosis

1. Introduction

Congenital anomalies of the kidney and urinary tract (CAKUT) are the most common congenital malformations, with a frequency of 3–6 per 1000 live births. They include: isolated kidney malformations (agenesis, hypo-dysplasia, multicystic renal disease, ureteropelvic junction obstruction) and urinary tract malformations (megaureters, megacystis, posterior urethral valve (PUV), urethral atresia/obstruction, urogenital sinus and cloacal malformations, obstructive ureterocele). CAKUT have also been reported in Prune-Belly syndrome (PBS) and associated genetic syndromes, mainly 13, 18 and 21 trisomy [1].

The fetal bladder may be viewed and evaluated by ultrasound from the 12th gestational week, as a pelvic, oval, anechogen structure less than 6 mm of sagittal diameter.

An increased sagittal diameter of the fetal bladder has been considered as megacystis, regardless of etiologic factors and macroscopic features. Therefore, prenatal megacystis may be considered mainly an ultrasound diagnosis [1,2].

We aimed to evaluate the structural and histological differences between two megacystis diagnosed by routine prenatal ultrasound screening in the Obstetrical and Gynecological Clinic, University of

Catania, Italy, and examined in the Pathologic Anatomy Section of G.F. Ingrassia Department, University of Catania.

2. Materials and Methods

Two fetuses with urinary tract malformations were examined in the Pathologic Anatomy Section of the G.F. Ingrassia Department, University of Catania, Italy. The study was conducted in accordance with with the Declaration of Helsinki, and the protocol was approved by the Ethics Committee of Catania 1 (48102 of 7 November, according to national legislation about osservational studies, 20 March 2008, AIFA).

Case 1: 19th week termination of pregnancy (TOP); male, 330 gr; total length 24 cm; crown–rump (CR) length 15.3 cm; medial length of foot 3 cm; cranial circumference 15.5 cm; thoracic circumference 13 cm; abdominal circumference 11 cm. Ruby red skin; perforated orifices. Umbilical cord stump 10 × 0.7 cm; edema of penis. The anatomic relationship of thoracic organs was normal: heart in situs solitus with atrium–ventricular and ventricular–vascular concordance and lung development coherent with gestational age. Examination of the abdominal cavity showed: megacystis (25 mm sagittal diameter) with thickened wall (6 mm), megaureter with stenosis of ureteral orifices in the bladder, and bilateral hydronephrotic kidneys (both 18 mm maximum diameter).

Ecographic diagnosis: urinary obstruction syndrome due to posterior urethral valve (PUV). The US (ultrasonographic) examination showed a megacystis with a maximum diameter of 44 mm and mild hydroureteronephrosis with bright hyperechogenic kidneys. The bladder had the so-called "key hole sign", suggesting a possible PUV. Fetal biometry and amniotic fluid were appropriate for gestational age (GA). No other major abnormalities were detected (Figure 1).

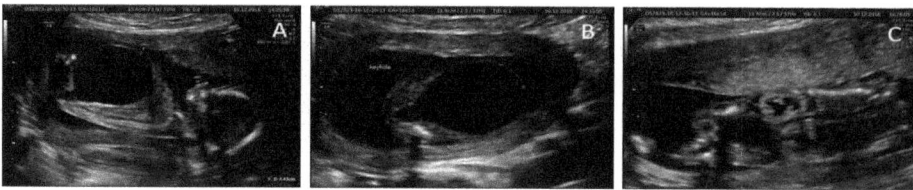

Figure 1. Case 1, US (ultrasonographic). (**A**) Sagittal view of the entire fetus with megacystis. (**B**) Coronal view of the bladder with the keyhole sign. (**C**) Coronal view of the hyperechogenic kidneys. Courtesy of Dr. G. Giunta.

Case 2: 15th week TOP; XXY karyotype; 40 gr; total length 11 cm; crown–rump (CR) length 8.5 cm; medial length of foot 1.5 cm; cranial circumference 7 cm; thoracic circumference 6 cm; abdominal circumference 7 cm. Ruby red skin; imperforated orifices. Turricephal and anencephal skull, prognathism, prominent ocular bulbs and low implant of the ears. The abdominal wall was flaccid due to the incomplete development of the diaphragm and ribs. The abdominal organs were herniated in the thoracic cavity and in the neck across the skin. Megacystis (65 mm sagittal diameter) with a thinned wall (2 mm) occupied the abdominal and thoracic cavities; both kidneys and surrenal glands were underdeveloped (both with a maximum diameter of 10 mm).

Ecographic diagnosis: Prune-Belly syndrome, PBS. The ultrasonographic (US) examination was very difficult due to maternal BMI > 35 and the anhydramnios—absence of amniotic fluid. The fetus showed a megacystis with a maximum diameter of 38 mm. The whole fetal body had a very uncommon posture and it was impossible to assess other fetal structures because of the anhydramnios (Figure 2).

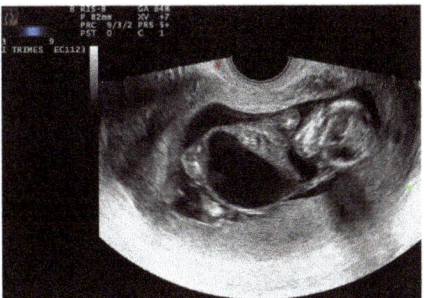

Figure 2. Case 2, US. Megacystis and anhydramnios. Courtesy of Dr. G. Giunta.

The organs of both fetuses were carefully dissected, separated from each other, fixed in 10% buffered formalin and processed until paraffin embedding. 5 μm sections were stained with hematoxylin-eosin (EE). Additional immunohistochemical stainings with smooth muscular actin (SMA, Clone 1A4, Dako, Glostrup, Denmark, Dil: 1:100), S100 protein (polyclonal, Dako, Glostrup, Denmark, Dil: 1:100) and WT1c (clone WT 6F-H2, Dako, Glostrup, Denmark, prediluted) were performed on bladder and bowel slides. Bladder and bowel samples from a fetus of XXI gestational age were considered as a normal control.

3. Results

3.1. Normal Control

Bladder: SMA staining marked longitudinal and transversal muscular layers intersected by embryonal mesenchyme; nervous plexuses were evaluated with S100 protein, showing their arrangement among the muscular layers; WT1c was poorly marked in ganglion cells, neural cells and their cytoplasmic extensions (Figure 3).

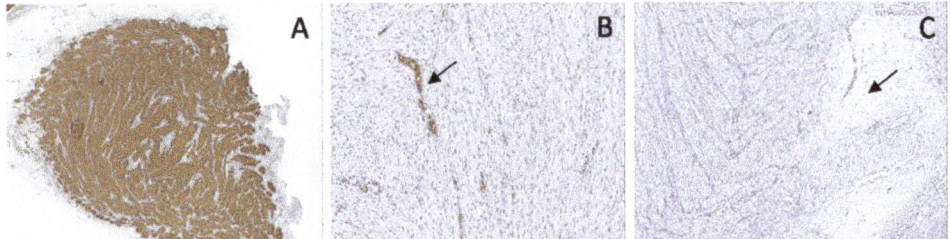

Figure 3. Normal bladder. Immunohistochemical staining shows smooth muscular actin (SMA) (**A**) in longitudinal and transversal muscular layers, S100 (**B**) in nervous plexuses (arrow) among the muscular layers and WT1c in ganglion cells (arrow) and neural cells (**C**).

Large and small bowel: SMA stained longitudinal and transverse muscular layers and interposed embryonal mesenchyme; S100 protein marked submucosal and myenteric plexuses with neural and ganglion cells; WT1c was shown in ganglion cells and their cytoplasmic extensions (Figure 4).

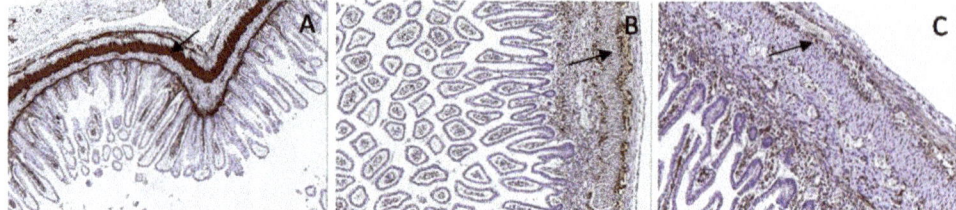

Figure 4. Normal bowel. Immunohistochemical staining shows: SMA (**A**) in longitudinal and transverse muscular layers (arrow), S100 (**B**) in submucosal and myenteric plexuses (arrow) and WT1c (**C**) in ganglion cells (arrow).

3.2. Case 1 PUV

Bladder: SMA highlighted muscular fiber disarray (shredded-carrots-like) with interposed embryonal mesenchyme; S100 staining showed hyperplastic neural plexus with irregular arrangement among muscular fibers; WT1c was poorly expressed in ganglion cells and in their cytoplasmic extensions (Figure 5).

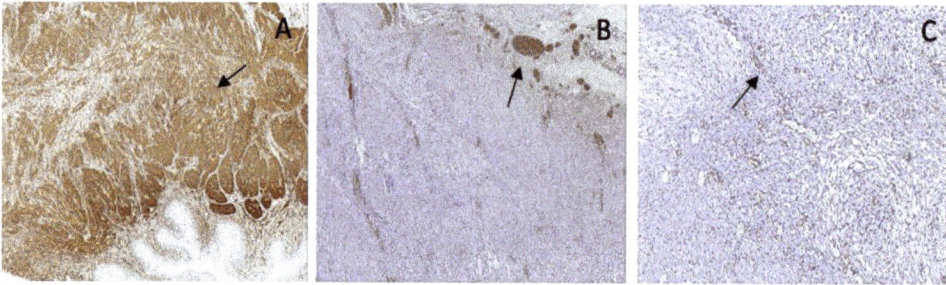

Figure 5. Case 1, posterior urethral valve (PUV). Immunohistochemical staining in bladder shows: SMA (**A**) in disarrayed muscular fibers (arrow), S100 (**B**) in hyperplastic neural plexus (arrow) and WT1c (**C**) poorly expressed in ganglion cells (arrow).

Large and small bowel: as in the normal control, SMA highlighted two muscular layers and interposed embryonal mesenchyme, S100 marked submucosal and myenteric plexuses with neural and ganglion cells, and WT1c was shown in ganglion cells and in their cytoplasmic extensions (Figure 6).

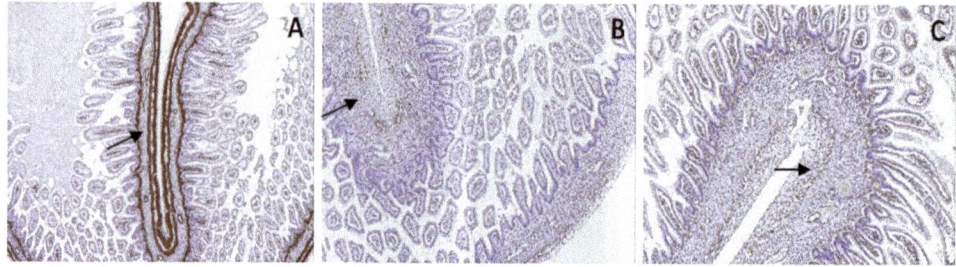

Figure 6. Case 1, PUV. Immunohistochemical staining in bowel: SMA (**A**) in the muscular layers (arrow), S100 (**B**) in submucosal and myenteric plexuses (arrow) and WT1c in ganglion cells (**C**) (arrow).

3.3. Case 2 (PBS)

Bladder: SMA highlighted a thin, longitudinal, muscular layer with disarray of muscular fibers (shredded-carrots-like) and poor interposed embryonal mesenchyme; S100 was shown only in peripheral nervous fibers and WT1c was negative (Figure 7).

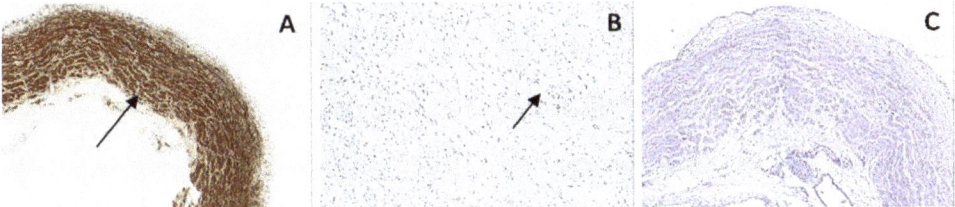

Figure 7. Case 2, Prune-Belly syndrome (PBS). Immunohistochemical staining in bladder: SMA (**A**) in a thin, longitudinal, muscular layer (arrow), S100 (**B**) only in peripheral nervous fibers (arrow), WT1c (**C**) negative.

Large and small bowel: SMA highlighted two longitudinal side-by-side muscular layers, without interposed embryonal mesenchyme; S100 protein and WT1c were not expressed (Figure 8).

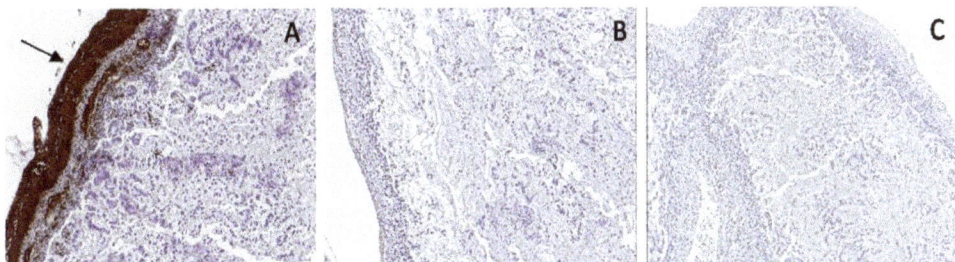

Figure 8. Case 2, PBS. Immunohistochemical staining in bowel: SMA (**A**) in two longitudinal side-by-side muscular layers (arrow), S100 (**B**) and WT1c (**C**) were not expressed.

4. Discussion

The kidney and urinary tract develops from two different embryonal sheets: kidneys, ureters and bladder trigone from the mesodermal sheet, and bladder and urethra from the endodermal sheet. The bladder develops from the fourth to seventh week of gestational age from the urogenital sinus. At the ninth week, after the involution of cloaca, the urogenital sinus opens into the amniotic cavity. CAKUT represent up to 20%–30% of all major congenital pre and postnatal defects [3], including both sporadic and familial cases and associated anomalies, such as syndromic malformations.

Among all CAKUT, our paper focuses on mainly bladder and urethral malformations. Isolated bladder anomalies, such as bladder agenesis, complete/incomplete duplication or bladder extrophy, are rare. Instead, morphologic bladder anomalies, known as megacystis, are more frequent and related to urethral or neuromuscular anomalies.

Fetal bladder is defined as megacystis if its longitudinal diameter is >10% of crown–rump length in different gestational ages. In the first trimester, the longitudinal diameter may be more than 6 mm.

Prenatal detection of a larger bladder could suggest an outlet obstruction, mainly due to urethral obstruction, but also other congenital complex malformations of the kidney and urinary tract. Moreover, in the case of megacystis, microcolon syndrome as well as neuro-muscular malformations should be considered.

PUV has been considered the most common cause of urethral obstruction in newborn males, while obstruction of the anterior urethral valve is less common and its complications are less severe than PUV.

Three types of PUV have been described: type 1, the most common (95%), with two mucosal folds from the bottom of veromontanum to the membranous urethra; type 2, with mucosal folds extending along posterolateral urethral wall from the ureteric orifice to the veromontanum; type 3, with a circular diaphragm with a central opening in the membranous urethra. In any type of urethral obstruction, the high intravesical pressure leads to defects in the muscular differentiation, with fibrotic tissue interposed among muscular fibers and a thickened bladder wall [1,2].

PBS occurs mainly in baby or infant males (97%) and is characterized by atrophy of the anterior abdominal wall due to muscular absence, anomalies in the urinary tract, such as megaureters and bilateral hydronephrosis, and testicular agenesis or cryptorchidism. More often, the bladder shows thickened walls with dilated ureteral orifices in the vesical trigone and vesicoureteral reflux. However, bladder histology is variable, showing both increased and decreased muscular fibers, with or without interposed connective tissue. In a previous study, Volmar et al. [4] described PBS with increased muscular thickness of the bladder in a case of intravesical obstruction, while a more recent work [5] reported PBS with decreased muscular thickness of the bladder in a case of urethral obstruction. In the latter case, the higher intravesical pressure, together with atrophy of the abdominal wall, could cause decreased muscular thickness, increased fibroblastic activity and overproduction of collagen type I, inhibiting muscular contractility and electrical impulse diffusion through the muscular layers.

Megacystis/megaureter syndrome is characterized by megacystis with thinned walls, vesicoureteral reflux, bilateral hydroureters and hydronephrosis and, often, dysplastic kidneys. It is frequently associated with microcolon and functional obstruction of the gastrointestinal and urinary tracts [6].

However, gestational age and vesical longitudinal diameter may be considered the main prognostic factors: it has been reported [2] that mild megacystis (8–12 mm) in early pregnancy (10–14 weeks) could spontaneously resolve, while severe megacystis (>17 mm) had a poor prognosis at any gestational age. Moreover, the ultrasound "keyhole sign", which is more frequently but not exclusively linked to PUV, has been considered the only important discriminant criteria. Some surgical therapies have been suggested to treat fetal megacystis, including amnioinfusion, vesicoamniotic shunting and vescicocentesis, but their outcome has been considered uncertain because fetal megacystis is often associated with other adverse prognostic factors.

Our two cases showed different gestational age (19 and 15 weeks), severe megacystis (25 mm and 85 mm) and, above all, different development of the muscular layers (thickened and thinned muscular layers).

Due to the heterogeneity in the definition of megacystis, in bladder development evaluation, and in future outcomes, we proposed to evaluate the histological differences and potential relationship with enteric nervous system development.

The immunohistochemical expression of S100 protein, SMA and WT1c was assessed and their expression in the bladder and in the small and large bowel from normal fetus and fetuses with megacystis were compared.

Comparing normal bladder with the bladder in PUV, SMA staining highlighted a disarray of muscular fibers and increased embryonal mesenchyme, due to the higher intravesical pressure, while in PBS, it showed thinned muscular layers with only longitudinal fibers and poor interposed embryonal mesenchyme (Figure 9).

To our knowledge, for the first time, the distribution of neural components among muscular fibers using S100 protein and WT1c has been assessed in the bladder [7].

In the normal bladder, S100 protein showed small ganglionic plexuses running parallel to the muscular fibers. In PUV, S100 staining showed small and giant hyperplastic ganglionic structures running parallel to the muscular fibers, while in PBS, S100 was negative (Figure 10).

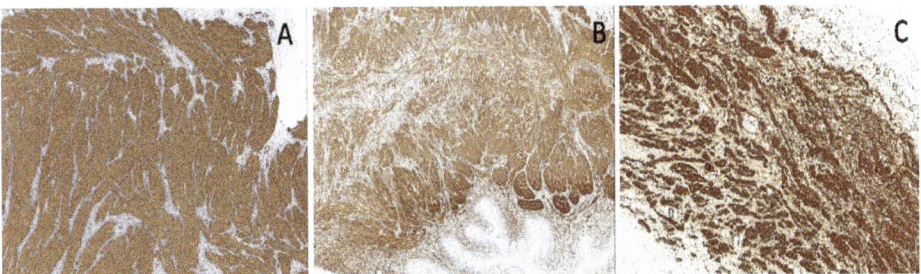

Figure 9. Comparative SMA expression in normal bladder (**A**), PUV (**B**) and PBS (**C**).

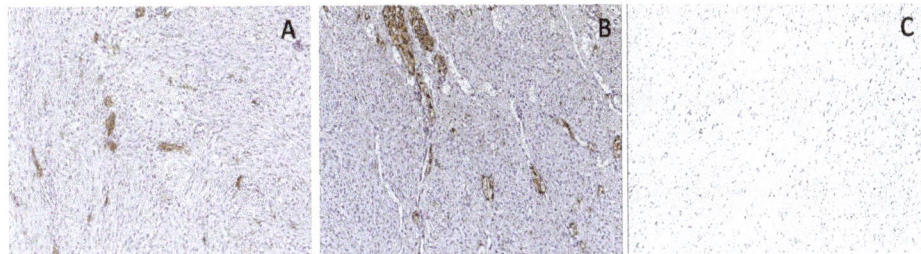

Figure 10. Comparative S100 expression in normal bladder (**A**), PUV (**B**) and PBS (**C**).

As concerns WT1c expression, normal bladder and PUV showed poor positivity in ganglion cells, in neural cells and in their cytoplasmic extensions, while WT1c was negative in PBS (Figure 11).

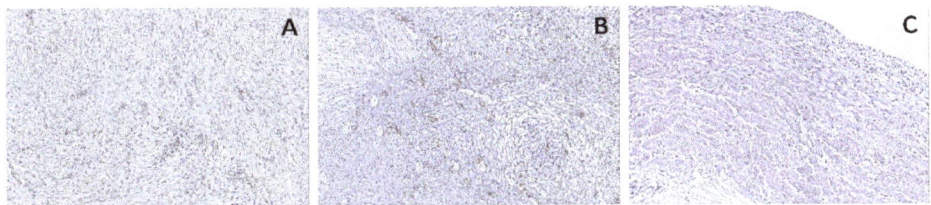

Figure 11. Comparative WT1c expression in normal bladder (**A**), PUV (**B**) and PBS (**C**).

Considering the relationship between the enteric nervous system and urinary tract development [6], SMA, S100 and WT1c expressions were also assessed in the enteric wall of the fetuses in order to to prove or deny their relationship and, above all, the pre or postnatal outcome as well as life expectancy.

In the normal fetus and PUV, SMA showed a double muscular layer and muscularis mucosae with interposed embryonal mesenchyme; in PBS, a single thickened muscular layer and disrupted muscularis mucosae are shown (Figure 12).

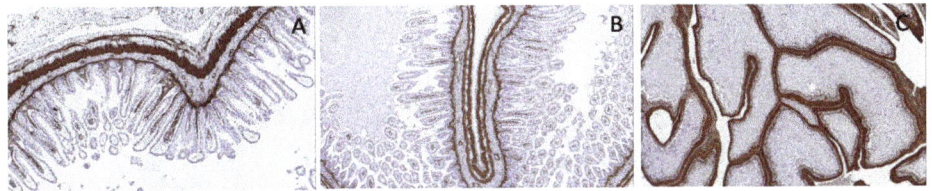

Figure 12. Comparative SMA expression in normal bowel (**A**), PUV (**B**) and PBS (**C**).

S100 and WT1c expression are shown in myenteric and submucosal plexuses in the normal bowel and in PUV; both antibodies were not expressed in PBS, proving the same neuromuscular defect in the bladder and bowel (Figures 13 and 14).

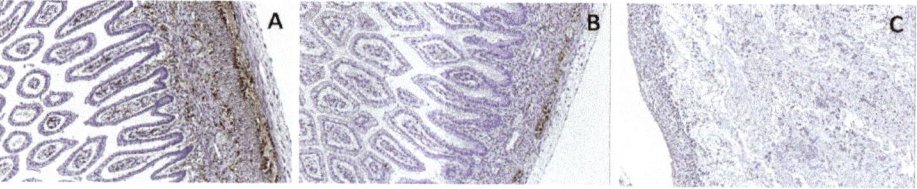

Figure 13. Comparative S100 expression in normal bowel (**A**), PUV (**B**) and PBS (**C**).

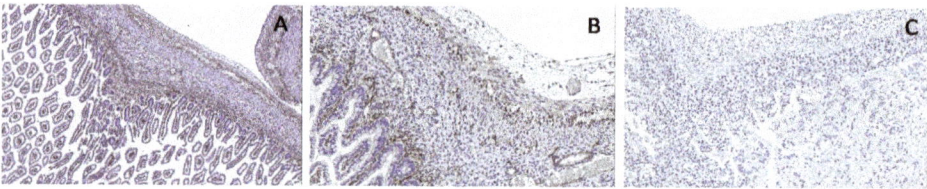

Figure 14. Comparative WT1c expression in normal bowel (**A**), PUV (**B**) and PBS (**C**).

Recent literature reports interesting data about the relationship between the intrinsic enteric nervous system (ENS) and the central nervous system, communicating through the gut–brain axis. Both systems develop from the neural crest progenitor and are regulated by the interactions among enteric neurons, glia and enteric-endocrine cells [8]. We hypothesized the same embryologic nature in enteric and vesical neural plexuses. Therefore, S100 and WT1c expression were evaluated in bladder and bowel muscular layers. Both markers were not expressed in the bladder and bowel of PBS associated with anencephaly, confirming a close relationship between encephalic and peripheral neural development.

In conclusion, megacystis could be considered only a macroscopic definition, concerning the size of the fetal bladder rather than the embryologic origin [9]. A larger bladder may be a single malformation or multiple malformations associated with the bowel and/or encephalic malformations, which decide the outcome and prognosis in fetal megacystis.

Author Contributions: Conceptualization, L.P., L.S. and G.G.; Data curation, R.C., A.C., L.S.; Methodology, L.P., L.S., G.G.; Resources, A.C. and R.C.; Writing—original draft, L.P.; Writing—review & editing, L.S. and R.C.

Funding: This research received no external funding

Acknowledgments: We wish to thank the Scientific Bureau of the University of Catania for language support.

Conflicts of Interest: The authors declare no conflict of interest.

References

1. Khong, Y.T.; Malcomson Roger, D.G. The urinary system. In *Keeling's Fetal and Neonatal Pathology*, 5th ed.; Springer Verlag: Berlin, Germany, 2015; pp. 643–651.
2. Taghavi, K.; Sharpe, C.; Stringer, M.D. Fetal megacystis: A systematic review. *J. Pediatr. Urol.* **2017**, *13*, 7–15. [CrossRef] [PubMed]
3. Rosenblum, S.; Pal, A.; Reidy, K. Renal development in the fetus and premature infant. *Semin. Fetal Neonatal Med.* **2017**, *22*, 58–66. [CrossRef] [PubMed]

4. Vollmar, K.E.; Fritsch, M.K.; Perlman, E.J.; Hutchins, G.M. Patterns of congenital lower urinary tract obstructive uropathy: Relation to abnormal prostate and bladder development and the prune belly syndrome. *Pediatr. Dev. Pathol.* **2001**, *4*, 467–472. [CrossRef] [PubMed]
5. Julio Junior Helce, R.; Costa Suelen, F.; Costa Waldemar, S.; Barcellos Sampaio, F.J.; Favorito Luciano, A. Structural study of the bladder in fetuses with prune belly syndrome. *Neurourol. Urodyn.* **2017**, *37*, 148–152. [CrossRef]
6. Hofmann, A.D.; Duess, J.W.; Puri, P. Congenital anomalies of the kidney and urinary tract (CAKUT) associated with Hirschsprung's disease: A systematic review. *Pediatr. Surg. Int.* **2014**, *30*, 757–761. [CrossRef]
7. Parenti, R.; Salvatorelli, L.; Musumeci, G.; Parenti, C.; Giorlandino, A.; Motta, F.; Magro, G. Wilms'tumor 1 (WT1) protein expression in human developing tissues. *Acta Histochem.* **2015**, *117*, 386–396. [CrossRef]
8. Kulkarni, S.; Ganz, J.; Bayrer, L.; Bogunovic, M.; Rao, M. Advances in enteric neurobiology: The "brain" in the gut in health and disease. *J. Neurosci.* **2018**, *38*, 9346–9354. [CrossRef] [PubMed]
9. Fontanella, F.; Maggio, L.; Verheij, J.B.G.M.; Duin, L.K.; Adama Van Scheltema, P.N.; Cohen-Overbeek, T.E.; Pajkrt, E.; Bekker, M.; Willekes, C.; Bax, C.J.; et al. Fetal megacystis: A lot more than LUTO. *Ultrasound Obstet. Gynecol.* **2019**, *53*, 779–787. [CrossRef] [PubMed]

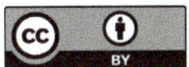

© 2019 by the authors. Licensee MDPI, Basel, Switzerland. This article is an open access article distributed under the terms and conditions of the Creative Commons Attribution (CC BY) license (http://creativecommons.org/licenses/by/4.0/).

Article

Identification of Novel Markers of Prostate Cancer Progression, Potentially Modulated by Vitamin D

Rosario Caltabiano [1], Paola Castrogiovanni [2], Ignazio Barbagallo [3], Silvia Ravalli [2], Marta Anna Szychlinska [2], Vincenzo Favilla [4], Luigi Schiavo [5], Rosa Imbesi [2], Giuseppe Musumeci [2] and Michelino Di Rosa [2,*]

[1] Department G.F. Ingrassia, Section of Anatomic Pathology, University of Catania, 95123 Catania, Italy; rocaltab@unict.it
[2] Department of Biomedical and Biotechnological Sciences, Human Anatomy and Histology Section, School of Medicine, University of Catania, 95123 Catania, Italy; pacastro@unict.it (P.C.); silviaravalli@gmail.com (S.R.); marta.sz@hotmail.it (M.A.S.); roimbesi@unict.it (R.I.); giumusu@gmail.com (G.M.)
[3] Department of Drug Sciences, University of Catania, Viale A. Doria 6, 95125 Catania, Italy; ibarbag@unict.it
[4] Department of Surgery, Urology Section, University of Catania, 95123 Catania, Italy; favillavincenzo@gmail.it
[5] Obesity Unit, CETAC Medical and Research Center, 81100 Caserta, Italy; luigi.schiavo@unicampania.it
* Correspondence: mdirosa@unict.it

Received: 27 August 2019; Accepted: 13 November 2019; Published: 15 November 2019

Abstract: Prostate cancer (PCa) is one of the most common cancers in men. The main risk factors associated with the disease include older age, family history of the disease, smoking, alcohol and race. Vitamin D is a pleiotropic hormone whose low levels are associated with several diseases and a risk of cancer. Here, we undertook microarray analysis in order to identify the genes involved in PCa. We analyzed three PCa microarray datasets, overlapped all genes significantly up-regulated, and subsequently intersected the common genes identified with the down-regulated genes transcriptome of LNCaP cells treated with $1\alpha,25(OH)_2D_3$, in order to identify the common genes involved in PCa and potentially modulated by Vitamin D. The analysis yielded 43 genes potentially involved in PCa and significantly modulated by Vitamin D. Noteworthy, our analysis showed that six genes (PRSS8, SOX4, SMYD2, MCCC2, CCNG2 and CD2AP) were significantly modulated. A Pearson correlation analysis showed that five genes out of six (SOX4 was independent), were statistically correlated with the gene expression levels of KLK3, and with the tumor percentage. From the outcome of our investigation, it is possible to conclude that the genes identified by our analysis are associated with the PCa and are potentially modulated by the Vitamin D.

Keywords: Vitamin D; prostate cancer; immunohistochemistry

1. Introduction

Vitamin D is synthesized in the body through a complex series of steps beginning in the skin, under the influence of ultraviolet light, where a cholesterol precursor molecule (7-dehydrocholesterol) is transformed into the Vitamin D hormone precursor, *cholecalciferol* (also known as Vitamin D3). Vitamin D3 is subsequently hydroxylated in the liver by the 25-hydroxycholecalciferol and transformed in *calcidiol* or *calcifediol* ($25(OH)D_3$ or $25D_3$), and this latter is subjected, in the kidney, to an hydroxylation, to yield the most active hormone form of these compounds, *calcitriol* (1,25-dihydroxycholecalciferol or $1,25(OH)_2D_3$ or $1,25D_3$) [1]. The three main stages in Vitamin D metabolism, 25-hydroxylation, 1α-hydroxylation and 24-hydroxylation, are all performed by cytochrome P450 mixed-function oxidases (CYPs).

These enzymes are distributed either in the endoplasmic reticulum (ER) (CYP2R1) or in the mitochondria (CYP27A1, CYP27B1 and CYP24A1). The 24-hydroxylase (CYP24A1) and 1-hydroxylase

(CYP27B1) enzymes are considered to be pivotal determinants of the local concentration of active vitamin D. When Vitamin D3 is transferred to the liver, it is hydroxylated (by CYP27A1) and then converted to 25-hydroxyvitamin D3, which is the major form of vitamin D present in the blood. In this form it is also hydroxylated in other tissues, predominantly the kidney, through 1-α hydroxylase (CYP27B1), which is then converted to 1,25-dihydroxyvitamin D3. This form is able to bind to vitamin D-binding proteins (VBP) in the bloodstream and modulate the transcription of its target gene through binding to the vitamin D receptor (VDR) in tissues. The last steps of Vitamin D3 catabolism are played by the catalytic enzyme, 24-hydroxylase, encoded by CYP24A1 and responsible for vitamin D catabolism, which is then metabolized to calcitroic acid, a bile secretion [2].

Serum 25(OH)D_3 is the barometer for Vitamin D status. Serum calcitriol provides no information about Vitamin D status, and it is often at physiological or even elevated due to secondary hyperparathyroidism associated with Vitamin D deficiency.

The Vitamin D plays a relevant role in bone formation, activates the immune cells [3–5], regulates the host defense against microbial and virus infections [6–8], inhibits several tumor pathways, such as the proliferation and angiogenesis [9] and it has been hypothesized that it is able to reduce prostate cancer (PCa) risk [10]. In this regard, it has been shown that a 'U' shaped relationship may exist between Vitamin D status (*cholecalciferol, calcidiol, calcitriol and calcitroic acid*) and PCa, and that the optimal range of circulating 25(OH)D_3 for PCa prevention may be narrow [11].

Prostate cancer (PCa) is one of the most common causes of morbidity and mortality in men. Several factors have been linked to the incidence of PCa and its aggressiveness. Among these, age, race and family history are some of the strongest [12]. The incidence rate is high in men 65–74 years of age with a median age at diagnosis of 66. The percent of PCa deaths is highest among men between 75 to 84 years old with a median age at death of 80 [13] Epidemiologic studies regarding PCa showed that there are significant differences in geographical distribution and race. The African-American race, for example, experiences an incidence rate of 60% compared to Caucasian men, other than more aggressive forms and worse treatment management, leading to increased mortality [14]. Interestingly, one of the major correlations between Vitamin D levels and PCa is based on studies on African-American men. In these individuals, 25(OH)D_3 levels are often low (probably for the effect of skin pigmentation on the synthesis of Vitamin D), and PCa risks are clearly higher than those of Caucasian men. Nowadays, the mechanisms for this association are still unclear.

There are a large number of epidemiologic studies linking Vitamin D and prostate cancer risk and outcomes. The high serum vitamin D3 levels, estimated by measuring 25(OH)D_3, play important roles in the prevention of various forms of cancer, including prostate cancer [15]. An in vitro study using prostate cancer LNCaP cells reported that a potent analog of 1,25(OH)$_2$D$_3$ (EB108928) plays an inhibitory role on the growth of cancer cells [16]. In another study in immortalized human prostate cell lines (PZ-HPV-7 cells), 10 nM of 25(OH)D_3 was reported to have growth inhibitory activity [16]. In 2018, a meta-analysis study, composed of seven eligible cohort studies with 7808 participants, suggested that higher 25(OH)D_3 level was associated with a reduction of mortality in prostate cancer patients, suggesting that Vitamin D can be considered an important protective factor in the progression and prognosis of prostate cancer [17]. Recently, it has been shown that dietary Vitamin D causes a dose-dependent increase in serum 25(OH)D_3 levels and a reduction in the percentage of mice with adenocarcinoma, but it did not improve bone mass. In contrast, high calcium did suppress serum 1,25(OH)$_2$D$_3$ levels, leading to an increased incidence of adenocarcinoma and improved bone mass. These data support the hypothesis that the loss of Vitamin D signaling accelerates the early stages of prostate carcinogenesis [18]. Furthermore, it is important to note that several factors could influence the anticancer action played by Vitamin D on PCa, such as the polymorphism of its receptor (VDR) [19] or the expression of the enzymes (CYP24A1 and CYP27B1) that regulate its metabolism [20].

The aim of this study was to find new target genes of PCa, and those potentially modulated by the action of Vitamin D (1,25D_3 and 25D_3). We explored several microarray datasets in order to investigate and identify possible cancer gene pathways hypothetically modulated by the action of Vitamin D.

2. Materials and Methods

2.1. Dataset Selection

In our analysis, we have selected several microarray datasets based on mRNA expression profiling available on the NCBI GEODataset (https://www.ncbi.nlm.nih.gov/gds/). Mesh terms "Prostate cancer" and "Vitamin D" were used to identify potential datasets of interest. We sorted the obtained datasets by the number of samples (High to Low) and for clinical data made available by the authors. Three dataset of PCa and two of the LNCaP cell line were selected: GSE70770 [21,22], GSE62872 [23], GSE6919 [24,25], GSE64657, and GSE107438 [26].

The GSE70770 (platform GPL10558), was composed by 293 prostate biopsies samples obtained by 74 matched benign tissue (indicated as healthy) and 219 patients subjected to robotic radical prostatectomy (RRP) surgery. As regards the GSE62872 (platform GPL19370), the overall design included 160 normal prostate tissue samples from the Health Professionals Follow-up Study (indicated as healthy) and 264 with a prostate tumor. In the GSE6919 (platform GPL8300), we selected 18 adjacent normal prostate tissue biopsies free of any pathological alteration (indicated as healthy) and 65 primary prostate tumor biopsies from patients subjected to prostatectomy. Furthermore, our study included a further one dataset (GSE64657, platform GPL4133) of an in-vitro model of the PCa cell line (*LNCaP*) after 24 h treatment with different nuclear receptor ligands, and with time-matching control. We have decided to consider only the data coming from the *LNCaP* treatment with Vitamin D (100 nM $1,25D_3$ for 24 h), the natural ligand for VDR. There is no publication available for this dataset. The experimental details are recoverable on the following link (https://www.ncbi.nlm.nih.gov/geo/query/acc.cgi?acc=GSE64657). In order to verify the gene pathways modulation by Vitamin D in prostate cancer, we analyzed the GSE107438 dataset, composed by LNCaP cells line transfected with control siRNA (siCT), siRNA for CYP27B1 (siCYP27B1) or siRNA for VDR (siVDR) followed by 100 nM of 25(OH)D3 (25D3) or $1,25(OH)_2D3$ ($1,25D_3$) treatment for another 24 h. Complete experimental details are available in the following publication [26].

Complete demographic data of patients and healthy controls can be obtained from the relative publication cited above.

2.2. Data Processing

To process and identify significant differentially expressed genes (SDEG) in data sets, we used the MultiExperiment Viewer (MeV) software (The Institute for Genomic Research (TIGR), J. Craig Venter Institute, Rockville, MD, USA). In cases where multiple genes probes have insisted on the same GeneID NCBI, we have used those with the highest variance. The significance threshold level for all data sets was $p < 0.05$. The genes with $p < 0.05$ were selected for further analysis. For all datasets we performed a statistical analysis with GEO2R, applying a Benjamini & Hochberg (False discovery rate) to adjust p values for multiple comparisons [27–29]. From GSE70770, we identified, respectively, 2279 and 9785 genes that were significantly up-regulated and down-regulated, comparing the prostate biopsies samples of healthy vs. tumor patients. Regarding GSE62872, we obtained a total of 2312 and 1060, respectively, of significantly up-regulated and down-regulated genes, comparing the prostate biopsies samples of healthy vs. tumor patients. The analysis of GSE6919 produced 1747 and 1060 genes, respectively, that were significantly up-regulated and down-regulated in prostate biopsies samples of healthy vs. tumor patients. Furthermore, the analysis of GSE64657 produced 995 up-regulated and 2196 down-regulated and significantly expressed genes, comparing the LNCaP cells line treated with vehicle (ethanol) and $1,25D_3$ (100 nM) for 24 h. All data analysis are available in Table S1.

In order to identify genes commonly modulated between the four GSEs, we performed a Venn diagram analysis, using the web-based utility Venn Diagram Generator (http://bioinformatics.psb.ugent.be/webtools/Venn/). To analyze a 2 × 2 contingency table, a chi-square with Yates correction was performed by GraphPad Prism software (http://graphpad.com/quickcalcs/contingency1.cfm). The association between rows (groups) and columns (outcomes) with $p < 0.01$ was considered to be statistically significant.

The genes Ontology analysis was performed using the web utility GeneMANIA (http://genemania.org/, http://genemania.org/) [30] and the GATHER (Gene Annotation Tool to Help Explain Relationships) (http://changlab.uth.tmc.edu/gather/) [31]. The GeneMANIA was also used for built the weighted gene networks commonly modulated. GeneMANIA searches publicly-available genomics and proteomics data, including data from gene and protein expression profiling studies and primary and curated molecular interaction networks and pathways, to find related genes. The network weighting method is 'Gene-Ontology (GO)-based weighting, Biological Process-based'. This weighting method assumes the input gene list is related in terms of biological processes (as defined by GO).

GHATER (Gene Annotation Tool to Help Explain Relationships) (http://changlab.uth.tmc.edu/gather/) is an online tool that explains the function of a group of genes, such as a cluster of co-regulated genes from microarrays. The tool is a comprehensive system that combines gene function, ontology, pathways and statistical tools that enable researchers to analyze large-scale, genome-wide data from sequencing, proteomics or gene expression experiments. The analysis of gene ontology is based on the Bayes factor. This is a measure of the strength of the evidence supporting an association of an annotation with your gene list. Higher Bayes factors indicate stronger evidence that the annotation is relevant to your genes. The p value restituted during the analysis is calculated based on the probability of seeing a Bayes factor of a particular magnitude in a query. Complete explanation of the online tool can be retrieved in the following publication [31] and in the following online website (http://changlab.uth.tmc.edu/gather/FAQ.html).

2.3. The Immunohistochemistry (IHC) Analysis by the Human Atlas Project

The analysis of the data from the microarray provided results about the mRNA expression levels. To confirm these results, we decided to use the web utility "The Human Protein Atlas" (https://www.proteinatlas.org/) [32–34]. This web site is licensed under the Creative Commons Attribution-ShareAlike 3.0 International License (https://creativecommons.org/licenses/by-sa/3.0/) for all copyrightable parts (https://wiki.creativecommons.org/wiki/Data) of the database. We selected the immunohistochemistry analysis available on the web site. For each antibody, the observed staining has been assigned a validation score. The validation score is based on the result of two different validations that are separately evaluated. The different levels of validation score are Supported, Approved or Uncertain (https://www.proteinatlas.org/about/antibody+validation#ifv). Annotation parameters include an evaluation of *staining intensity* (SI) (negative, weak, moderate or strong), *fraction of stained cells* (rare, <25%, 25–75% or >75%) and *subcellular localization* (nuclear and/or cytoplasmic/membranous). The reliability scores are based on the following criteria:

Supportive: Two independent antibodies yielding similar or partly similar staining patterns; two independent antibodies yielding dissimilar staining patterns, both supported by experimental gene/protein characterization data; one antibody yielding a staining pattern supported by experimental gene/protein characterization data; one antibody yielding a staining pattern with no available experimental gene/protein characterization data, but supported by other assay within the protein atlas; one or more independent antibodies yielding staining patterns not consistent with experimental gene/protein characterization data, but supported by siRNA assay.

Uncertain: Two independent antibodies yielding partly similar staining patterns, but not consistent with experimental protein/gene characterization data; two independent antibodies yielding dissimilar staining patterns with no available, or partly supportive/partly conflicting, experimental gene/protein characterization data; one antibody yielding a staining pattern with no available, or partly supportive/partly conflicting experimental gene/protein characterization data.

Details of analysis performed are available in Table S1.

2.4. Statistical Analysis

For statistical analysis, Prism 7 software (GraphPad Software, San Diego, California, USA) was used. Based on the Shapiro-Wilk test, almost all data were skewed, so nonparametric tests were used. Significant differences between groups were assessed using the Mann–Whitney U test, and a Kruskal-Wallis test was performed to compare data between all groups followed by Dunn's post hoc test. Correlations were determined using Spearman's ϱ correlation. All tests were two-sided and significance was determined at $p < 0.05$. To analyze a 2 × 2 contingency table, a Chi-square with Yates correction was performed by GraphPad Prism software (http://graphpad.com/quickcalcs/contingency1.cfm). The association between rows (groups) and columns (outcomes) with $p < 0.0001$ was considered to be extremely statistically significant.

The analysis of microarray data by Z-score transformation was used in order to allow the comparison of microarray data independent of the original hybridization intensities [35].

3. Results

3.1. The Vitamin D Is Able to Modulate 43 Key Genes in PCa

The comparison of the three human PCa datasets (GSE70770, GSE62872 and GSE6919) produced 276 common significantly up-regulated genes (458 down-regulated genes) (Figure 1A) (Table S1).

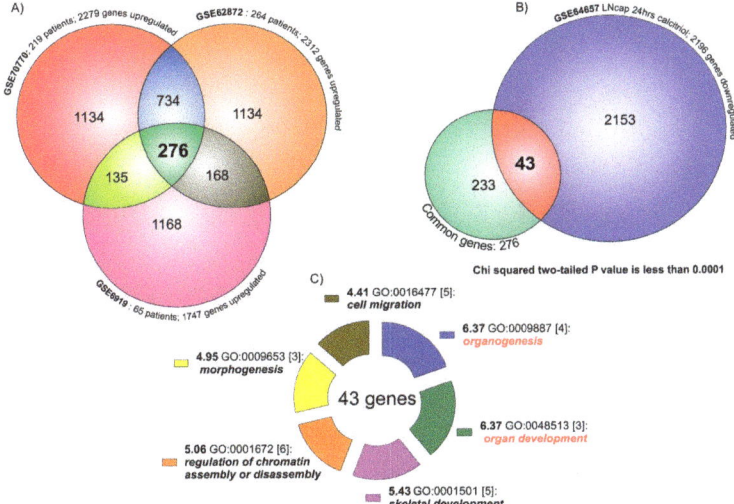

Figure 1. Venn diagram analysis of PCa transcriptome. (**A**) The three PCa datasets (GSE70770, GSE62872 and GSE6919) overlapping produced 276 common significantly up-regulated key genes. The overlapping between GSE70770 (2279 SUG) vs. GSE62872 (2312 SUG) showed 1010 genes in common (the sum of 276 and 734). As regard GSE6919 (1747 SUG) vs. GSE70770 overlapping, we identified 411 genes. Similar results were obtained when we compared GSE6919 vs. GSE62872 (444 genes in common). (**B**) The analysis of the intersection between the transcriptome of genes common up-regulated in the three PCa datasets (276) and the transcriptome of the down-regulated genes in LNCaP cell line treated with Vitamin D for 24 h (2196 SUG), showed 43 (almost 15%) significantly common regulated (chi-squared, $p < 0.0001$). (**C**) When we loaded the 43 genes in the GATHER browser, we showed that the biological process most significantly regulated by these genes were organogenesis, organ development, skeletal development, chromatin assembly, morphogenesis and cell migration.

These common regulated key genes were compared to significantly down-regulated genes in GSE64657, composed by the transcriptome of the LNCaP cell line, treated for 24 h with 100 nM of 1,25D$_3$ (Figure 1B). The data overlapping produced 43 genes significantly in common between the dataset (chi-square $p < 0.0001$), namely meaning being virtually modulated by the action of Vitamin D in PCa. Gene Ontology (GO) analysis of the 43 genes belonging to the common group modulated by Vitamin

D identified six main molecular functions as statistically significant: *organogenesis* (GO:0009887)(neg ln(p value) = 6.37); *organ development* (GO:0048513)(neg ln(p value) = 6.37); *skeletal development* (GO:0001501)(neg ln(p value) = 5.43); *regulation of chromatin assembly or disassembly* (GO:0001501)(neg ln(p value) = 5.06); *morphogenesis* (GO:0009653)(neg ln(p value) = 4.95); *cell migration* (GO:0016477)(neg ln(p value) = 4.41) (Figure 1C). Complete annotation, significance and genes involved are available in Table S1, section Gather Analysis.

We also overlapped the common down-regulated key genes in PCas obtained by the Venn analysis of the three datasets, with the significantly up-regulated genes in GSE64657. The overlap produced 41 genes significantly in common between the dataset (chi-square p < 0.0001), also modulated by Vitamin D (Table S1).

In this study, we decided to focus our analysis only to the 43 key genes in common obtained overlapping the up-regulated genes in cancer and the genes down-regulated by the Vitamin D. We used these 43 genes to generate a network analysis by GeneMania web utility software (Figure 2A).

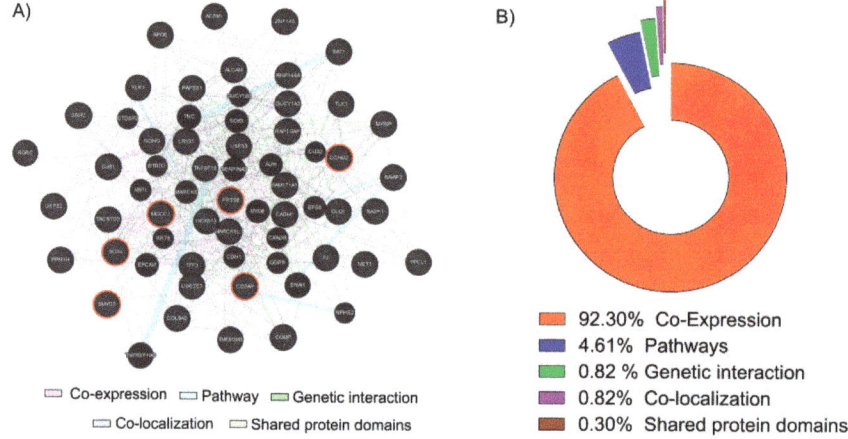

Figure 2. Network and GO analysis by GeneMania. (**A**) The 43 key genes up-regulated in PCa biopsies and down-regulated in the LNCaP cell line treated with Vitamin D (100 nM for 24 h) were loaded into GeneMania, in order to generate a GO and a Regulatory molecular network. Red circle genes represent the six most significantly up-regulated in PCa and down-regulated by the action of Vitamin D in our LNCaP cell line (**B**). The analysis showed that 92.30% of genes resulted co-expressed, 4.61% belonging to the same pathways, 1.97% present a genetic interaction, 0.82% were co-localized and 0.30% shared the same protein domains.

The 92.30% of genes resulted co-expressed, 4.61% belonging to the same pathways, 1.97% present a genetic interaction, 0.82% were co-localized and 0.30% shared the same protein domains (Figure 2B). Complete data report is available in Table S2. Belonging to among the 43 key genes, we selected the six most significantly up-regulated in PCa and down-regulated by the action of Vitamin D in LNCaP cell line: *serine protease 8* (PRSS8); *SRY-box 4* (SOX4); *SET and MYND domain containing 2* (SMYD2); *methylcrotonoyl-CoA carboxylase 2* (MCCC2); *cyclin G2* (CCNG2); *CD2 associated protein* (CD2AP). We decided to perform a Z-score transformation in order to allow the comparison of microarray data independent of the original hybridization intensities.

The three microarray dataset clustering (GSE70770, GSE62872 and GSE6919) allowed us to obtain a large number of samples (251 healthy control and 548 PCa samples). Complete demographic data of patients and healthy controls can be retrieved from the relative publication and in the Table S1. The samples were homogeneous for the age (Table S1). We showed that all genes increased significantly with respect to the single dataset (Figure 3A) (Figure S1).

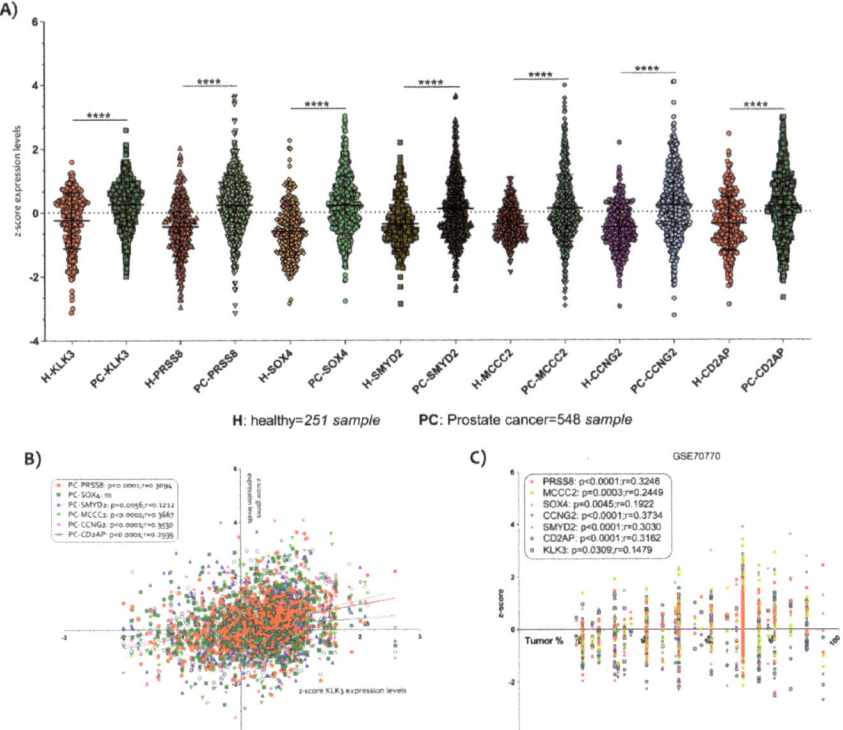

Figure 3. Selection of six key genes modulated in PCa. (**A**) In order to allow the comparison of microarray datasets independent of the original hybridization intensities, we decided to apply a Z score transformation. The normalization allowed us to applicate a Z test for the six genes most significantly up-regulated in PCa and down-regulated by the action of Vitamin D in the LNCaP cell line. We obtained 251 healthy subjects and 548 PCa samples. All genes selected (KLK3, PRSS8, SOX4, SMYD2, MCCC2, CCNG2 and CD2AP) resulted significantly up-regulated in PCa biopsies compared to prostate biopsies of healthy subject ($p < 0.0001$) (**B**). A significantly positive correlation was observed between all six key genes selected and KLK3 expression levels. (**C**) Similar results were obtained when we analyze the correlation between the six genes' z-score expression levels and the tumor percent. Data are expressed as z-score intensity expression levels and presented as vertical scatter dot plots. p values < 0.05 were considered to be statistically significant **** $p < 0.00005$).

In order to verify a possible correlation between the selected genes and the PCa tumor progression, we correlate the z-score intensity expression levels of all six genes highlighted with the genes expression of *kallikrein related peptidase 3* (KLK3). The KLK3 is a serine protease produced by epithelial cells in the prostate and its protein is also known as *PSA* (prostate *specific antigen*). It is largely demonstrated that the serum levels of PSA increase in the presence of cancer [36]. We showed a significantly positive correlation between all genes and KLK3 gene expression (Figure 3B). SOX4 was an exception (Table S1).

Interesting data were obtained when we decided to analyze the correlation between the z-score expression levels of the six genes and the histological parameter of tumor percent, available in the datasets. We showed that all genes were significantly positively correlated to the tumor % ($p < 0.0001$ with $r = 0.3246$ for PRSS8; $p = 0.0003$ with $r = 0.2449$ for MCCC2; $p = 0.0045$ with $r = 0.1922$ for SOX4; $p < 0.0001$ with $r = 0.3734$ for CCNG2; $p < 0.0001$ with $r = 0.3030$ for SMYD2; $p < 0.0001$ with $r = 0.3162$

for CD2AP) (Figure 3C) (Table S1), particularly, we identified that CCNG2 was the most correlated to the tumor %.

Furthermore, we also hypothesized that the genes involved in the production and inactivation of Vitamin D could be modulated in PCa patients. The expression levels analysis of the *cytochrome P450 family 27 subfamily B member 1* (CYP27B1), the *cytochrome P450 family 24 subfamily A member 1* (CYP24A1), the *cathelicidin antimicrobial peptide* (CAMP) and the *vitamin D receptor* (VDR) showed interesting results (Figure 4).

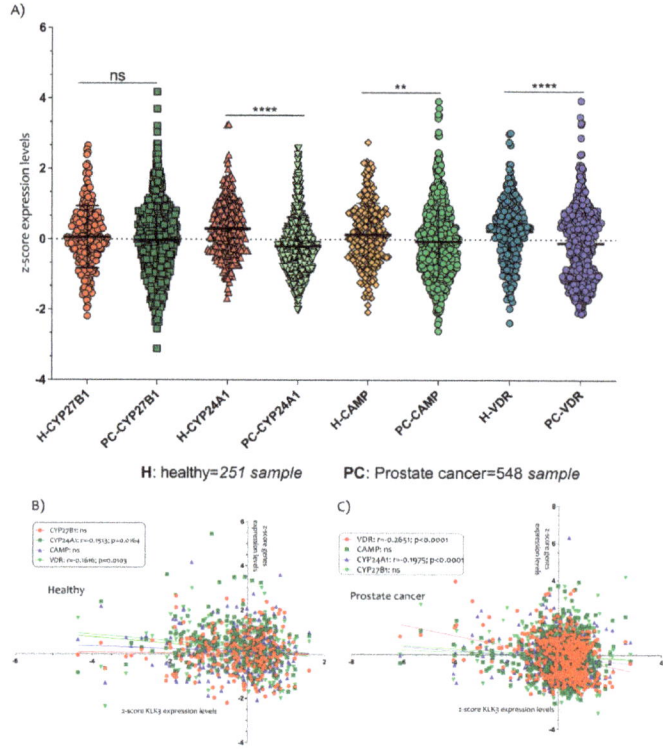

Figure 4. The Vitamin D metabolism genes modulated in PCa patients. (**A**) The expressions of CYP24A1, CAMP and VDR were significantly down-regulated in PCa patients compared to healthy controls subjects. Also, the expression levels of VDR and CYP24A1 were correlated negatively with KLK3 in healthy (**B**) and in PCa patients (**C**). Data are expressed as expression levels and presented as vertical bars. p values < 0.05 were considered to be statistically significant (** p < 0.005; **** p < 0.00005).

All genes, except CYP27B1 (p = ns), were downregulated in PCa patients compared to healthy controls subjects (CYP24A1 p < 0.0001; CAMP p < 0.0001; VDR p< 0.0001) (Figure 4A). In addition, we showed that the expression levels of VDR and CYP24A1 were negatively correlated with KLK3 in healthy (CYP24A1 with r = −0.1513 and p = 0.0164; VDR with r = −0.1616 and p = 0.0103) (Figure 4B) and in PCa patients (CYP24A1 with r = −0.1975 and p < 0.0001; VDR with r = −0.2651 and p < 0.0001) (Figure 4C).

3.2. PCa Related Genes Were Modulated by Vitamin D in LNCaP Cell Line

In the LNCaP cell line, the 1,25D$_3$ played significant modulatory effect on the expression levels of PRSS8 (p = 0.0006), SOX4 (p = 0.0004), SMYD2 (p = 0.0049), MCCC2 (p = 0.0002), CCNG2 (p = 0.0074) and CD2AP ($p = 0.0048$). Indeed, all genes were significantly down-regulated by the 1,25D$_3$ (100 nM for 24 h) (Figure 5A).

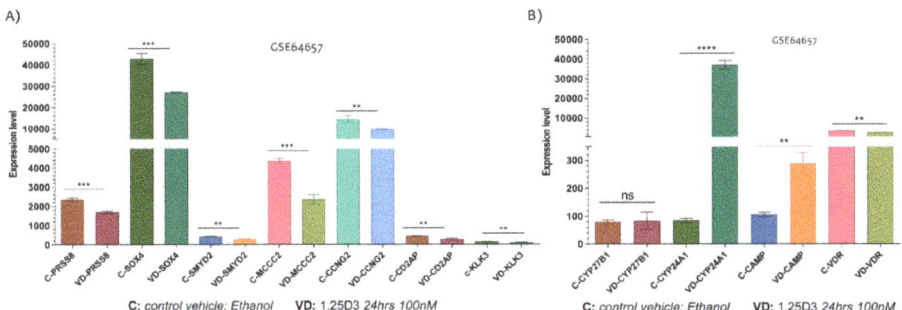

Figure 5. The Vitamin D-modulated PCa related genes. (**A**) The expression of PRSS8, SOX4, SMYD2, MCCC2, CCNG2 and CD2AP were significantly down-regulated in this LNCaP cell line at 24 h after exposition to 100 nM of 1,25D$_3$. (**B**) In addiction, the expression levels of Vitamin D metabolism genes were significantly modulated in LNCaP cells line under 1,25D$_3$ exposition (no significant modulation was observed for CYP27B1) (Data are expressed as expression levels and presented as vertical bars. p values < 0.05 were considered to be statistically significant ** $p < 0.005$; *** $p < 0.0005$; **** $p < 0.00005$).

Noteworthy, we investigated the expression levels of Vitamin D target genes such as CYP27B1, CYP24A1, VDR and CAMP, and we showed that CYP24A1 ($p < 0.0001$) and CAMP ($p = 0.0015$) were significantly up-regulated in LNCaP cells treated with 1,25D$_3$ for 24 h (no significantly modulation was observed for CYP27B1, $p = 0.8430$) (Figure 5B). Conversely, the VDR gene expression levels were significantly downregulated by 1,25D$_3$ treatment ($p = 0.0012$) (Figure 5B).

3.3. The Vitamin D Regulatory Mechanism on the Six PCa Genes Selected

In order to explain how Vitamin D plays a role in the modulation of the marker genes highlighted in our study, we analyzed a new dataset (GSE107438) composed of LNCaP cells transfected with control siRNA (siCT), siRNA for CYP27B1 (siCYP27B1) or siRNA for VDR (siVDR), followed by 100 nM of 25D$_3$ or 1,25D$_3$ treatment for a further 24 h. The analysis of genes belonging to the Vitamin D pathway such as CAMP, VDR, CYP27B1 and CYP24A1 demonstrated that in this LNCaP cell line, the 1,25D$_3$ reduced the expression levels of CYP27B1 and CAMP, and on the contrary, increased the expression levels of CYP24A1. No variation was observed for VDR expression levels (Figure 6A,B).

These results showed accordance with the analysis previously effectuated (Figure 5, GSE64657). In addition, the 25D$_3$ LNCaP cell treatment strongly increases CAMP and CYP24A1 expression levels. The siCYP27B1 and siVDR LNCaP cells treatment have demonstrated that CYP24A1 and CAMP are regulated principally by 25D$_3$ in LNCaP cells via CYP27B1 and VDR. As regards the PCa genes highlighted in our analysis, we have demonstrated that all genes were sensitive to the effect of 1,25D$_3$ and 25D$_3$ at the dose of 100 nM for 24 h (were an exception the expression levels of MCC2) (Figure 6C,D). Furthermore, the siCYP27B1 and siVDR LNCaP cells treatment showed that the downregulation of KLK3 depends strictly on the CYP27B1 gene transcription. More mildly, the PRSS8 and SMYD2 genes expression also depends on the transcription of the CYP27B1 gene. Co-silencing of the CYP27B1 and VDR genes was determinant in the transcription of the CCNG2, PRSS8, SMYD2 and SOX4 genes (Figure 6C,D).

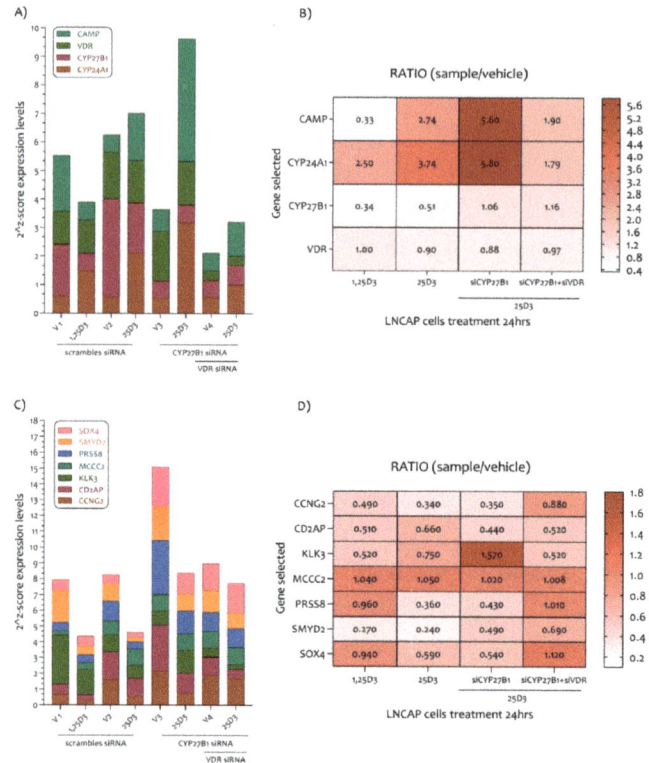

Figure 6. PCa-related genes modulated in the LNCaP cell line under $1,25D_3$ and $25D_3$ treatment. (**A**) In the LNCaP cell line the $1,25D_3$ reduced the expression levels of CYP27B1 and CAMP, and on the contrary increased the expression levels of CYP24A1. An exception were VDR expression levels. (**B**) The CYP24A1 and CAMP expression levels are regulated by $25D_3$ in LNCaP cells via CYP27B1 and VDR. (**C**) All PCa related genes were sensitive to the effect of $1,25D_3$ and $25D_3$ (an exception was MCC2). (**D**) The siCYP27B1 and siVDR LNCaP cells treatment showed a strong modulation of KLK3 gene transcription.

We showed that all selected genes were modulated by $1,25D_3$ and its precursor $25D_3$. In addition, $25D_3$ downregulates KLK3 and SMYD3 genes expression with CYP27B1 activity. Furthermore, $25D_3$ modulates the expression levels of CCNG2, CD2AP, PRSS8, SMYD2 and SOX4 via VDR transcription (Figure 6).

3.4. Immunohistochemistry Analysis of the Six PCa Genes Selected

In order to evaluate the protein expression levels of PRSS8, SOX4, SMYD2, MCCC2, CCNG2 and CD2AP in heathy subjects and PCa patients, we explored the Human Atlas project portal. Aware that the number of biopsies available on The Human Protein Atlas database was small (Table 1), taking into consideration the limits related to this, but in order to verify our hypothesis, we decided to proceed by analyzing the histological biopsies of healthy and pathological tissue with protein staining of the six genes that were the object of our study. For all protein detected, we found a potentially increased staining in prostate adenocarcinoma with High grade compared to healthy prostate tissue biopsies, except for SMYD2 which did not present changes in intensity between the healthy and pathological prostate tissue (Figure 7).

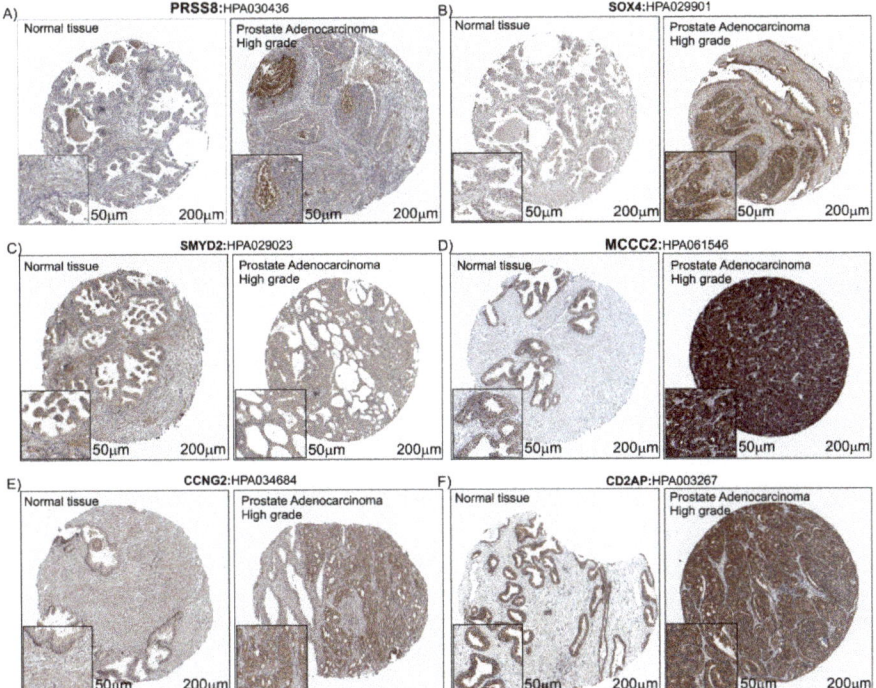

Figure 7. IHC of the six PCa-selected genes. Immunostaining for PRSS8 (**A**), SOX4 (**B**), SMYD2 (**C**), MCCC2 (**D**), CCNG2 (**E**) and CD2AP (**F**) in Prostate Adenocarcinoma High grade compared to normal prostate tissue (Control) (see the text for the details). The images downloaded from the Human Atlas Project (https://www.proteinatlas.org/) have been re-adapted using CorelDraw. The original files web site links are available as well as the complete analyzes, in Table 1 and Table S1.

Particularly, MCCC2, CD2AP and SOX4 presented an higher intensity staining in adenocarcinoma with High grade compared to healthy prostate tissue biopsies (Figure 7B,D,F) (Table 1).

The immunostaining details are reported in Table 1 and in Table S1. However, as regards CD2AP and MCCC2, the protein expression levels seemed quite high in normal epithelium; the higher staining observed in cancer is probably due to the higher number of epithelial cells in cancer tissue.

Table 1. Immunostaining details recovered from The Human Atlas Project.

Protein	State	Antibody	Staining	Intensity	Quantity	Localization	Cells	Biopsies	Patient ID
PRSS8	Healthy	HPA030436	Low	Moderate	<25%	Cytoplasmic/membranous	Glandular cells	3	2472
	HGPAC		Medium	Moderate	75%–25%	Cytoplasmic/membranous	Tumor cells	4	3563
SOX4	Healthy	HPA029901	Low	Weak	75%–25%	Nuclear	Glandular cells	3	2472
	HGPAC		Medium	Moderate	>75%	Cytoplasmic/membranous/nuclear	Tumor cells	7	3570
SMYD2	Healthy	HPA029023	Medium	Moderate	>75%	Cytoplasmic/membranous	Glandular cells	3	2472
	HGPAC		Low	Weak	75%–25%	Cytoplasmic/membranous	Tumor cells	1	2825
MCCC2	Healthy	HPA061546	High	Strong	>75%	Cytoplasmic/membranous	Glandular cells	3	2472
	HGPAC		High	Strong	>75%	Cytoplasmic/membranous	Tumor cells	12	2816
CCNG2	Healthy	HPA034684	Low	Moderate	<25%	Cytoplasmic/membranous	Glandular cells	3	2472
	HGPAC		Medium	Moderate	>75%	Cytoplasmic/membranous	Tumor cells	2	3978
CD2AP	Healthy	HPA003267	High	Strong	>75%	Cytoplasmic/membranous	Glandular cells	3	2053
	HGPAC		High	Strong	>75%	Cytoplasmic/membranous	Tumor cells	15	250

HGPAC: High grade prostatic adenocarcinoma. Healthy: normal prostate tissue biopsies. The % indicates the fraction of stained cells (rare, <25%, 25–75% or >75%).

4. Discussion

In this paper, we undertook an analysis to identify the key genes involved in PCa. We analyzed three PCa microarray datasets (GSE70770, GSE62872 and GSE6919), merged all the genes significantly up-regulated and subsequently, intersected the common genes identified (n = 276) with the transcriptome of genes down-regulated in the *LNCaP cell line* treated with Vitamin D, in order to identify the common key genes involved in PCa and potentially modulated by the action of Vitamin D. The analysis yielded 43 genes involved in PCa significantly modulated by Vitamin D. These genes were involved in different molecular processes, among which the most interesting were *organogenesis, morphogenesis and cell migration*, all mechanisms involved in the genesis and in the tumor progression. Noteworthy, our analysis showed that six genes (PRSS8, SOX4, SMYD2, MCCC2, CCNG2 and CD2AP) were significantly modulated in both PCa biopsies and in the *LNCaP cell line* treated with Vitamin D. A literature investigation showed that all these genes were involved in different tumor progressions. Furthermore, a Z-score transformation of all datasets allowed us to group all the healthy prostate samples (n = 251) and PCa (n = 548), thus significantly increasing the court of subjects included in the study. A Spearman's ϱ correlation analysis showed that five genes out of six (PRSS8, SMYD2, MCCC2, CCNG2 and CD2AP), were positively and statistically correlated with the gene expression levels of KLK3 and with the tumor %. Contrary note, SOX4 expression levels were positively correlated only with the tumor %, but not with KLK3 gene expression levels. Furthermore, the analysis of the data deriving from GSE107438, the treatment of LNCaP cell line with siCYP27B1 and siVDR, showed that a downregulation of KLK3 expression levels depends strictly on the CYP27B1 gene transcription. More mildly, the PRSS8 and SMYD2 genes expression also depends on the transcription of the CYP27B1 gene. Co-silencing of the CYP27B1 and VDR genes was determinant in the transcription of the CCNG2, PRSS8, SMYD2 and SOX4 genes. Our results have been in part confirmed by the immunostaining obtained by the Human Atlas Project portal. The immunohistochemistry analysis showed that *five* genes (PRSS8, SOX4, MCCC2, CCNG2 and CD2AP) out of six appeared more expressed in PCa biopsies compared to healthy prostate tissue. No difference was observed for SYMD2.

Prostasin (PRSS8) is a serine protease, mainly expressed in normal prostate epithelia, the prostate gland and in seminal fluid [37]. This protein is implicated in epithelial sodium channel regulation and essential for terminal epithelial differentiation [38]. Nowadays, the role played by this molecule in cancer is unclear. It was shown that it may be related to tumor promoter mechanisms [39] as well as tumor suppression [40–42]. In several studies it has been shown that PRSS8 plays a role as a tumor suppressor in various malignancies, such as in hepatocellular carcinoma [43]. In 2016 Tamir et al. showed that abundant amounts of secreted prostasin found in the sera of early stage ovarian cancer (OVC) can potentially be used as a minimally invasive screening biomarker for early stage OVC [44]. As regarding the role of PRSS8 and PCa, there is no large bibliography. Noteworthy, in 2003, Takahashi and colleagues demonstrated that in 54 patients (Japanese), the PRSS8 mRNA expression levels, measured by northern blot analysis, were not correlated with the clinical stage of human PCa. Furthermore, almost in all cases of metastatic and hormone-refractory cancers, these demonstrated a down-regulation of *prostasin* expression. The authors at the end of their manuscript suggested that *prostasin* cannot be regarded as a prognostic indicator for human PCa, although it may be a useful marker for tumor differentiation [45]. In light of this, our results are totally contrasting with the results obtained by Takahashi in 2003. It must be kept in mind that the samples analyzed in this study come from different ethnic groups, and there was also a difference in the number of the subjects recruited (54 with respect the 548 present in our analysis) and the control samples, healthy, were subjects with benign prostatic hyperplasia (BPH). This difference could be the basis for the different results obtained in the study.

In any case, the increase in mRNA levels in prostate tumor biopsies, their positive correlation with the tumor percentage and the messenger of KLK3 and their modulation by Vitamin D, need further confirmation from an in vitro experimental point of view.

As regard SOX4, in our analysis we showed that the expression levels were increased in PCa patients' biopsies compared to the healthy prostate subjects. These results are totally in agreement with the recent bibliography [46,47]. SOX4 is a transcription factor involved in the regulation of embryonic development. SOX4 is highly expressed in several human cancers of epithelial origin and is associated with a poor clinical outcome. It has been related with the loss of epithelial features and the gain of mesenchymal traits, including cell migration and invasion [48]. SOX4 knockdown repressed the cell proliferation and migration ability. Moreover, inhibition of SOX4 could reverse the epithelial-mesenchymal transition processes through up-regulation of adhesion molecules such as E-cadherin and the down-regulation of vimentin [47]. In our analysis we showed that Vitamin D was able to reduce significantly the expression of SOX4 in the *LNCaP cell line*. Noteworthy, it has been shown that the Vitamin D is able to induce E-cadherin expression in breast cancer cells by promoter demethylation [49]. Taking all of this into consideration, the Vitamin D could be able to reduce the tumor cell migration and invasion, via SOX4 down-regulation and consequently up-regulation of E-Cadherin.

SMYD2 (SET and MYND domain-containing protein 2) is a histone lysine methyltransferase enzyme, belonging to the family that contains five enzymes that share two highly conserved domains (the catalytic SET domain and the MYND domain) [50]. This enzyme is highly expressed in a variety of cancers [51,52]. Recently, it has been shown that SMYD2 inhibits tumor suppressor proteins p53 [53] and PTEN [54]. However, to date, there has been no report on the clinical and prognostic significance of SMYD2 in patients with PCa. In our analysis, we showed that mRNA of SYMD2 is over-expressed in PCa and the treatment of the *LNCaP cell line* with Vitamin D reduces the expression levels, but this result was not confirmed by the PCa biopsies observation. Consequently, the Vitamin D could increase PTEN expression via a down-regulation of SYMD2, and inhibit cell proliferation in PCa. In support of this hypothesis, it has been shown that the Vitamin D plays an inhibitory effect on the hepatocellular carcinoma cells proliferation through the down-regulation of HDAC2 and up-regulation of PTEN [55].

The expression analysis of MCCC2 in PCa biopsies, showed an over-expression on mRNA and a positive correlation with KLK3 gene expression levels and tumor %. This enzyme catalyzes the carboxylation of 3-methylcrotonyl-CoA to form 3-methylglutaconyl-CoA. There is evidence that mutations of this gene is associated with 3-Methylcrotonylglycinuria, an autosomal recessive disorder of leucine catabolism [56]. As regards its role in cancer, there exist only two reports that bind it to tumor development. These two reports identified MCCC2 over-expression linked to LNM PCa tissues [57] and to low-grade PCa [58]. Our results could be a good start to investigate the role of MCCC2 in cancer.

In our analysis, another interesting molecule identified as potentially a marker of PCa was CCNG2. This molecule belongs to the cyclin family, and its expression is significantly higher in cell cycle-arrest [59]. The current literature suggests that CCNG2 plays an important inhibitory role in cancer initiation and progression [60]. It has been shown that CCNG2 dysregulation is related to cancer progression and could play an important role in cell transformation and the early stages of cancer development [60,61]. Seemingly, our findings would seem to contrast with the role played by CCNG2 in cancer. Recently, Canovas et al. demonstrated that primary prostate tumors show a significantly higher expression of PTOV1, CCNG2 and MYC compared to benign tissue [62]. Furthermore, in this set of tumors, the expression of CCNG2 significantly correlates with prostate tumor aggressiveness. The authors concluded their study, hypothesizing that CCNG2 is as potential markers of metastasis and bad prognosis when detected in primary prostate tumors. These results are in good agreement with our finding. Moreover, it has been shown that the Vitamin D plays an anti-proliferative effect in the *LNCaP cell line* reducing the cyclin-dependent kinase 2 activity [63].

The CD2AP is a protein closely associated with the cytoskeleton structure. This protein interacts with the filamentous actin and a variety of cell membrane proteins. Its expression is involved in kidney diseases, including nephrin and polycystin-2 [64]. Although several studies have indicated that CD2AP regulates cell shape and movements, little attention has been paid to the cancer [65]. To date, there has been no report on CD2AP expression levels in PCa. To our knowledge, this is the first study which suggests the role of CD2AP in PCa.

5. Conclusions

Investigating the target genes, significantly up-regulated in the present analysis and down-regulated by the Vitamin D action, may help to discover the molecular mechanisms involved in PCa progression. The large cohort of our analysis allowed us to improve the diagnostic meaning of our results. Further IHC analysis on a much broader court than the one analyzed in our study could further confirm our results. From the outcome of our investigation, it is possible to conclude that the mechanism involved during the PCa progression could be modulated by Vitamin D. Further research on the role played by the Vitamin D on PCa key genes is necessary to extend our results and to try an answer to the several questions which still remain to be addressed.

Supplementary Materials: The following are available online at http://www.mdpi.com/2076-3417/9/22/4923/s1. Figure S1: The six key genes expression levels in GSE70770, GSE62872 and GSE6919. Table S1: Contains the complete analyzes used for the realization of this manuscript. Table S2: The GeneMania-report of the 43 key genes selected.

Author Contributions: M.D.R.; Data curation, S.R. and M.D.R.; Formal analysis, V.F. and M.D.R.; Funding acquisition, R.C.; Investigation, R.C.; L.S. and R.I.; Methodology, I.B.; Project administration, R.C.; Resources, S.R.; Software, M.D.R.; Supervision, M.D.R.; Validation, P.C.; Visualization, M.A.S. and G.M.; Writing—original draft, M.D.R.; Writing—review & editing, I.B. and G.M.

Funding: This research gained the support of the University Research Project Grant (Triennial Research Plan 2016-2018), Department of Biomedical and Biotechnological Sciences (BIOMETEC), University of Catania, Italy.

Acknowledgments: We would like to show our gratitude to the authors of microarray datasets made available online, for consultation and re-analysis.

Conflicts of Interest: The authors declare no conflict of interest.

References

1. Trump, D.L.; Aragon-Ching, J.B. Vitamin D in prostate cancer. *Asian J. Androl.* **2018**, *20*, 244–252. [CrossRef] [PubMed]
2. Bikle, D.D. Vitamin D metabolism, mechanism of action, and clinical applications. *Chem. Biol.* **2014**, *21*, 319–329. [CrossRef] [PubMed]
3. Pinzone, M.R.; Di Rosa, M.; Celesia, B.M.; Condorelli, F.; Malaguarnera, M.; Madeddu, G.; Martellotta, F.; Castronuovo, D.; Gussio, M.; Coco, C.; et al. LPS and HIV gp120 modulate monocyte/macrophage CYP27B1 and CYP24A1 expression leading to vitamin D consumption and hypovitaminosis D in HIV-infected individuals. *Eur. Rev. Med Pharmacol. Sci.* **2013**, *17*, 1938–1950. [PubMed]
4. Di Rosa, M.; Malaguarnera, L.; Nicolosi, A.; Sanfilippo, C.; Mazzarino, C.; Pavone, P.; Berretta, M.; Cosentino, S.; Cacopardo, B.; Pinzone, M.R.; et al. Vitamin D3: An ever green molecule. *Front. Biosci.* **2013**, *5*, 247–260. [CrossRef] [PubMed]
5. Malaguarnera, L.; Marsullo, A.; Zorena, K.; Musumeci, G.; Di Rosa, M. Vitamin D3 regulates LAMP3 expression in monocyte derived dendritic cells. *Cell. Immunol.* **2017**, *311*, 13–21. [CrossRef] [PubMed]
6. Nunnari, G.; Fagone, P.; Lazzara, F.; Longo, A.; Cambria, D.; Di Stefano, G.; Palumbo, M.; Malaguarnera, L.; Di Rosa, M. Vitamin D3 inhibits TNFalpha-induced latent HIV reactivation in J-LAT cells. *Mol. Cell. Biochem.* **2016**, *418*, 49–57. [CrossRef] [PubMed]
7. Jimenez-Sousa, M.A.; Martinez, I.; Medrano, L.M.; Fernandez-Rodriguez, A.; Resino, S. Vitamin D in Human Immunodeficiency Virus Infection: Influence on Immunity and Disease. *Front. Immunol.* **2018**, *9*, 458. [CrossRef]
8. Pinzone, M.R.; Di Rosa, M.; Malaguarnera, M.; Madeddu, G.; Foca, E.; Ceccarelli, G.; d'Ettorre, G.; Vullo, V.; Fisichella, R.; Cacopardo, B.; et al. Vitamin D deficiency in HIV infection: An underestimated and undertreated epidemic. *Eur. Rev. Med. Pharmacol. Sci.* **2013**, *17*, 1218–1232.
9. Di Rosa, M.; Malaguarnera, M.; Zanghi, A.; Passaniti, A.; Malaguarnera, L. Vitamin D3 insufficiency and colorectal cancer. *Crit. Rev. Oncol. Hematol.* **2013**, *88*, 594–612. [CrossRef]

10. Gilbert, R.; Martin, R.M.; Beynon, R.; Harris, R.; Savovic, J.; Zuccolo, L.; Bekkering, G.E.; Fraser, W.D.; Sterne, J.A.; Metcalfe, C. Associations of circulating and dietary vitamin D with prostate cancer risk: A systematic review and dose-response meta-analysis. *Cancer Causes Control CCC* **2011**, *22*, 319–340. [CrossRef]
11. Kristal, A.R.; Till, C.; Song, X.; Tangen, C.M.; Goodman, P.J.; Neuhauser, M.L.; Schenk, J.M.; Thompson, I.M.; Meyskens, F.L., Jr.; Goodman, G.E.; et al. Plasma vitamin D and prostate cancer risk: Results from the Selenium and Vitamin E Cancer Prevention Trial. *Cancer Epidemiol. Biomark. Prev. A Publ. Am. Assoc. Cancer Res. Cosponsored By Am. Soc. Prev. Oncol.* **2014**, *23*, 1494–1504. [CrossRef]
12. Patel, A.R.; Klein, E.A. Risk factors for prostate cancer. *Nat. Clin. Pract. Urol.* **2009**, *6*, 87–95. [CrossRef] [PubMed]
13. Siegel, R.L.; Miller, K.D.; Jemal, A. Cancer statistics, 2018. *CA A Cancer J. Clin.* **2018**, *68*, 7–30. [CrossRef] [PubMed]
14. Odedina, F.T.; Akinremi, T.O.; Chinegwundoh, F.; Roberts, R.; Yu, D.; Reams, R.R.; Freedman, M.L.; Rivers, B.; Green, B.L.; Kumar, N. Prostate cancer disparities in Black men of African descent: A comparative literature review of prostate cancer burden among Black men in the United States, Caribbean, United Kingdom, and West Africa. *Infect. Agents Cancer* **2009**, *4* (Suppl. 1), S2. [CrossRef] [PubMed]
15. Trump, D.L.; Deeb, K.K.; Johnson, C.S. Vitamin D: Considerations in the continued development as an agent for cancer prevention and therapy. *Cancer J.* **2010**, *16*, 1–9. [CrossRef]
16. Munetsuna, E.; Kawanami, R.; Nishikawa, M.; Ikeda, S.; Nakabayashi, S.; Yasuda, K.; Ohta, M.; Kamakura, M.; Ikushiro, S.; Sakaki, T. Anti-proliferative activity of 25-hydroxyvitamin D3 in human prostate cells. *Mol. Cell. Endocrinol.* **2014**, *382*, 960–970. [CrossRef] [PubMed]
17. Song, Z.Y.; Yao, Q.; Zhuo, Z.; Ma, Z.; Chen, G. Circulating vitamin D level and mortality in prostate cancer patients: A dose-response meta-analysis. *Endocr. Connect.* **2018**, *7*, R294–R303. [CrossRef]
18. Fleet, J.C.; Kovalenko, P.L.; Li, Y.; Smolinski, J.; Spees, C.; Yu, J.G.; Thomas-Ahner, J.M.; Cui, M.; Neme, A.; Carlberg, C.; et al. Vitamin D Signaling Suppresses Early Prostate Carcinogenesis in TgAPT121 Mice. *Cancer Prev. Res.* **2019**, *12*, 343–356. [CrossRef]
19. Singh, P.K.; Doig, C.L.; Dhiman, V.K.; Turner, B.M.; Smiraglia, D.J.; Campbell, M.J. Epigenetic distortion to VDR transcriptional regulation in prostate cancer cells. *J. Steroid Biochem. Mol. Biol.* **2013**, *136*, 258–263. [CrossRef]
20. Farhan, H.; Wahala, K.; Cross, H.S. Genistein inhibits vitamin D hydroxylases CYP24 and CYP27B1 expression in prostate cells. *J. Steroid Biochem. Mol. Biol.* **2003**, *84*, 423–429. [CrossRef]
21. Ross-Adams, H.; Lamb, A.D.; Dunning, M.J.; Halim, S.; Lindberg, J.; Massie, C.M.; Egevad, L.A.; Russell, R.; Ramos-Montoya, A.; Vowler, S.L.; et al. Corrigendum to "Integration of Copy Number and Transcriptomics Provides Risk Stratification in Prostate Cancer: A Discovery and Validation Cohort Study" [EBioMedicine 2 (9) (2015) 1133–1144]. *EBioMedicine* **2017**, *17*, 238. [CrossRef]
22. Whitington, T.; Gao, P.; Song, W.; Ross-Adams, H.; Lamb, A.D.; Yang, Y.; Svezia, I.; Klevebring, D.; Mills, I.G.; Karlsson, R.; et al. Gene regulatory mechanisms underpinning prostate cancer susceptibility. *Nat. Genet.* **2016**, *48*, 387–397. [CrossRef] [PubMed]
23. Penney, K.L.; Sinnott, J.A.; Tyekucheva, S.; Gerke, T.; Shui, I.M.; Kraft, P.; Sesso, H.D.; Freedman, M.L.; Loda, M.; Mucci, L.A.; et al. Association of prostate cancer risk variants with gene expression in normal and tumor tissue. *Cancer Epidemiol. Biomark. Prev. A Publ. Am. Assoc. Cancer Res. Cosponsored By Am. Soc. Prev. Oncol.* **2015**, *24*, 255–260. [CrossRef] [PubMed]
24. Chandran, U.R.; Ma, C.; Dhir, R.; Bisceglia, M.; Lyons-Weiler, M.; Liang, W.; Michalopoulos, G.; Becich, M.; Monzon, F.A. Gene expression profiles of prostate cancer reveal involvement of multiple molecular pathways in the metastatic process. *BMC Cancer* **2007**, *7*, 64. [CrossRef] [PubMed]
25. Yu, Y.P.; Landsittel, D.; Jing, L.; Nelson, J.; Ren, B.; Liu, L.; McDonald, C.; Thomas, R.; Dhir, R.; Finkelstein, S.; et al. Gene expression alterations in prostate cancer predicting tumor aggression and preceding development of malignancy. *J. Clin. Oncol. Off. J. Am. Soc. Clin. Oncol.* **2004**, *22*, 2790–2799. [CrossRef]
26. Susa, T.; Iizuka, M.; Okinaga, H.; Tamamori-Adachi, M.; Okazaki, T. Without 1alpha-hydroxylation, the gene expression profile of 25(OH)D3 treatment overlaps deeply with that of 1,25(OH)2D3 in prostate cancer cells. *Sci. Rep.* **2018**, *8*, 9024. [CrossRef]
27. Xiao, J.; Cao, H.; Chen, J. False discovery rate control incorporating phylogenetic tree increases detection power in microbiome-wide multiple testing. *Bioinformatics* **2017**, *33*, 2873–2881. [CrossRef]

28. Smyth, G.K. Linear models and empirical bayes methods for assessing differential expression in microarray experiments. *Stat. Appl. Genet. Mol. Biol.* **2004**, *3*, 3. [CrossRef]
29. Davis, S.; Meltzer, P.S. GEOquery: A bridge between the Gene Expression Omnibus (GEO) and BioConductor. *Bioinformatics* **2007**, *23*, 1846–1847. [CrossRef]
30. Zuberi, K.; Franz, M.; Rodriguez, H.; Montojo, J.; Lopes, C.T.; Bader, G.D.; Morris, Q. GeneMANIA prediction server 2013 update. *Nucleic Acids Res.* **2013**, *41*, W115–W122. [CrossRef]
31. Chang, J.T.; Nevins, J.R. GATHER: A systems approach to interpreting genomic signatures. *Bioinformatics* **2006**, *22*, 2926–2933. [CrossRef]
32. Uhlen, M.; Fagerberg, L.; Hallstrom, B.M.; Lindskog, C.; Oksvold, P.; Mardinoglu, A.; Sivertsson, A.; Kampf, C.; Sjostedt, E.; Asplund, A.; et al. Proteomics. Tissue-based map of the human proteome. *Science* **2015**, *347*, 1260419. [CrossRef] [PubMed]
33. Thul, P.J.; Akesson, L.; Wiking, M.; Mahdessian, D.; Geladaki, A.; Ait Blal, H.; Alm, T.; Asplund, A.; Bjork, L.; Breckels, L.M.; et al. A subcellular map of the human proteome. *Science* **2017**, *356*. [CrossRef] [PubMed]
34. Uhlen, M.; Zhang, C.; Lee, S.; Sjostedt, E.; Fagerberg, L.; Bidkhori, G.; Benfeitas, R.; Arif, M.; Liu, Z.; Edfors, F.; et al. A pathology atlas of the human cancer transcriptome. *Science* **2017**, *357*. [CrossRef] [PubMed]
35. Cheadle, C.; Vawter, M.P.; Freed, W.J.; Becker, K.G. Analysis of microarray data using Z score transformation. *J. Mol. Diagn. JMD* **2003**, *5*, 73–81. [CrossRef]
36. Jyoti, S.K.; Blacke, C.; Patil, P.; Amblihalli, V.P.; Nicholson, A. Prostate cancer screening by prostate-specific antigen (PSA); a relevant approach for the small population of the Cayman Islands. *Cancer Causes Control CCC* **2018**, *29*, 87–92. [CrossRef] [PubMed]
37. Yu, J.X.; Chao, L.; Chao, J. Prostasin is a novel human serine proteinase from seminal fluid. Purification, tissue distribution, and localization in prostate gland. *J. Biol. Chem.* **1994**, *269*, 18843–18848. [PubMed]
38. Vallet, V.; Chraibi, A.; Gaeggeler, H.P.; Horisberger, J.D.; Rossier, B.C. An epithelial serine protease activates the amiloride-sensitive sodium channel. *Nature* **1997**, *389*, 607–610. [CrossRef]
39. Yu, J.X.; Chao, L.; Ward, D.C.; Chao, J. Structure and chromosomal localization of the human prostasin (PRSS8) gene. *Genomics* **1996**, *32*, 334–340. [CrossRef]
40. Chen, L.M.; Hodge, G.B.; Guarda, L.A.; Welch, J.L.; Greenberg, N.M.; Chai, K.X. Down-regulation of prostasin serine protease: A potential invasion suppressor in prostate cancer. *Prostate* **2001**, *48*, 93–103. [CrossRef]
41. Narikiyo, T.; Kitamura, K.; Adachi, M.; Miyoshi, T.; Iwashita, K.; Shiraishi, N.; Nonoguchi, H.; Chen, L.M.; Chai, K.X.; Chao, J.; et al. Regulation of prostasin by aldosterone in the kidney. *J. Clin. Investig.* **2002**, *109*, 401–408. [CrossRef]
42. Chen, L.M.; Chai, K.X. Prostasin serine protease inhibits breast cancer invasiveness and is transcriptionally regulated by promoter DNA methylation. *Int. J. Cancer. J. Int. Du Cancer* **2002**, *97*, 323–329. [CrossRef] [PubMed]
43. Zhang, L.; Jia, G.; Shi, B.; Ge, G.; Duan, H.; Yang, Y. PRSS8 is Downregulated and Suppresses Tumour Growth and Metastases in Hepatocellular Carcinoma. *Cell. Physiol. Biochem. Int. J. Exp. Cell. Physiol. Biochem. Pharmacol.* **2016**, *40*, 757–769. [CrossRef] [PubMed]
44. Tamir, A.; Gangadharan, A.; Balwani, S.; Tanaka, T.; Patel, U.; Hassan, A.; Benke, S.; Agas, A.; D'Agostino, J.; Shin, D.; et al. The serine protease prostasin (PRSS8) is a potential biomarker for early detection of ovarian cancer. *J. Ovarian Res.* **2016**, *9*, 20. [CrossRef] [PubMed]
45. Takahashi, S.; Suzuki, S.; Inaguma, S.; Ikeda, Y.; Cho, Y.M.; Hayashi, N.; Inoue, T.; Sugimura, Y.; Nishiyama, N.; Fujita, T.; et al. Down-regulated expression of prostasin in high-grade or hormone-refractory human prostate cancers. *Prostate* **2003**, *54*, 187–193. [CrossRef]
46. Liu, E.; Sun, X.; Li, J.; Zhang, C. miR30a5p inhibits the proliferation, migration and invasion of melanoma cells by targeting SOX4. *Mol. Med. Rep.* **2018**, *18*, 2492–2498. [CrossRef]
47. Liu, Y.; Zeng, S.; Jiang, X.; Lai, D.; Su, Z. SOX4 induces tumor invasion by targeting EMT-related pathway in prostate cancer. *Tumour Biol. J. Int. Soc. Oncodevelopmental Biol. Med.* **2017**, *39*, 1010428317694539. [CrossRef]
48. Lourenco, A.R.; Coffer, P.J. SOX4: Joining the Master Regulators of Epithelial-to-Mesenchymal Transition? *Trends Cancer* **2017**, *3*, 571–582. [CrossRef]
49. Lopes, N.; Carvalho, J.; Duraes, C.; Sousa, B.; Gomes, M.; Costa, J.L.; Oliveira, C.; Paredes, J.; Schmitt, F. 1Alpha,25-dihydroxyvitamin D3 induces de novo E-cadherin expression in triple-negative breast cancer cells by CDH1-promoter demethylation. *Anticancer Res.* **2012**, *32*, 249–257.

50. Spellmon, N.; Holcomb, J.; Trescott, L.; Sirinupong, N.; Yang, Z. Structure and function of SET and MYND domain-containing proteins. *Int. J. Mol. Sci.* **2015**, *16*, 1406–1428. [CrossRef]
51. Sakamoto, L.H.; Andrade, R.V.; Felipe, M.S.; Motoyama, A.B.; Pittella Silva, F. SMYD2 is highly expressed in pediatric acute lymphoblastic leukemia and constitutes a bad prognostic factor. *Leuk. Res.* **2014**, *38*, 496–502. [CrossRef]
52. Komatsu, S.; Ichikawa, D.; Hirajima, S.; Nagata, H.; Nishimura, Y.; Kawaguchi, T.; Miyamae, M.; Okajima, W.; Ohashi, T.; Konishi, H.; et al. Overexpression of SMYD2 contributes to malignant outcome in gastric cancer. *Br. J. Cancer* **2015**, *112*, 357–364. [CrossRef] [PubMed]
53. Huang, J.; Perez-Burgos, L.; Placek, B.J.; Sengupta, R.; Richter, M.; Dorsey, J.A.; Kubicek, S.; Opravil, S.; Jenuwein, T.; Berger, S.L. Repression of p53 activity by Smyd2-mediated methylation. *Nature* **2006**, *444*, 629–632. [CrossRef] [PubMed]
54. Nakakido, M.; Deng, Z.; Suzuki, T.; Dohmae, N.; Nakamura, Y.; Hamamoto, R. Dysregulation of AKT Pathway by SMYD2-Mediated Lysine Methylation on PTEN. *Neoplasia* **2015**, *17*, 367–373. [CrossRef] [PubMed]
55. Huang, J.; Yang, G.; Huang, Y.; Zhang, S. Inhibitory effects of 1,25(OH)2D3 on the proliferation of hepatocellular carcinoma cells through the downregulation of HDAC2. *Oncol. Rep.* **2017**, *38*, 1845–1850. [CrossRef]
56. Morscher, R.J.; Grunert, S.C.; Burer, C.; Burda, P.; Suormala, T.; Fowler, B.; Baumgartner, M.R. A single mutation in MCCC1 or MCCC2 as a potential cause of positive screening for 3-methylcrotonyl-CoA carboxylase deficiency. *Mol. Genet. Metab.* **2012**, *105*, 602–606. [CrossRef]
57. Pang, J.; Liu, W.P.; Liu, X.P.; Li, L.Y.; Fang, Y.Q.; Sun, Q.P.; Liu, S.J.; Li, M.T.; Su, Z.L.; Gao, X. Profiling protein markers associated with lymph node metastasis in prostate cancer by DIGE-based proteomics analysis. *J. Proteome Res.* **2010**, *9*, 216–226. [CrossRef]
58. Marques, R.B.; Dits, N.F.; Erkens-Schulze, S.; van Ijcken, W.F.; van Weerden, W.M.; Jenster, G. Modulation of androgen receptor signaling in hormonal therapy-resistant prostate cancer cell lines. *PLoS ONE* **2011**, *6*, e23144. [CrossRef]
59. Horne, M.C.; Goolsby, G.L.; Donaldson, K.L.; Tran, D.; Neubauer, M.; Wahl, A.F. Cyclin G1 and cyclin G2 comprise a new family of cyclins with contrasting tissue-specific and cell cycle-regulated expression. *J. Biol. Chem.* **1996**, *271*, 6050–6061. [CrossRef]
60. Kim, Y.; Shintani, S.; Kohno, Y.; Zhang, R.; Wong, D.T. Cyclin G2 dysregulation in human oral cancer. *Cancer Res.* **2004**, *64*, 8980–8986. [CrossRef]
61. Hasegawa, S.; Nagano, H.; Konno, M.; Eguchi, H.; Tomokuni, A.; Tomimaru, Y.; Wada, H.; Hama, N.; Kawamoto, K.; Kobayashi, S.; et al. Cyclin G2: A novel independent prognostic marker in pancreatic cancer. *Oncol. Lett.* **2015**, *10*, 2986–2990. [CrossRef]
62. Canovas, V.; Punal, Y.; Maggio, V.; Redondo, E.; Marin, M.; Mellado, B.; Olivan, M.; Lleonart, M.; Planas, J.; Morote, J.; et al. Prostate Tumor Overexpressed-1 (PTOV1) promotes docetaxel-resistance and survival of castration resistant prostate cancer cells. *Oncotarget* **2017**, *8*, 59165–59180. [CrossRef] [PubMed]
63. Zhuang, S.H.; Burnstein, K.L. Antiproliferative effect of 1alpha,25-dihydroxyvitamin D3 in human prostate cancer cell line LNCaP involves reduction of cyclin-dependent kinase 2 activity and persistent G1 accumulation. *Endocrinology* **1998**, *139*, 1197–1207. [CrossRef] [PubMed]
64. Lehtonen, S.; Ora, A.; Olkkonen, V.M.; Geng, L.; Zerial, M.; Somlo, S.; Lehtonen, E. In vivo interaction of the adapter protein CD2-associated protein with the type 2 polycystic kidney disease protein, polycystin-2. *J. Biol. Chem.* **2000**, *275*, 32888–32893. [CrossRef] [PubMed]
65. Rizvi, H.; Paterson, J.C.; Tedoldi, S.; Ramsay, A.; Calaminici, M.; Natkunam, Y.; Lonardi, S.; Tan, S.Y.; Campbell, L.; Hansmann, M.L.; et al. Expression of the CD2AP adaptor molecule in normal, reactive and neoplastic human tissue. *Pathologica* **2012**, *104*, 56–64.

© 2019 by the authors. Licensee MDPI, Basel, Switzerland. This article is an open access article distributed under the terms and conditions of the Creative Commons Attribution (CC BY) license (http://creativecommons.org/licenses/by/4.0/).

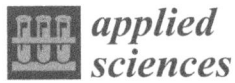

Article

Epigallocatechin-3-Gallate (EGCG), An Active Constituent of Green Tea: Implications in the Prevention of Liver Injury Induced by Diethylnitrosamine (DEN) in Rats

Saleh A. Almatroodi, Mohammed A. Alsahli, Hanan Marzoq Alharbi, Amjad Ali Khan and Arshad Husain Rahmani *

Department of Medical Laboratories, College of Applied Medical Sciences, Qassim University, Buraidah 52571, Saudi Arabia; smtrody@qu.edu.sa (S.A.A.); shly@qu.edu.sa (M.A.A.); han21han22@gmail.com (H.M.A.); akhan@qu.edu.sa (A.A.K.)
* Correspondence: AH.RAHMANI@QU.EDU.SA

Received: 14 October 2019; Accepted: 5 November 2019; Published: 11 November 2019

Featured Application: EGCG, an active constituent of green tea acts as a hepatoprotectant by reducing the serum levels of liver functional enzymes, increasing total anti-oxidative capacity, reducing pathological changes and apoptosis. Moreover, EGCG displayed a powerful hepatoprotective additive as it considerably mitigates the liver toxicity and apoptosis induced by DEN.

Abstract: Liver diseases are one of the most detrimental conditions that may cause inflammation, leading to tissue damage and perturbations in functions. Several drugs are conventionally available for the treatment of such diseases, but the emergence of resistance and drug-induced liver injury remains pervasive. Hence, alternative therapeutic strategies have to be looked upon. Epigallocatechin-3-gallate (EGCG) is a naturally occurring polyphenol in green tea that has been known for its disease-curing properties. In this study, we aimed to evaluate its anti-oxidative potential and protective role against diethylnitrosamine (DEN)-induced liver injury. Four different groups of rats were used for this study. The first group received normal saline and served as the control group. The second group received DEN (50 mg/kg body wt) alone and third group received DEN plus EGCG (40 mg/kg body wt) only. The fourth group were treated with EGCG only. The liver protective effect of EGCG against DEN toxicity through monitoring the alterations in aspartate transaminase (AST), and alanine transaminase (ALT) and alkaline phosphatase (ALP) activities, serum level of pro-inflammatory mediators and anti-oxidant enzymes, histopathological alterations, measurement of cellular apoptosis, and cell cycle analysis was examined. The rats that were given DEN only had a highly significantly elevated levels of liver enzymes and pro-inflammatory cytokines, highly decreased anti-oxidative enzymes, and histological changes. In addition, a significant elevation in the percentage of apoptotic nuclei and cell cycle arrest in the sub- G1 phase was detected. EGCG acts as a hepatoprotectant on DENs by reducing the serum levels of liver functional enzymes, increasing total anti-oxidative capacity, reducing pathological changes and apoptosis, as well as causing the movement of cells from the sub G1 to S or G2/M phase of the cell cycle. In conclusion, EGCG displayed a powerful hepatoprotective additive as it considerably mitigates the liver toxicity and apoptosis induced by DEN.

Keywords: DEN; liver; inflammation; ultra-structural changes; oxidative stress; EGCG

1. Introduction

The liver is one of the important organs of our body, having a vital role in the processes of metabolism and detoxification [1]. Around 10% of the world population is oppressed by liver disease [2]. Diseases, such as non-alcoholic fatty liver disease, are actively correlated with obesity, alcoholic steatosis, fibrosis, cirrhosis, and diabetes mellitus. Metabolic syndrome, chronic hepatitis, and hepatocellular carcinoma are some of the most comprehensive and colloquial liver diseases, drawing considerable attention from medical professionals and scientists [3,4]. In chronic liver injury, a large number of pro-inflammatory cytokines are released from injured cells, which stimulate cells, such as Kupffer cells, to deliver more inflammatory mediators and various types of free radicals. This signal is further amplified by the recruitment of neutrophils to the site of injury. Free radicals' release is known to induce cell/tissue damage via lipid peroxidation. As a result, the wound healing process is also induced to maintain homeostasis, wherein hepatic stellate cells are activated to release fibrogenic mediators accountable for the degradation of damaged cells and construction of new cells. However, Liver fibrosis results from chronic damage to the liver in conjunction with the accumulation of ECM proteins, which is a characteristic of most types of chronic liver diseases during persistent injury, wound healing is disturbed, and the degradation process is constrained. Subsequently, a large amount of collagen accumulates and causes fibrosis or cirrhosis [5].

Treatment methods involve the use of drugs, such as corticosteroids, anti- tumor necrosis factor (TNF) antibodies, and other antioxidants [6]. Several drugs are directly or indirectly linked to drug-induced liver injury and exhibit trivial adverse drug reactions, such as cell swelling, degeneration, necrosis, inflammation, hemorrhages, and fatty changes. Drug toxicity is a major issue of the available therapeutic drugs against liver disease. Despite these adverse reactions, a large mass of drugs shows stunted incidences of detrimental hepatic reactions. Consequently, liver injury is predominantly diagnosed only after extensive clinical applications of drugs. Antibiotics, statins, non-steroidal anti-inflammatory drugs, antiepileptics, and tuberculostatics are the most common causes of drug-induced liver injury [7]. Similarly, N-nitroso compounds, such as diethylnitrosamine (DEN) and dimethylnitrosamine (DMN), bear hepatotoxic and carcinogenic effects. These compounds are biotransformed to alkylating metabolites that causes DNA adduct formation. This biotransformation is mediated by a cyto-chrome P450 enzyme-dependent pathway, mainly including the enzyme CYP2E1. Parenteral or oral administration of modest quantities of DEN or DMN may cause extensive liver damage, including fibrosis, intense neutrophilic infiltration, extensive centrilobular hemorrhagic necrosis, and bridging necrosis, ultimately resulting in hepatocarcinogenesis. The tenacity of hepatic alterations induced via DEN have allowed it to be used in the establishment of a provocative experimental model for studies in anticipation of pathogenic alterations in hepatocarcinogenesis [8–10].

Although prerogative methods of treatment exist for maximum liver diseases, many types still remain immedicable and the emergence of drug resistance is most prevalent [2]. Also, drug-induced liver injury remains a challenge in diagnosis. Therefore, other safe, inexpensive, effective, and more reliable strategies for treatment are needed to control liver-associated diseases. Alternative medicines based on natural products are being increasingly used in the treatment of various diseases without any adverse effects on normal physiological processes. Natural products and their related products are being used as alternatives to conventional drugs in the management of various diseases. They are normally associated with secondary metabolites produced by an organism, which are actively involved in stimulating defense mechanisms against microorganisms, insects, and competing plants. A large number of plant products, including flowers, bark, leaves, and stem, are still commonly used in healthcare management worldwide. They have engendered a rich origin of structurally diverse substances with an expanded range of biological activities that may lead to the development of alternative therapies [11–14].

Green tea is one type of tea that is made from *Camellia sinensis* leaves and is frequently used as a beverage worldwide, including in Saudi Arabia. Green tea is mixture of various compounds and is also rich in polyphenols, which are powerful antioxidants [15,16]. Among the various polyphenolic substances, epigallocatechin-gallate (EGCG) is usually measured as a primary antioxidant in green tea extract [17], which has been proposed as being responsible for many of the potential promoting effects of tea [18,19]. EGCG is supposed to mitigate inflammatory processes and oxidative stress, thereby reducing liver injury [16,20–22]. Considering the importance and essentiality of the pathogenesis of liver diseases and its increasing incidence worldwide, we have made this study. Henceforth, an experimental study was performed to evaluate the liver protective effect of EGCG against nitrosodimethylamine-induced liver injury in rats.

2. Materials and Methods

2.1. Animal Model and Sample Collection

Rats (male Wistar 200 ± 25 g), aged 6 weeks, were collected from King Saud University, Saudi Arabia and were acclimatized for one week. The animal house was suitably ventilated with a 12-h cycle of day as well as night light conditions and the temperature was maintained at around 25 °C. The animals were fed a standard rodent pellet diet and had ad libitum access to water. All protocols concerning current study were in compliance with the ethical guidelines of the institute. The animals were categorized into four groups (a total number of eight rats in each group): Group 1: control; group 2: DEN (50 mg/kg bw in vehicle solution, oral gavage); group 3: DEN + EGCG (40 mg/kg bw in vehicle solution, oral gavage); and group 4: EGCG only, Table 1. All animals were sacrificed after 10 weeks of treatment and samples, such as blood and tissue, were collected for further analysis to achieve the objectives of the study. The serum was collected from the blood by centrifugation for 10 min at 1500× g and stored at a low temperature of −80 °C until further biochemical analysis. The aim of the study was achieved through the measurement of liver enzyme levels, levels of pro-inflammatory markers, expression of Phosphatase and tensin homolog (PTEN) protein through immunohistochemistry, and identification of apoptosis by Terminal deoxynucleotidyl transferase dUTP nick end labeling (TUNEL) staining. To provide greater insight into the subject, flow cytometry and transmission electron microscopy were done to evaluate the cell cycle and ultra-structural changes of the tissue. The research methodologies were directed towards the following landmark in a stepwise manner.

Table 1. Animal grouping.

Experimental Group	Group Number	Treatment	Number of Animals Per Group (n)
Negative control	1	Normal rats administered with vehicle solution	08
Disease control	2	DEN administered via oral gavage	08
Treatment	3	DEN and EGCG	08
Treatment	4	EGCG with vehicle solution	08

2.2. Determination of Liver Function (ALT, ALP, and AST) Enzymes, SOD, CAT, and GPx Antioxidant Enzymes and Total Antioxidant Capacity

Aspartate transaminase (AST), alanine transaminase (ALT), and alkaline phosphatase (ALP) levels were measured in serum. Total antioxidant capacity (TAC), superoxide dismutase (SOD), Glutathione peroxidase (GPx) and catalase (CAT) were assayed to measure the levels of hepatic injury, according to the instructions provided by the manufacturer (Abcam, UK).

2.3. Determination of C-Reactive Protein, Interleukin-6 (IL-6), and Tumor necrosis factor-α (TNF-α)

Serological analysis was performed to measure the serum levels of C-reactive protein (CRP), IL-6, and TNF-α. Specific rat ELISA kits (Abcam, UK) were used for the measurement of serum C- reactive protein (CRP), IL-6, and TNF-α according to the instructions provided by the manufacturer.

2.4. Histopathological Analysis

Liver tissues were collected and fixed in 10% formalin solution (neutral buffered saline) and processed for histopathological analysis as per the standardized procedure [23]. A paraffin block was sectioned using a rotary microtome, sections were placed onto glass slides, and then dried overnight. Thin paraffin sections (5 µm) were prepared and then stained with hematoxylin and eosin (H&E) dyes and observed under a light microscope, and photomicrographs were taken by pathologists who were blinded to the control and treatment groups.

2.5. Immunohistochemical Analysis

Expression of PTEN protein was analyzed through immunochemistry as per the method previously described [24,25]. Briefly, tissue sections were deparaffinized in xylene, and treated with 3% hydrogen peroxide for 15 to 20 min to block endogenous peroxidase activity. Antigen retrieval was made in citrate buffer, pH 6.0, for 25 min and then tissues were blocked in 5% normal serum for 30 min. Slides were incubated with primary antibody as PTEN monoclonal mouse antihuman antibody followed by secondary biotinylated antibody. Sections were then washed in phosphate buffer and incubated with streptavidin peroxidase for 20 to 25 min. Lastly, diaminobenzidine (DAB) was used as chromogen and then sections were counterstained with hematoxylin stain, a photograph was captured, and the results were interpreted accordingly.

Scoring Method

PTEN protein showing less than or equal to 10% of cells showing positivity was considered a negative case. If more than 10% of cells were positive for PTEN, this was considered as a positive case. The expression positivity was applied, +1 for 10% to 30% expression was considered as weak expression, +2 for 31% to 70% expression was moderate positivity, and +3 for more than 71% was considered strong expression. A total of 5 fields from each tissue were selected, and 100 cells from each field were counted and the result was interpreted

2.6. TUNEL Assay

Apoptosis in liver tissues was detected by the terminal deoxynucleotidyl transferase-mediated dUTP nick end-labelling (TUNEL) kit (Abcam, UK) following the manufacturer's protocol. Concisely, terminal deoxynucleotidyl transferase (TdT) attached to 3′-OH ends of DNA fragments generated and catalyzed the addition of biotin-labeled deoxynucleotides. Moreover, biotinylated nucleotides were bound with a streptavidin-horseradish peroxidase conjugate. Finally, diaminobenzidine (DAB) reacted with the horseradish peroxidase-labelled sample to generate a colored (brown) substrate at the site of DNA fragmentation. Apoptotic activity was quantified by the apoptotic index, which represented the percentage of apoptotic epithelial cells in each tissue. Apoptosis was measured by counting the percentage of positive cells and a photograph was taken, and the result was interpreted.

2.7. Transmission Electron Microscopy (TEM)

Transmission electron microscopy was performed using the method previously described [16] with little modifications. Briefly, around a 3 to 5 mm piece of liver tissue was fixed in freshly prepared 3% glutaraldehyde at 4 °C for 24 h. The samples were washed in phosphate buffer and stored at 4 °C for further processing. After fixation, the samples were washed in 1% osmium tetroxide, dehydrated via ethanol series and cleared using propylene oxide, and then embedded in resin. Round 50-nm thick sections were cut using ultramicrotome and sections were stained through uranyl acetate and lead citrate, photographed with transmission electron microscopy, and the results were interpreted accordingly.

2.8. Cell Cycle Analysis

Flow cytometry using propidium iodide (PI) staining was used to identify the cell distribution during the various phases of the cell cycle according to the manufacturer's instructions. Concisely, cells were harvested and washed in phosphate buffer saline, and fixed in cold ethanol for 25 to 30 min at a low temperature of 4 °C. In addition, cells were washed two times in phosphate buffer saline and centrifuged and the RNase was added. Finally, 150–200 µL of propidium iodide was added and forward scatter and side scatter were measured to identify single cells. This is usually determined by their frequency histogram, which offers information about the relative frequency of cells in the phases of the cell cycle.

2.9. Statistical Analysis

Data from each treated group are expressed as means ± SEM. Statistical comparison between groups was made using SPSS software by matching analysis of variance. A p-value < 0.05 was considered as statistically significant.

3. Results

3.1. EGCG Reduces the Serum Level of Biochemical Enzymes

In liver injury, alterations occur in the transportation function of hepatocytes, thus triggering leakage in the plasma membrane and henceforth causing an increase of serum levels of liver enzymes. The levels of liver function enzymes, including alanine transaminase (ALT), alkaline phosphatase (ALP), and aspartate transaminase (AST), were measured in all experimental groups. The levels of enzymes, including ALT, ALP, and AST, were significantly higher in the DEN only-treated group (disease control) than the normal control group ($p < 0.05$). Moreover, DEN with EGCG-treated group demonstrated significantly lower levels of all tested enzymes in comparison to the DEN-only group ($p < 0.05$) (Figure 1).

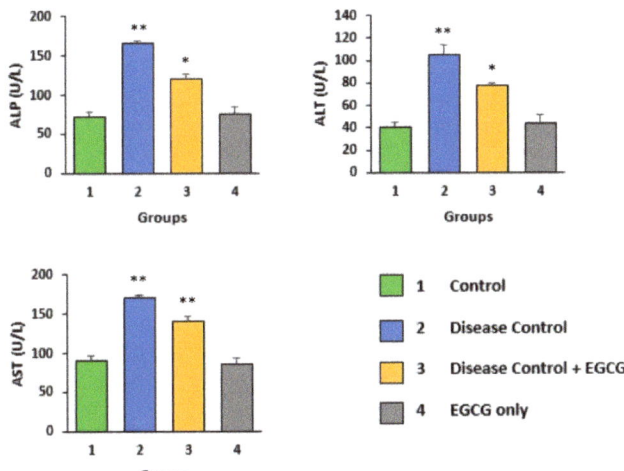

Figure 1. Effect of EGCG on Alanine aminotransferase (ALT), Alkaline phosphatase (ALP), and Aspartate transaminase (AST) activity in DEN-induced liver injury. Enzyme levels, including ALT, ALP, and AST, were significantly higher in the DEN-treated group than the normal control group. Moreover, the DEN + EGCG group revealed considerably lower ALT, ALP, and AST values than the DEN-only group. Statistical significances are compared between control versus DEN-treated groups only ($p < 0.01$), and DEN-treated versus DEN plus EGCG ($p < 0.05$).

3.2. Antioxidant Activity of EGCG

The antioxidant activity of EGCG was analyzed by measuring the serum levels of hepatic antioxidant enzymes, including SOD, CAT, and GPx. The activities of antioxidant enzymes, such as SOD, CAT, and GPx, were found to be significantly decreased in the DEN only-treated group compared to the control group (Figure 2). Furthermore, the activities of SOD, CAT, and GPx meaningfully increased in the DEN + EGCG group ($p < 0.005$). Moreover, the total antioxidant capacity was significantly decreased in the DEN only-treated group as compared to the control group. However, the total antioxidant capacity was found to be significantly increased in the DEN + EGCG group ($p < 0.005$) (Figure 2). This result clearly demonstrated that EGCG plays a vital role in liver damage protection by improving antioxidant enzyme levels.

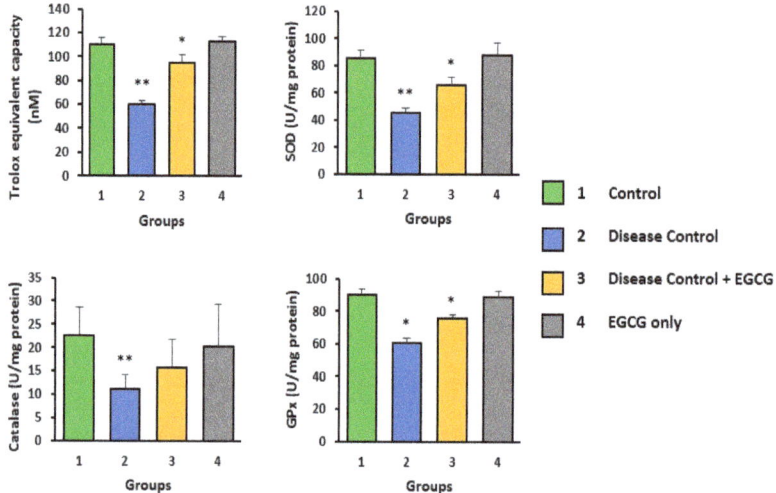

Figure 2. Effect of EGCG on antioxidant enzymes Superoxide Dismutase (SOD), Catalase (CAT), and Glutathione peroxidase (GPx) and total antioxidant capacity in DEN-induced liver injury. The levels of antioxidant enzymes were significantly lower in the DEN only-treated group than the control group. The DEN + EGCG group displayed significantly higher antioxidant enzyme levels than the DEN-only group ($p < 0.01$). Total antioxidant capacity was also found to be significantly increased in the DEN + EGCG group ($p < 0.05$).

3.3. EGCG Reduces the Serum Levels of CRP and Pro-Inflammatory Mediators—TNF-α and IL-6

DEN treatment increases the levels of pro-inflammatory cytokines TNF-α and IL-6 in the serum of animals, as compared to the serum of animals without any treatment (control) ($p < 0.05$). On the other hand, treatment with EGCG significantly decreased their levels ($p < 0.05$). The level of CRP was high in the serum of animals of the DEN only-treated group, as compared to the serum of animals without any treatment, and treatment with EGCG significantly decreased the level of CRP (Figure 3).

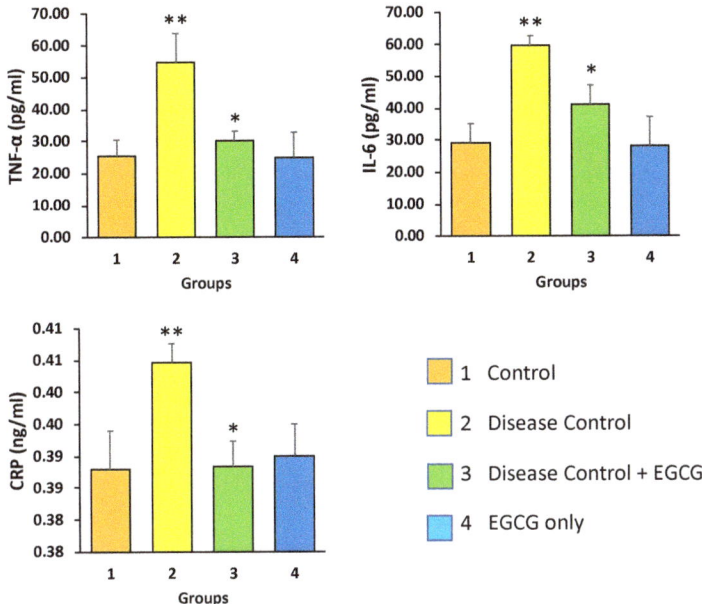

Figure 3. Effect of EGCG on the serum levels of TNF-α, CRP, and IL-6. EGCG treatment significantly decreases the levels of Tumour Necrosis Factor alpha (TNF-α), c-reactive protein (CRP), and Interleukin 6 (IL-6) in the DEN + EGCG group ($p < 0.05$) as compared to the DEN-treated group ($p < 0.01$).

3.4. EGCG Reduces Hepatic Histological Alterations

Liver tissues from all the experimental groups were analyzed through H&E staining and histological findings were compared accordingly (Figure 4a–e). The DEN only-treated group displayed altered liver tissues, including dilate and congested central vein, hemorrhage and increased inflammatory cells in the portal tract, hemorrhage, and necrosis. However, these alterations were found to be significantly mild/lower in the EGCG-treated group ($p < 0.05$).

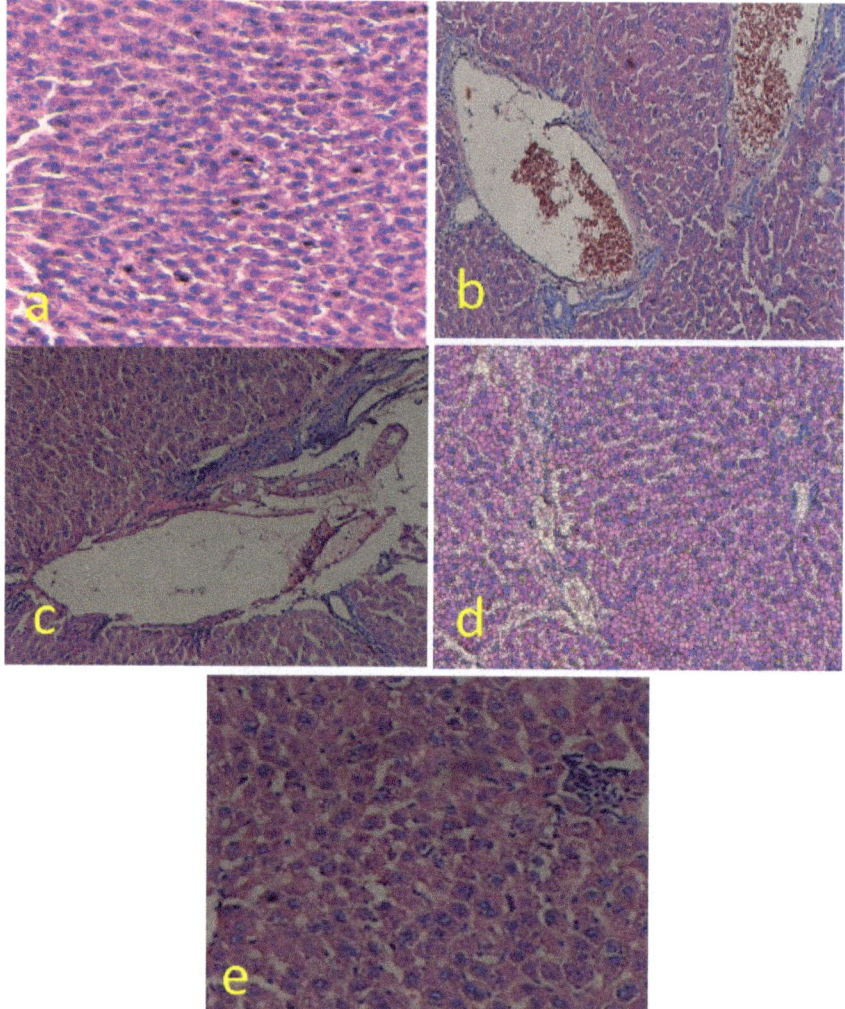

Figure 4. Histopathological analysis. H&E (X40) stained photomicrographs of liver tissues showing (**a**) the normal architecture of hepatocytes—control group. (**b–d**) DEN only-treated tissues displaying dilate and congested central vein, hemorrhage, and increased inflammatory cells in the portal tract, hemorrhage, and necrosis. (**e**) EGCG-treated tissue, where the liver tissue alteration was significantly lowered compared to the disease control group (DEN only-treated group).

3.5. Immunohistochemical Analysis

Expression of PTEN protein was evaluated in the tissues of different groups via immunohistochemistry staining. PTEN protein expression was noticed in all groups (Figure 5a–d) and loss of PTEN protein expression was not observed in any of the groups. The expression pattern of PTEN protein among different groups was found to be statistically insignificant ($p > 0.05$).

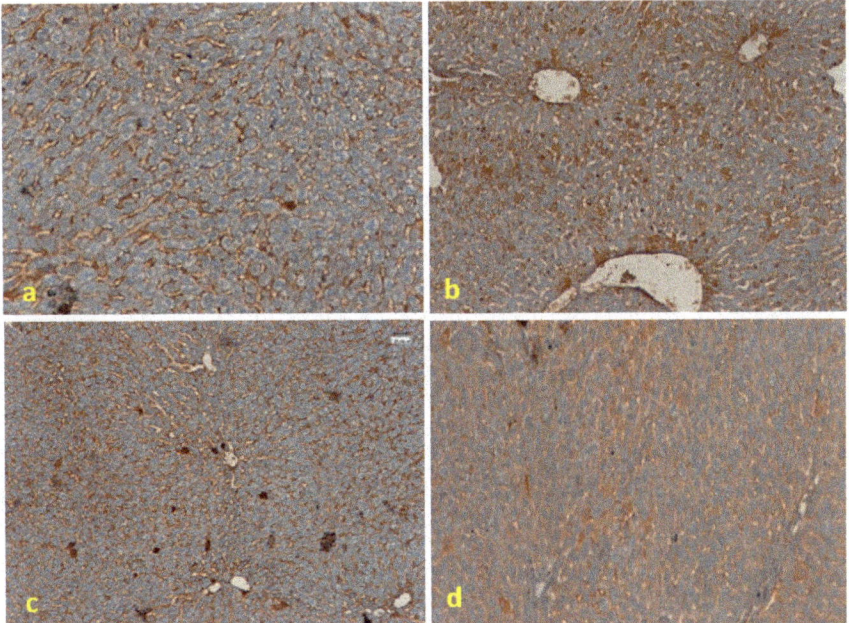

Figure 5. Immunohistochemical analysis. Phosphatase and tensin homolog (PTEN) protein expression was evaluated in different treatment groups (**a–d**). (**a**) The control group showed high PTEN expression; (**b**) the DEN-treated group also displayed a high expression of PTEN; (**c**). PTEN expression was also noted in the DEN + EGCG treated group and (**d**) EGCG-only group.

3.6. Evaluation of Apoptotic Bodies Via TUNEL Assay

Control tissue, EGCG-treated group, and DEN + EGCG group tissue did not possess apoptotic nuclei as indicated by the TUNEL assay. However, some positive TUNEL cells were observed in the DEN only-treated group (Figure 6a–d).

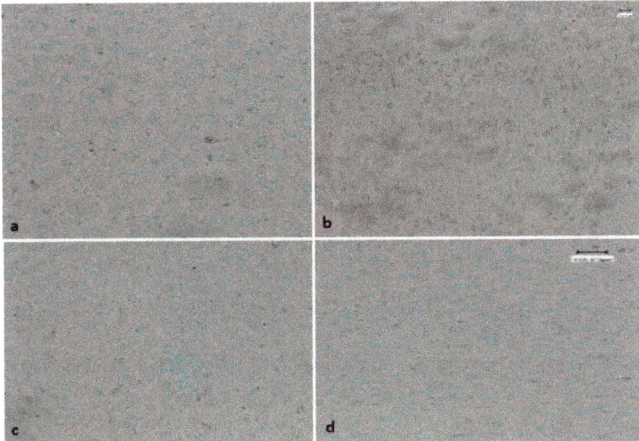

Figure 6. TUNEL Assay. Apoptotic nuclei were absent in (**a**) the liver tissue of the control group; (**c**) tissue from the DEN + EGCG group and (**d**) tissue from the EGCG only-treated group. However, (**b**) the liver tissue of DEN only-treated group indicated the presence of some positive apoptotic nuclei.

3.7. Effect of EGCG on Ultrastructure Changes of Liver

An electron microscopy-based experiment was performed to analyze the ultrastructure of liver tissue. The hepatocytes of the liver tissue of the normal control group demonstrated normal mitochondria and most of the mitochondria were spherical or round-shaped, dense granulated cytoplasm, smooth endoplasmic reticulum tubules with cristae normally present and normal rough endoplasmic reticulum whereas the observation of hepatocytes in the DEN-treated group showed extensive cellular damage. It was seen that a swollen and reduced number of mitochondria, distorted shape mitochondria, large clumps of glycogen surrounding cell organelles, broken SER tubules, and dilation of the rough endoplasmic reticulum ($p < 0.05$). A number of damaged hepatocytes were found in the DEN-only treatment group, and the majority of the cytoplasmic organelles in these cells were degraded. The hepatocytes of liver tissue of the DEN plus EGCG-treated group showed a reduction of the damage in hepatocytes. Mitochondria are spherical or round-shaped but the presence of some dilated mitochondria, presence of glycogen clump, well-developed SER-ER tubule, and few lysosomes. The normal hepatocytes were seen in the EGCG only-treated group (Figure 7a–d).

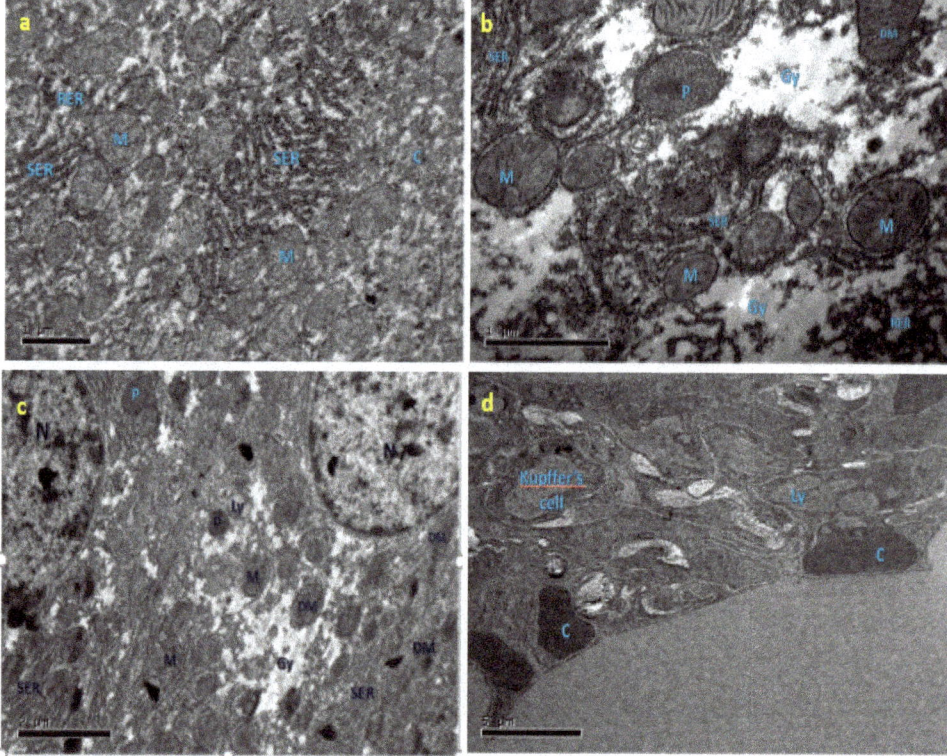

Figure 7. Ultrastructural changes of liver. Electron microscopy was used to observe the ultrastructure of hepatic cells. (**a**) Hepatocytes of the liver tissue of the control group revealed normal mitochondria and most of the mitochondria are spherical or round-shaped, smooth endoplasmic reticulum tubules with cristae normally present, and normal rough endoplasmic reticulum; (**b**) DEN only-treated tissues displaying extensive cellular damage. Swollen and reduced number of mitochondria, distorted shape mitochondria, large clumps of glycogen surrounding cell organelles, broken SER tubules, and dilation of the rough endoplasmic reticulum was seen. (**c**) EGCG plus DEN-treated tissue—where the liver tissue alteration was significantly reduced as compared to the disease control group ($p < 0.05$) (DEN only-treated group). (**d**) EGCG only-treated group exhibited normal hepatocytes.

3.8. Effect of EGCG on the Cell Cycle

Cell cycle analysis was done using flow cytometry. A relative frequency of cells in different phases of the cell cycle were calculated. The control group (a) contained around 80% of cells in the S and G2/M phase. However, cells were arrested in the sub-G1 phase in tissues treated with DEN only (b). On the other hand, the EGCG plus DEN (c) treatment allowed the cells to move from the sub-G1 phase to the G1 and S phase as indicated by an increased frequency of cells in the S and G2/M phase (~93%). (d) The EGCG only-treated group (Figures 8a–d and 9a–d).

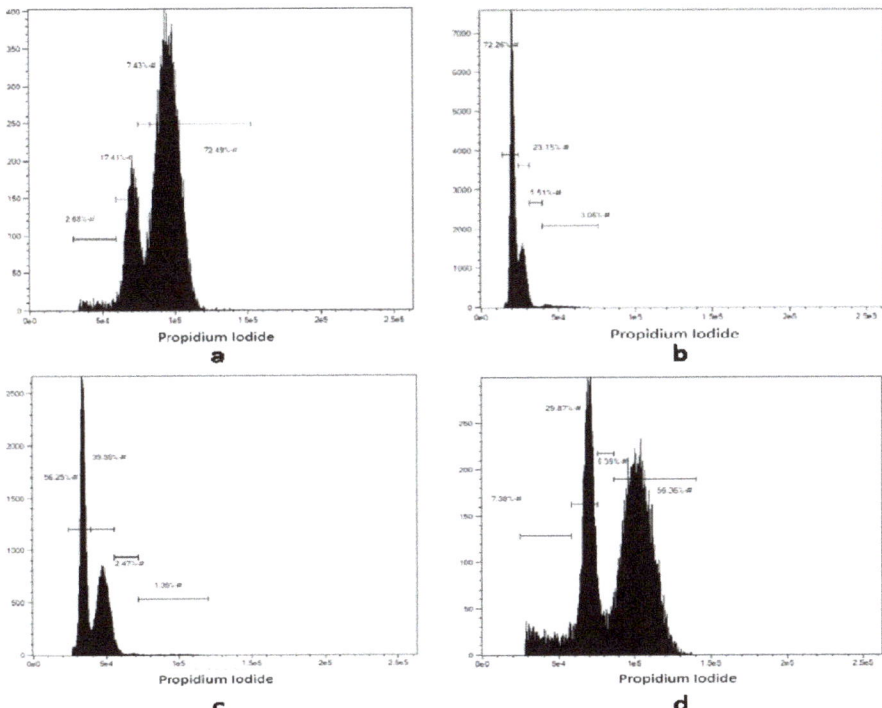

Figure 8. Cell cycle analysis. Relative frequencies of cells in different phases of the cell cycle in The control group (**a**) contained around 80% of cells in the S and G2/M phase. However, cells were arrested in the sub-G1 phase in tissues treated with DEN only (**b**). On the other hand, the EGCG plus DEN (**c**) treatment allowed the cells to move from the sub-G1 phase to the G1 and S phase as indicated by an increased frequency of cells in the S and G2/M phase. (**d**) The EGCG only-treated group.

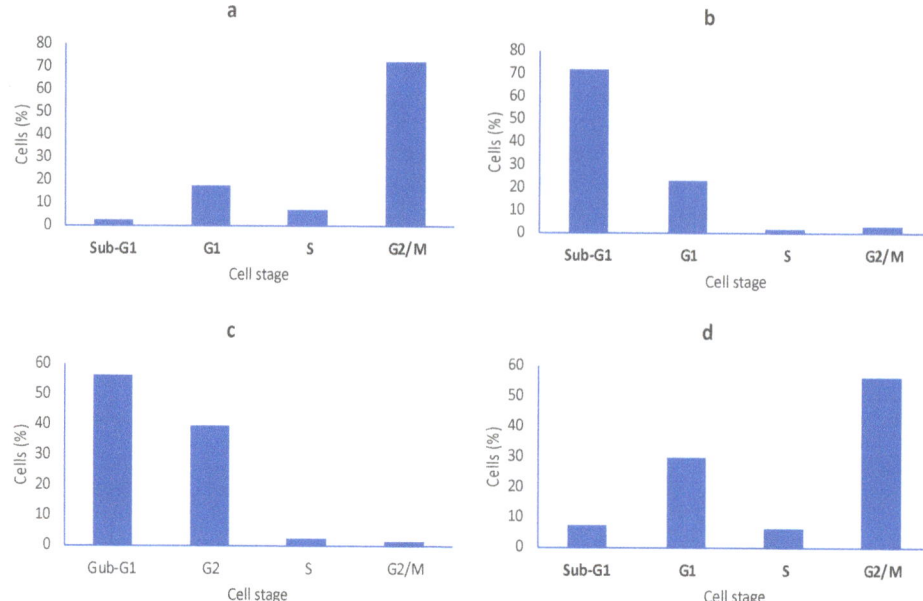

Figure 9. Cell cycle significance analysis between the groups using a bar diagram. Relative frequencies of cells in different phases of the cell cycle in (**a**) control, (**b**) DEN only-treated, (**c**) DEN + EGCG-treated, and (**d**) EGCG only-treated groups.

4. Discussion

The current study results provide evidence of the role of EGCG in the regulation of apoptosis, antioxidant production, and inflammatory cytokines in rat liver damage with the concept of mitochondrial homeostasis. Significantly, the current study results also advocate for an argument for further analysis of EGCG or structurally related molecules as inhibitors of TNF-α and IL-6 synthesis and possibly other cytokine-regulated diseases. The anti-inflammatory, tumor-suppressing, and anti-oxidative effects of EGCG have been studied formerly. Howbeit, its antioxidant effect is the most imperative one [26,27]. During liver injury, the generation of free radicals and reactive oxygen species plays a critical role in the augmentation of tissue damage. As the injury proceeds, inflammatory cascades are activated, leading to the release of pro-inflammatory cytokines and free radicals, which finally causes activation of inflammatory Kupffer cells and recruitment of neutrophils at the site of injury. Stimulated inflammatory cells are accountable for the generation of more free radicals and provoked secretion of pro-inflammatory mediators. A large amount of released free radicals induce lipid peroxidation in the cellular phospholipid bilayer, which can damage the cytosol and other cellular organelles [5]. Thoughtfully, the anti-oxidative effects of EGCG come into action through activation of anti-oxidation protective signaling, thus reducing injury [28,29]. Similarly, other studies have shown anti-oxidative and preventive effects of EGCG on different hepatic injury animal models [30,31].

In the current study, DEN-induced liver injury in a rat model was characterized by an increase in the secretion of pro-inflammatory cytokines, including IL-6 and TNF-α. This study shows that EGCG ameliorated liver injury along with a decrease of IL-6 and TNF-α levels in serum. These results are supported by previous studies in which IL-6 deficiency or IL-6R blockade ameliorated hepatocyte damage, indicating that the control of IL-6 production may produce a valuable outcome in liver injury [32,33]. A previous study by Jamal et al. [34] showed that administration of green tea polyphenols showed a role in the prevention of acute liver injury in mice by reducing CRP, IL-6, and TNF-α. However, this study specifically provides insight into one of the potential mechanisms of EGCG's liver protective activity.

Moreover, EGCG treatment also increases the levels of anti-oxidative enzymes SOD, CAT, and GPx, suggesting the activation of anti-oxidation protective signaling pathways to provide protection against oxidative damage. The upregulation of serum levels of AST, ALP, and ALT is a strong indication of the manifestation of oxidative stress in DEN-induced liver injury. The current study result demonstrates that EGCG reduces oxidative stress by reducing the serum levels of these liver functionality enzymes. It has been reported that oxidative stress regulates the apoptotic signaling pathway in cells. This result agrees with a previous finding that treatment with EGCG plays a significant role in the reduction of liver injury, oxidative stress, and the inflammatory response [5]. Moreover, EGCG also significantly attenuated the severity of CCl (4)-induced liver injury and the progression of liver fibrosis. Another study reported that in vitro model of oxidative stress induced by ethanol provided evidence that EGCG prevented some aspect of liver cell injury caused by ethanol [35].

PTEN is one of the tumor suppressor genes and it is located in the 10q23 region encoding for a 403-amino acid multifunctional protein that comprises lipid and protein phosphatase activities [36]. The overexpression/altered expression of PTEN protein has been noticed in tumors [37]. Several studies have suggested a role for PTEN in hepatic injury [38,39], but the expression pattern of PTEN protein among different groups was statistically insignificant in the current study.

Mitochondria are the major source of endogenous reactive oxygen species, and altering mitochondrial homeostasis is a known mechanism for toxic compounds, including DEN [40,41]. EGCG treatment significantly improves mitochondrial health and number as determined by our TEM study; several studies [42–44] with EGCG are in accordance with our study. Further studies are needed to fully investigate this mechanism.

Previous study have suggested that PARP is a family of proteins involved in a number of cellular processes including DNA repair and apoptosis [45]. This has been evidently established by an increase in apoptotic nuclei upon DEN-induced liver injury. However, EGCG decreases the presence of apoptotic nuclei as demonstrated by the TUNEL assay. Therefore, the present data advocate that administration of EGCG plays a role in the reduction of liver injury-related cell apoptosis, possibly by decreasing cleaved caspase-3 and cleaved caspase-9 levels. Thus, the accumulation of DEN in the liver caused several damaging effects, including marked pathological changes in liver enzyme activities, generation of reactive oxygen species, and DNA damage, as well as apoptosis. These effects were reversed by administration of EGCG. Additionally, EGCG administration displayed a clear effect on the cell cycle, accompanied by a decrease in the sub-G1 population (indicating apoptosis) and a significant increase in S or G2/M (indicating cell proliferation), the mechanism of which needs to be further elucidated. A previous finding was in accordance with the current finding and the study reported negative regulators of the protein kinases and cyclins, thus arresting the cell cycle at the eG_0/G_1 phase [46], and EGCG, a chief compound of green tea, inhibited DNA synthesis and arrested the cell cycle at the $G0/G_1$ phase [47].

In conclusion, the result of the current study demonstrates that EGCG treatment reduced the amount of DEN-induced hepatic injury by decreasing mitochondrial oxidative stress and cellular apoptosis. Furthermore, it was also revealed that EGCG inhibits CRP, TNF-α, and IL-6 production and suppresses the inflammation process. Hence, EGCG can be used as a plausible therapeutic tool against liver injury and other liver-associated diseases.

Author Contributions: Conceptualization, S.A.A. and A.H.R.; Formal analysis, M.A.A.; Methodology, H.M.A.; Supervision, H.M.A.; Validation, A.A.K.; Writing—original draft, S.A.A. and A.H.R.; Writing—review & editing, M.A.A., A.A.K. and A.H.R.

Funding: This work was funded and supported by Qassim University Research Deanship Grants # cams1-2018-1-14-S-3360.

Conflicts of Interest: There are no conflict of interest regarding this study.

Data Availability: The data used to support the findings of the current study are included within the article.

References

1. Samuel, A.J.S.J.; Mohan, S.; Chellappan, D.K.; Kalusalingam, A.; Ariamuthu, S. *Hibiscus vitifolius* (Linn.) root extracts shows potent protective action against anti-tubercular drug induced hepatotoxicity. *J. Ethnopharmacol.* **2012**, *141*, 396–402. [CrossRef] [PubMed]
2. Mishra, B.B.; Tiwari, V.K. Natural products: An evolving role in future drug discovery. *Eur. J. Med. Chem.* **2011**, *46*, 4769–4807. [CrossRef] [PubMed]
3. Gao, M.; Nettles, R.E.; Belema, M.; Snyder, L.B.; Nguyen, V.N.; Fridell, R.A.; Serrano-Wu, M.H.; Langley, D.R.; Sun, J.H.; O'Boyle, D.R., II; et al. Chemical genetics strategy identifies an HCV NS5A inhibitor with a potent clinical effect. *Nature* **2010**, *465*, 96. [CrossRef] [PubMed]
4. Ghosh, N.; Ghosh, R.; Mandal, V.; Mandal, S.C. Recent advances in herbal medicine for treatment of liver diseases. *Pharm. Biol.* **2011**, *49*, 970–988. [CrossRef] [PubMed]
5. Tipoe, G.L.; Leung, T.M.; Liong, E.C.; Lau, T.Y.H.; Fung, M.L.; Nanji, A.A. Epigallocatechin-3-gallate (EGCG) reduces liver inflammation, oxidative stress and fibrosis in carbon tetrachloride (CCl_4)-induced liver injury in mice. *Toxicology* **2010**, *273*, 45–52. [CrossRef] [PubMed]
6. Louvet, A.; Mathurin, P. Alcoholic liver disease: Mechanisms of injury and targeted treatment. *Nat. Rev. Gastroenterol. Hepatol.* **2015**, *12*, 231. [CrossRef] [PubMed]
7. Björnsson, E. Drug-induced liver injury in clinical practice. *Aliment. Pharmacol. Ther.* **2010**, *32*, 3–13. [CrossRef] [PubMed]
8. Park, D.H.; Shin, J.W.; Park, S.K.; Seo, J.N.; Li, L.; Jang, J.J.; Lee, M.J. Diethylnitrosamine (DEN) induces irreversible hepatocellular carcinogenesis through overexpression of G1/S-phase regulatory proteins in rat. *Toxicol. Lett.* **2009**, *191*, 321–326. [CrossRef] [PubMed]
9. Magee, P.N.; Barnes, J. The production of malignant primary hepatic tumours in the rat by feeding dimethylnitrosamine. *Br. J. Cancer* **1956**, *10*, 114. [CrossRef] [PubMed]
10. Verna, L.; Whysner, J.; Williams, G.M. N-nitrosodiethylamine mechanistic data and risk assessment: Bioactivation, DNA-adduct formation, mutagenicity, and tumor initiation. *Pharmacol. Ther.* **1996**, *71*, 57–81. [CrossRef]
11. Paterson, I.; Anderson, E.A. The renaissance of natural products as drug candidates. *Science* **2005**, *310*, 451–453. [CrossRef] [PubMed]
12. Teuten, E.L.; Xu, L.; Reddy, C.M. Two abundant bioaccumulated halogenated compounds are natural products. *Science* **2005**, *307*, 917–920. [CrossRef] [PubMed]
13. Rollinger, J.; Langer, T.; Stuppner, H. Strategies for efficient lead structure discovery from natural products. *Curr. Med. Chem.* **2006**, *13*, 1491–1507. [CrossRef] [PubMed]
14. Majeed, R.; Reddy, M.V.; Chinthakindi, P.K.; Sangwan, P.L.; Hamid, A.; Chashoo, G.; Saxena, A.K.; Koul, S. Bakuchiol derivatives as novel and potent cytotoxic agents: A report. *Eur. J. Med. Chem.* **2012**, *49*, 55–67. [CrossRef] [PubMed]
15. Beecher, G.R.; Warden, B.A.; Merken, H. Analysis of tea polyphenols. *Proc. Soc. Exp. Biol. Med.* **1999**, *220*, 267–270. [PubMed]
16. Salah, N.; Miller, N.J.; Paganga, G.; Tijburg, L.; Bolwell, G.P.; Riceevans, C. Polyphenolic flavanols as scavengers of aqueous phase radicals and as chain-breaking antioxidants. *Arch. Biochem. Biophys.* **1995**, *322*, 339–346. [CrossRef] [PubMed]
17. Isbrucker, R.A.; Bausch, J.; Edwards, J.A.; Wolz, E. Safety studies on epigallocatechin gallate (EGCG) preparations. Part 1: Genotoxicity. *Food Chem. Toxicol.* **2006**, *44*, 626–635. [CrossRef] [PubMed]
18. Lambert, J.D.; Yang, C.S. Mechanisms of cancer prevention by tea constituents. *J. Nutr.* **2003**, *133*, 3262S–3267S. [CrossRef] [PubMed]
19. Wolfram, S.; Wang, Y.; Thielecke, F. Anti-obesity effects of green tea: From bedside to bench. *Mol. Nutr. Food Res.* **2006**, *50*, 176–187. [CrossRef] [PubMed]
20. Frei, B.; Higdon, J.V. Antioxidant activity of tea polyphenols in vivo: Evidence from animal studies. *J. Nutr.* **2003**, *133*, 3275S–3284S. [CrossRef] [PubMed]
21. Kundu, J.K.; Na, H.K.; Chun, K.S.; Kim, Y.K.; Lee, S.J.; Lee, S.S.; Lee, O.S.; Sim, Y.C.; Surh, Y.J. Inhibition of Phorbol Ester–Induced COX-2 Expression by Epigallocatechin Gallate in Mouse Skin and Cultured Human Mammary Epithelial Cells. *J. Nutr.* **2003**, *133*, 3805S–3810S. [CrossRef] [PubMed]

22. Yang, F.; Oz, H.S.; Barve, S.; De Villiers, W.J.; McClain, C.J.; Varilek, G.W. The green tea polyphenol (−)-epigallocatechin-3-gallate blocks nuclear factor-κB activation by inhibiting IκB kinase activity in the intestinal epithelial cell line IEC-6. *Mol. Pharmacol.* **2001**, *60*, 528–533. [PubMed]
23. Bancroft, J.D.; Gamble, M. *Theory and Practice of Histological Techniques*, 6th ed.; Churchill Livingstone, Elsevier: London, UK, 2008.
24. Rahmani, A.; Alzohairy, M.; Khadri, H.; Mandal, A.K.; Rizvi, M.A. Expressional evaluation of vascular endothelial growth factor (VEGF) protein in urinary bladder carcinoma patients exposed to cigarette smoke. *Int. J. Clin. Exp. Pathol.* **2012**, *5*, 195–200. [PubMed]
25. Rahmani, A.H.; Babiker, A.Y.; AlWanian, W.M.; Elsiddig, S.A.; Faragalla, H.E.; Aly, S.M. Association of cytokeratin and vimentin protein in the genesis of transitional cell carcinoma of urinary bladder patients. *Dis. Mark.* **2015**, *2015*, 204759. [CrossRef] [PubMed]
26. Singh, B.N.; Shankar, S.; Srivastava, R.K. Green tea catechin, epigallocatechin-3-gallate (EGCG): Mechanisms, perspectives and clinical applications. *Biochem. Pharmacol.* **2011**, *82*, 1807–1821. [CrossRef] [PubMed]
27. Yang, C.S.; Wang, X. Green tea and cancer prevention. *Nutr. Cancer* **2010**, *62*, 931–937. [CrossRef] [PubMed]
28. Thangapandiyan, S.; Miltonprabu, S. Epigallocatechin gallate effectively ameliorates fluoride-induced oxidative stress and DNA damage in the liver of rats. *Can. J. Physiol. Pharmacol.* **2013**, *91*, 528–537. [CrossRef] [PubMed]
29. Moravcová, A.; Cervinkova, Z.; Kucera, O.; Mezera, V.; Lotková, H. Antioxidative effect of epigallocatechin gallate against D-galactosamine-induced injury in primary culture of rat hepatocytes. *Acta Med.* **2014**, *57*, 3–8.
30. Yao, H.T.; Yang, Y.C.; Chang, C.H.; Yang, H.T.; Yin, M.C. Protective effects of (-)-epigallocatechin-3-gallate against acetaminophen-induced liver injury in rats. *Biomedicine* **2015**, *5*, 15. [CrossRef] [PubMed]
31. Tak, E.; Park, G.C.; Kim, S.H.; Jun, D.Y.; Lee, J.; Hwang, S.; Song, G.W.; Lee, S.G. Epigallocatechin-3-gallate protects against hepatic ischaemia-reperfusion injury by reducing oxidative stress and apoptotic cell death. *J. Int. Med. Res.* **2016**, *44*, 1248–1262. [CrossRef] [PubMed]
32. Karatayli, E.; Hall, R.A.; Weber, S.N.; Dooley, S.; Lammert, F. Effect of alcohol on the interleukin 6-mediated inflammatory response in a new mouse model of acute-on-chronic liver injury. *Biochim. Biophys. Acta Mol. Basis Dis.* **2019**, *1865*, 298–307. [CrossRef] [PubMed]
33. Farouk, S.; Sabet, S.; Zahra, F.A.A.; El-Ghor, A.A. Bone marrow derived-mesenchymal stem cells downregulate IL17A dependent IL6/STAT3 signaling pathway in CCl4-induced rat liver fibrosis. *PLoS ONE* **2018**, *13*, e0206130. [CrossRef] [PubMed]
34. Jamal, M.H.; Ali, H.; Dashti, A.; Al-Abbad, J.; Dashti, H.; Mathew, C.; Al-Ali, W.; Asfar, S. Effect of epigallocatechin gallate on uncoupling protein 2 in acute liver injury. *Int. J. Clin. Exp. Pathol.* **2015**, *8*, 649–654. [PubMed]
35. Oliva, J.; Bardag-Gorce, F.; Tillman, B.; French, S.W. Protective effect of quercetin, EGCG, catechin and betaine against oxidative stress induced by ethanol in vitro. *Exp. Mol. Pathol.* **2011**, *90*, 295–299. [CrossRef] [PubMed]
36. Milella, M.; Falcone, I.; Conciatori, F.; Cesta Incani, U.; Del Curatolo, A.; Inzerilli, N.; Nuzzo, C.; Vaccaro, V.; Vari, S.; Cognetti, F.; et al. PTEN: Multiple Functions in Human Malignant Tumors. *Front. Oncol.* **2015**, *5*, 24. [CrossRef] [PubMed]
37. Rahmani, A.; Alzohairy, M.; Babiker, A.Y.; Rizvi, M.A.; Elkarimahmad, H.G. Clinicopathological significance of PTEN and bcl2 expressions in oral squamous cell carcinoma. *Int. J. Clin. Exp. Pathol.* **2012**, *5*, 965–971. [PubMed]
38. Su, S.; Luo, D.; Liu, X.; Liu, J.; Peng, F.; Fang, C.; Li, B. miR-494 up-regulates the PI3K/Akt pathway via targetting PTEN and attenuates hepatic ischemia/reperfusion injury in a rat model. *Biosci. Rep.* **2017**, *37*. [CrossRef] [PubMed]
39. Cheng, Y.; Tian, Y.; Xia, J.; Wu, X.; Yang, Y.; Li, X.; Huang, C.; Meng, X.; Ma, T.; Li, J. The role of PTEN in regulation of hepatic macrophages activation and function in progression and reversal of liver fibrosis. *Toxicol. Appl. Pharmacol.* **2017**, *317*, 51–62. [CrossRef] [PubMed]
40. Chang, W.; He, W.; Li, P.P.; Song, S.S.; Yuan, P.F.; Lu, J.T.; Wei, W. Protective effects of Celastrol on diethylnitrosamine-induced hepatocellular carcinoma in rats and its mechanisms. *Eur. J. Pharmacol.* **2016**, *784*, 173–180. [CrossRef] [PubMed]

41. Sun, Q.; Long, Z.; Wu, H.; Liu, Y.; Wang, L.; Zhang, X.; Wang, X.; Hai, C. Effect of alcohol on diethylnitrosamine-induced hepatic toxicity: Critical role of ROS, lipid accumulation, and mitochondrial dysfunction. *Exp. Toxicol. Pathol.* **2015**, *67*, 491–498. [CrossRef] [PubMed]
42. James, K.D.; Kennett, M.J.; Lambert, J.D. Potential role of the mitochondria as a target for the hepatotoxic effects of (-)-epigallocatechin-3-gallate in mice. *Food Chem. Toxicol.* **2018**, *111*, 302–309. [CrossRef] [PubMed]
43. Shen, K.; Feng, X.; Su, R.; Xie, H.; Zhou, L.; Zheng, S. Epigallocatechin 3-gallate ameliorates bile duct ligation induced liver injury in mice by modulation of mitochondrial oxidative stress and inflammation. *PLoS ONE* **2015**, *10*, e0126278. [CrossRef] [PubMed]
44. Mezera, V.; Endlicher, R.; Kucera, O.; Sobotka, O.; Drahota, Z.; Cervinkova, Z. Effects of Epigallocatechin Gallate on Tert-Butyl Hydroperoxide-Induced Mitochondrial Dysfunction in Rat Liver Mitochondria and Hepatocytes. *Oxid. Med. Cell. Longev.* **2016**, *2016*, 7573131. [CrossRef] [PubMed]
45. Luo, X.; Kraus, W.L. On PAR with PARP: Cellular stress signaling through poly (ADP-ribose) and PARP-1. *Genes Dev.* **2012**, *26*, 417–432. [CrossRef] [PubMed]
46. Jiang, F.; Jiang, R.; Zhu, X.; Zhang, X.; Zhan, Z. Genipin inhibits TNF-alpha-induced vascular smooth muscle cell proliferation and migration via induction of HO-1. *PLoS ONE* **2013**, *8*, e74826.
47. Liu, P.L.; Liu, J.T.; Kuo, H.F.; Chong, I.W.; Hsieh, C.C. Epigallocatechin gallate attenuates proliferation and oxidative stress in human vascular smooth muscle cells induced by interleukin-1beta via heme oxygenase-1. *Mediat. Inflamm.* **2014**, *2014*, 523684. [CrossRef] [PubMed]

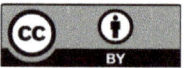

© 2019 by the authors. Licensee MDPI, Basel, Switzerland. This article is an open access article distributed under the terms and conditions of the Creative Commons Attribution (CC BY) license (http://creativecommons.org/licenses/by/4.0/).

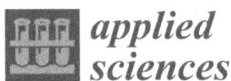 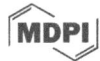

Article

Quantitative Immunomorphological Analysis of Heat Shock Proteins in Thyroid Follicular Adenoma and Carcinoma Tissues Reveals Their Potential for Differential Diagnosis and Points to a Role in Carcinogenesis

Alessandro Pitruzzella [1], Letizia Paladino [1], Alessandra Maria Vitale [1], Stefania Martorana [2], Calogero Cipolla [2], Giuseppa Graceffa [2], Daniela Cabibi [3], Sabrina David [1], Alberto Fucarino [1], Fabio Bucchieri [1], Francesco Cappello [1,4], Everly Conway de Macario [4,5], Alberto JL Macario [4,5] and Francesca Rappa [1,*]

1. Department of Biomedicine, Neuroscience and Advanced Diagnostics (BIND), Institute of Human Anatomy and Histology, University of Palermo, 90127 Palermo, Italy; alessandro.pitruzzella@unipa.it (A.P.); letizia.paladino@unipa.it (L.P.); alessandra.vitale92@gmail.com (A.M.V.); sabrina.david@unipa.it (S.D.); alberto.fucarino@unipa.it (A.F.); fabio.bucchieri@unipa.it (F.B.); francesco.cappello@unipa.it (F.C.)
2. Department of Surgical Oncological and Oral Sciences, University of Palermo, 90127 Palermo, Italy; stefania.martorana@unipa.it (S.M.); calogero.cipolla@unipa.it (C.C.); giuseppa.graceffa@unipa.it (G.G.)
3. Department "G. D'Alessandro", Pathology Institute, University of Palermo, 90127 Palermo, Italy; daniela.cabibi@unipa.it
4. Euro-Mediterranean Institute of Science and Technology (IEMEST), 90100 Palermo, Italy; econwaydemacario@som.umaryland.edu (E.C.deM.); AJLMacario@som.umaryland.edu (A.J.L.M.)
5. Department of Microbiology and Immunology, School of Medicine, University of Maryland at Baltimore-Institute of Marine and Environmental Technology (IMET), Baltimore, MD 21202, USA
* Correspondence: francyrappa@hotmail.com

Received: 17 September 2019; Accepted: 11 October 2019; Published: 15 October 2019

Abstract: Hsp27, Hsp60, Hsp70, and Hsp90 are chaperones that play a crucial role in cellular homeostasis and differentiation, but they may be implicated in carcinogenesis. Follicular neoplasms of the thyroid include follicular adenoma and follicular carcinoma. The former is a very frequent benign encapsulated nodule, whereas the other is a nodule that infiltrates the capsule, blood vessels and the adjacent parenchyma, with a tendency to metastasize. The main objective was to assess the potential of the Hsps in differential diagnosis and carcinogenesis. We quantified by immunohistochemistry Hsp27, Hsp60, Hsp70, and Hsp90 on thin sections of human thyroid tissue with follicular adenoma or follicular carcinoma, comparing the tumor with the adjacent peritumoral tissue. Hsp60, Hsp70, and Hsp90 were increased in follicular carcinoma compared to follicular adenoma, while Hsp27 showed no difference. Histochemical quantification of Hsp60, Hsp70, and Hsp90 allows diagnostic distinction between follicular adenoma and carcinoma, and between tumor and adjacent non-tumoral tissue. The quantitative variations of these chaperones in follicular carcinoma suggest their involvement in tumorigenesis, for instance in processes such as invasion of thyroid parenchyma and metastasization.

Keywords: Hsp27; Hsp60; Hsp70; Hsp90; molecular chaperone; chaperonopathies; thyroid; follicular adenoma; follicular carcinoma; differential diagnosis; carcinogenesis

---

1. Introduction

Thyroid tumors are the most frequent endocrine malignancies and their incidence is steadily increasing [1]. They are divided into epithelial and non-epithelial tumors. Follicular neoplasms of the thyroid gland include benign follicular adenoma (FA) and follicular carcinoma (FC) [2]. FA is the most common benign thyroid tumor and occurs in follicular cells. Macroscopically, it may appear as a single nodule, whose diameter can vary from a few millimetres to a few centimetres, surrounded by a single capsule. Microscopically, it is characterized by the proliferation of many follicles surrounded by a capsule and, depending on their size the adenomas can be sorted into normofollicular, microfollicular, macrofollicular, and solid-trabecular.

Among thyroid carcinomas, FC is the second most common epithelial tumor after papillary carcinoma, occurring late in life, with the fifth and sixth decades being the most affected, and is more aggressive than papillary carcinoma [3]. Macroscopically it appears as a thyroid nodule of variable diameter and may or may not possess a capsule. Microscopically, FC consists of a proliferation of follicles, similarly to FA, but the neoplastic follicles invade the tumor capsule when present, penetrating into blood vessels and/or the adjacent normal thyroid tissue, a feature that can only be appreciated with histological but not with cytological techniques [4].

Immunohistochemical analysis does not usually allow the differentiation between benign and malignant lesions and, as a consequence, the majority of patients with these lesions are referred to surgery without a precise diagnosis. For this reason, it is necessary to improve the preoperative diagnosis also because no clinical, radiological, or laboratory test currently available is sufficiently sensitive and specific to distinguish benign from malignant follicular lesions detected by fine-needle aspiration [5].

Molecular chaperones are the main components of the chaperoning system with canonical and non-canonical functions [6,7]. The former functions pertain to maintenance of protein homeostasis and include assisting in the: folding of nascent polypeptides as soon as they emerge from the ribosome and until they reach their native and biologically active tridimensional structure; prevention of protein misfolding and aggregation; translocation of proteins from one cell compartment to another; and driving damaged or unnecessary proteins toward degradation [8–12].

Many chaperones are heat shock proteins (Hsp) but although not all Hsp are chaperones the terms molecular chaperone (or chaperone in short) and Hsp are used as synonyms. Chaperones are classified according to molecular weight [7] and designated variously, which causes confusion, and because of this, attempts at nomenclature standardization have been made [13].

Although chaperones are considered essentially cytoprotective, it is now known that they can also be pathogenic if abnormal in structure, or location, or quantity, causing diseases named chaperonopathies, including several types of cancer [7,14].

Some chaperones are increased in various cancers with the magnitude of the increase being closely associated with prognosis and with resistance to anticancer therapy, the former being worse and the latter being higher as the chaperones increase is bigger [15,16].

There are few data in the literature on the role of Hsp in thyroid cancer, for example Hsp27 was increased in anaplastic carcinoma [17], and in papillary carcinoma, in which it was induced by 17 β-estradiol, which facilitates proliferation and confers resistance to apoptosis [18]. In this study, we performed immunomorphological analysis on samples of FA and FC to evaluate, for the first time to our knowledge, the tissue levels of Hsp27, Hsp60, Hsp70, and Hsp90. We focused on these chaperones based on the fact that they are implicated in chaperonopathies, including carcinogenesis [15,19].

2. Materials and Methods

2.1. Sample Collection

Formalin-fixed and paraffin-embedded thyroid tissue of human FA and FC (10 samples for each group) were retrieved from the archives of the Department of Human Pathology of the University of Palermo to perform immunohistochemical assays for Hsp27, Hsp60, Hsp70, and Hsp90. These samples were from patients who had undergone thyroidectomy surgery in the Department of Surgical, Oncological and Oral Sciences at the University of Palermo (Table 1). The experiments related to this study were conducted as part of the study project approved by the Ethics Committee of University Hospital AUOP Paolo Giaccone of Palermo (N° 05/2017 of 05/10/2017).

Table 1. Patient demographics and tumor characteristics.

Sex	Age (yrs)*	Localization	Thyroid Weight (g)	Nodules Size (mm)	
		FOLLICULAR ADENOMA			
M	27	Right lobe	35	17	
F	39	Right lobe	15	28	
F	69	Left lobe	30	24	
M	46	Right lobe	35	32	
F	73	Left lobe	120	30	
F	55	Left lobe	20	20	
F	67	Right lobe	40	22	
M	35	Left lobe	55	38	
F	29	Isthmus	60	42	
F	48	Right lobe	70	15	
		FOLLICULAR CARCINOMA			Stage (AJCC/TNM)
F	41	Left lobe	45	25	I
F	29	Right lobe	35	30	I
M	62	Right lobe	80	35	I
F	51	Right lobe	50	40	I
F	48	Isthmus	20	28	I
F	39	Left lobe	25	25	I
M	67	Right lobe	45	38	II
F	57	Right lobe	60	22	II
F	29	Left lobe	25	19	I
F	61	Right lobe	30	41	I

*Abbreviations. Yrs, years; M, male; F, female; AJCC, American Joint Committee on Cancer; TNM, Tumor-Nodes-Metastasis.

2.2. Immunohistochemistry

Immunohistochemical experiments were performed on 5-micron thick sections of paraffin-embedded tissue, obtained with a cutting microtome. The slides were dewaxed in xylene for 30 min at 60 °C and rehydrated, at 22 °C, by sequential immersion in a graded series of alcohols and transferred into distilled water for 5 min. Then, the sections were incubated for 8 min in Sodium Citrate Buffer (pH 6) at 95 °C for antigen unmasking and immersed for 8 min in acetone at −20 °C to prevent the detachment of the sections from the slide. After a wash of sections with PBS (Phosphate Buffered Saline pH 7.4) at 22 °C for 5 min, the experiments for Hsp60, Hsp70, and Hsp90 were performed applying a streptavidin–biotin complex method, using Histostain®-Plus 3rd Gen IHC Detection Kit (Life Technologies, Frederik, MD, USA; Cat. No. 85–9073). Therefore, the sections were treated for 5 min with Peroxidase Quenching Solution (reagent A of Histostain®-Plus 3rd Gen IHC Detection Kit, Life Technologies) to inhibit endogenous peroxidase activity, and after another wash with PBS at 22 °C for 5 min, were treated with blocking solution (reagent B of Histostain®-Plus 3rd Gen IHC Detection Kit, Life Technologies) for 10 min to block non-specific antigenic sites. Subsequently, the sections were incubated overnight at 22 °C, with a primary antibody against human Hsp60 (rabbit anti-Hsp60 polyclonal antibody, Santa Cruz Biotechnology, Inc., Santa Cruz, CA, USA, cat. N°: sc-13966, dilution 1:300), human Hsp70 (mouse anti-Hsp70 monoclonal antibody, clone W27, Santa Cruz Biotechnology, Inc, Santa Cruz, CA, USA, cat. N°: sc-24, dilution 1:200) and human Hsp90 (mouse anti-Hsp90 monoclonal antibody, clone F-8, Santa Cruz Biotechnology, Inc., Santa Cruz, CA, USA, cat. N°: sc-13119, dilution 1:200). Appropriate positive and negative (isotype) controls, were run concurrently. The following day, after a wash with PBS at 22 °C for 5 min, the sections were incubated with a universal biotinylated secondary antibody (Biotinylated Secondary Antibody reagent C Histostain®-Plus 3rd Gen IHC Detection Kit, Life Technologies) for 10 min. After a subsequent washing with PBS for 5 min, the sections were incubated with streptavidin-peroxidase complex (Streptavidin-Peroxidase Conjugate reagent D Histostain®-Plus 3rd Gen IHC Detection Kit, Life Technologies) for 10 min, and following a further washing in PBS for 5 min, the slides were incubated in the dark for 5 min with the DAB chromogen (diaminobenzidine) (DAB chromogen reagents E1 and E2 Histostain®-Plus 3rd Gen IHC Detection Kit, Life Technologies). The experiments for Hsp27 were performed using an IHC goat kit (Cell & Tissue Staining Kit, R&D Systems, Inc., Minneapolis, MN, USA, Cat N° CTS008). Sections, after deparaffinization, were treated at 22 °C for 5 min with Peroxidase Blocking Reagent (Cell & Tissue Staining Kit, R&D Systems, Inc.) to inhibit endogenous peroxidase activity and after another wash with PBS for 5 min, with a Serum Blocking Reagent D (Cell & Tissue Staining Kit, R&D Systems, Inc.) for 15 min to block non-specific antigenic sites. Since the detection is based on the formation of Avidin-Biotin complex, the sections were treated with Avidin Blocking Reagent (Cell & Tissue Staining Kit, R&D Systems, Inc.) at 22°C for 15 min. After a wash with PBS, the sections were incubated with Biotin Blocking Reagent for 15' (Cell & Tissue Staining Kit, R&D Systems, Inc.). After another wash with PBS, the sections were incubated at 22 °C overnight, with a primary antibody against human Hsp27 (goat anti-Hsp27 polyclonal antibody, Santa Cruz Biotechnology, Inc., Santa Cruz, CA, USA, cat. N°: sc-1048, dilution 1:150). For all samples, appropriate positive and negative (isotype) controls were run concurrently. So the samples were washed at 22 °C three times in PBS for 15 min/wash, and then the sections were incubated with Biotinylated Secondary Antibody (Cell & Tissue Staining Kit, R&D Systems, Inc.) for 40 min most often (the length of this incubation time varies depending on the thickness of the section). After that, the slides were washed three times in PBS for 15 min/wash. The high detection sensitivity of this method is obtained by using premium quality biotinylated secondary antibodies and High Sensitivity Streptavidin-conjugated HRP (HSS-HRP). HSS is a chemical analog of Streptavidin that interacts only with Biotin bound to secondary antibodies. The sections were incubated at 22 °C with HSS-HRP (Vial B, Cell & Tissue Staining Kit, R&D Systems, Inc.) for 30 min. For all samples, the visualization is based on enzymatic conversion of chromogenic substrates 3,3′ Diaminobenzidine (DAB) into a colored precipitate (brown), by horseradish peroxidase (HRP) at the sites of antigen localization, after two subsequent washing with PBS for 2 min/wash, the slides were incubated in the dark for 5 min with the DAB chromogen (200 µL of DAB chromogen solution were required to cover tissue section on a single slide). Two drops of DAB Crhomogen were added to 2 mL of DAB Chromogen Buffer (Cell & Tissue Staining Kit, R&D Systems, Inc.).

The nuclei were counterstained with hematoxylin (Hematoxylin aqueous formula, REF 05-06012/LN. Cat. S2020, Bio-Optica, Milano, Italy). Finally, the slides were mounted for observation with coverslips using a permanent mounting medium (Vecta Mount, H-5000, Vector Laboratories, Inc. Burlingame, CA, USA). The observation of the sections was carried out with an optical microscope (Leica DM 5000 B, Leica Microsystems Srl, Buccinasco (MI), Italy) connected to a digital camera (Leica DC 300F).

Two independent observers (F.C, and F.R) examined all specimens on two separate occasions and performed a quantitative analysis to quantify the percentage of epithelial cells positive for Hsp27, Hsp60, Hsp70, and Hsp90. All the observations were done at a magnification of 400× and the percentage of positive cells was calculated in a high-power field (HPF) and repeated for 10 HFP. The immunopositivity evaluation is expressed as average percentage of all immuno-quantifications performed in each case for each Hsp. Statistical analyses were carried out using the GraphPad Prism 4.0 package (GraphPad Inc., San Diego, CA, USA). One-way ANOVA analysis of variance with Bonferroni post-hoc multiple comparisons was used to detect significant statistical differences. All data are reported as the means ± SD, and the level of statistical significance was set at $p \leq 0.05$.

2.3. Results

The presence and levels of Hps27, Hsp60, Hps70 and, Hsp90 were determined in the tumor tissue itself and in the adjacent parenchyma (AP) of FA and FC. The immunopositivity for Hsp27 was observed in the cytoplasm and the nucleus in tumoral cells while only in the cytoplasm in the cells of the adjacent parenchyma. It was high in all specimens and it did not show significant quantitative differences between the specimens or tissue type: it was 73% in FA and 70% in its AP, and 68% in FC and 47% in its AP (Figure 1).

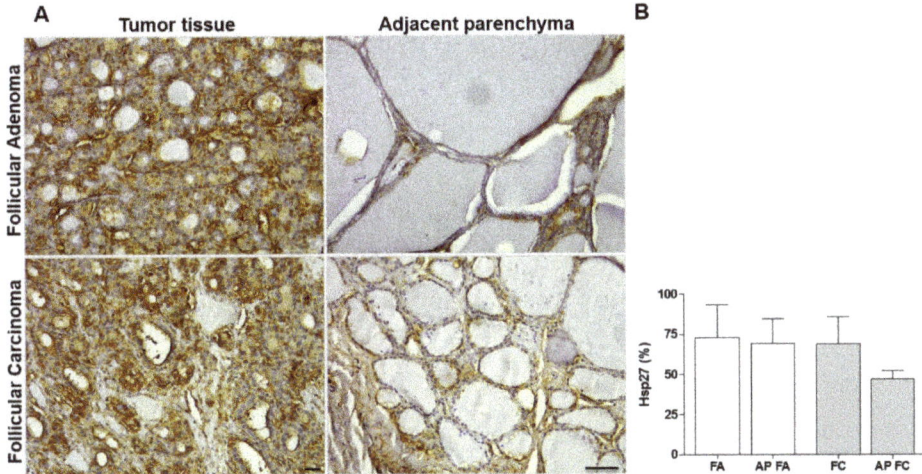

Figure 1. Hsp27 Immunohistochemistry. (**A**) Representative images of immunohistochemical results for Hsp27. Magnification 200×; scale bar 100 μm. (**B**) The histogram shows statistical results for the immunohistochemical evaluation for Hsp27 in follicular adenoma (FA), adjacent parenchyma of follicular adenoma (AP FA), follicular carcinoma (FC) and adjacent parenchyma of follicular carcinoma (AP FC). Data are presented as mean +SD.

The Hsp60 tissue levels were 33% in FA and 7% in its AP with a significant difference ($p \leq 0.01$), and in FC the immunopositivity was 74% and 6% in its AP with a significant difference ($p \leq 0.001$). In the FA and FC epithelial cells, the immunopositivity was diffuse in the cytoplasm while in the epithelial cells of the AP was also in the cytoplasm but mild and granular. Statistical analysis also, showed a significant difference between FA and FC ($p \leq 0.001$) (Figure 2).

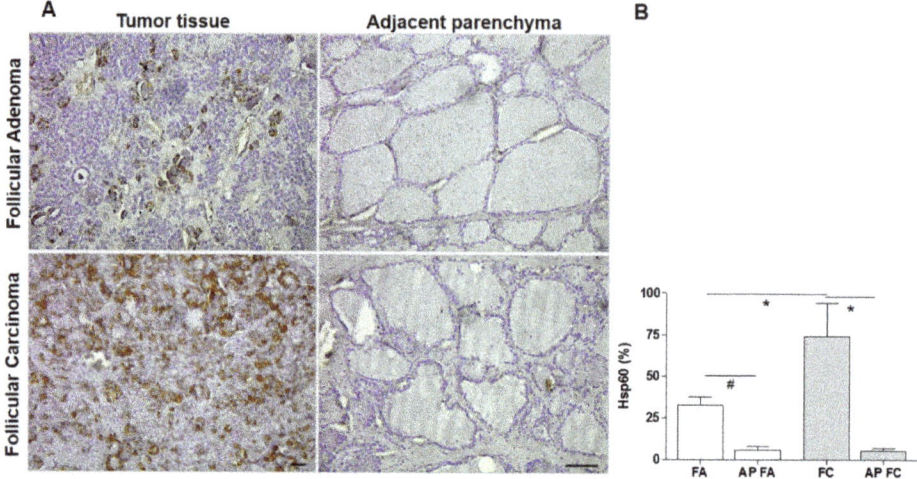

Figure 2. Hsp60 Immunohistochemistry. (**A**) Representative images of immunohistochemical results for Hsp60. Magnification 200X; scale bar 100 μm. (**B**) The histogram shows statistical results for the immunohistochemical evaluation for Hsp60 in follicular adenoma (FA), adjacent parenchyma of follicular adenoma (AP FA), follicular carcinoma (FC) and adjacent parenchyma of follicular carcinoma (AP FC). Data are presented as the mean +SD. * $p \leq 0.0001$, # $p \leq 0.01$.

The results for Hsp70 showed a positivity of 18% and 8% in FA and its AP, respectively, with no statistical difference, and of 55% and 7% in FC and its AP, respectively, with a statistical difference ($p \leq 0.001$). The epithelial cells of FC showed a high cytoplasmic positivity while those of FA and the AP of both neoformations, showed a mild and pointed immunopositivity. Statistical analysis also showed a significant difference between FA and FC ($p \leq 0.001$) (Figure 3).

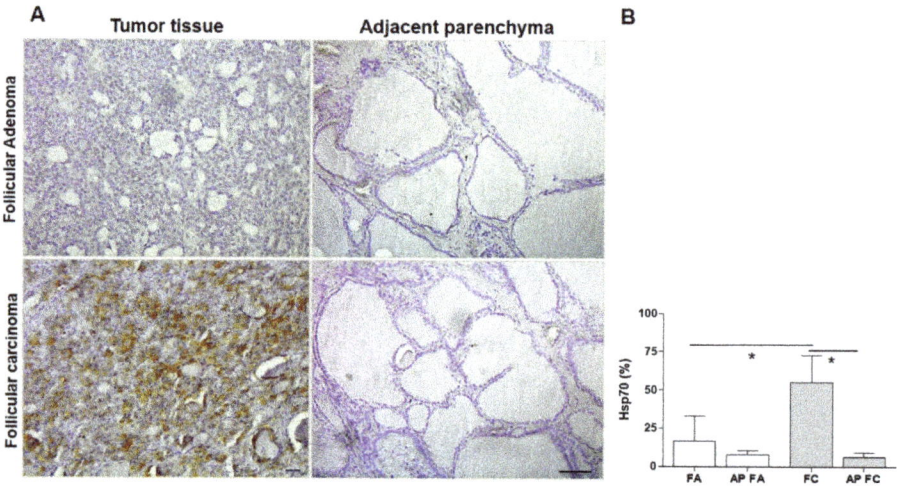

Figure 3. Hsp70 Immunohistochemistry. (**A**) Representative images of immunohistochemical results for Hsp70. Magnification 200×; scale bar 100 μm. (**B**) The histogram shows statistical results for the immunohistochemical evaluation for Hsp70 in follicular adenoma (FA), adjacent parenchyma of follicular adenoma (AP FA), follicular carcinoma (FC) and adjacent parenchyma of follicular carcinoma (AP FC). Data are presented as the mean +SD. * $p \leq 0.0001$.

The tissue levels of Hsp90 were 25% in FA and 15% in its AP, and were 56% in FC and 33% in its AP with no statistical difference. In all specimens the immunopositivity was cytoplasmic, intense in the FC and FA cells while mild in the cells of the AP. Statistical analysis also showed a significant difference between FA and FC ($p \leq 0.05$) (Figure 4).

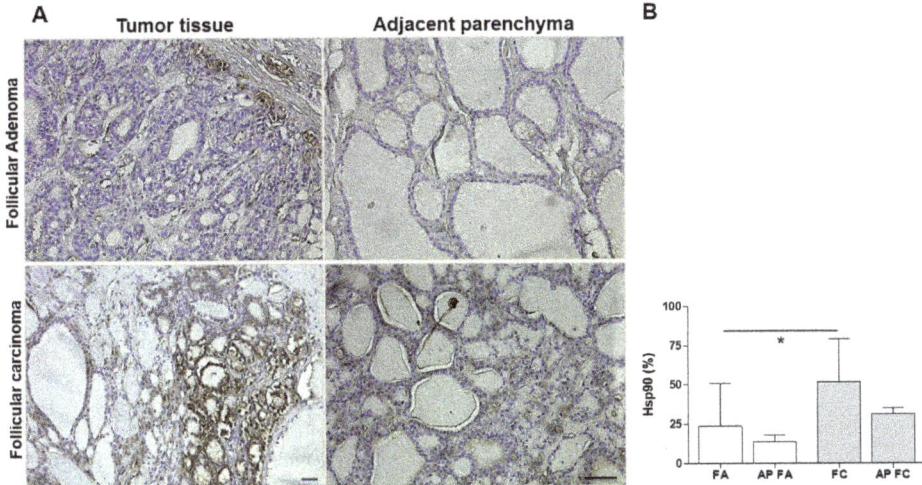

Figure 4. Hsp90 Immunohistochemistry: (**A**) Representative images of immunohistochemical results for Hsp90. Magnification 200×; scale bar 100 μm. (**B**) The histogram shows statistical results for the immunohistochemical evaluation for Hsp90 in follicular adenoma (FA), adjacent parenchyma of follicular adenoma (AP FA), follicular carcinoma (FC) and adjacent parenchyma of follicular carcinoma (AP FC). Data are presented as the mean +SD. * $p < 0.05$.

Our immunohistochemical observation was also dedicated to the evaluation of the intracellular localization of the Hsp immunopositivity. We observed an accumulation of Hsp60, Hsp70, and Hsp90 in the cytoplasm and of Hsp27 in the cytoplasm and in the nucleus.

3. Discussion

In this work, we studied the immunohistochemical levels of Hps27, Hsp60, Hps70, and Hsp90 in human thyroid tissue with follicular adenoma (FA) and follicular carcinoma (FC). FC is characterized by the ability to invade the tumor capsule when this is present and forcing its way inside blood vessels and in the adjacent normal thyroid tissue. This characteristic distinguishes FC from FA. In general, the pathological condition of cancer is characterized by an imbalance between cell proliferation and differentiation. A physiological balance between cell proliferation and differentiation is essential to ensure proper growth and development of multicellular organisms, and to maintain adult tissue and organ homeostasis. It is of fundamental interest in cancer pathology to understand the mechanisms underpinning the origin of the loss of cell differentiation capability and the induction of malignancy progression. Molecular chaperones play a key role in the maintenance of cellular and tissue homeostasis and in the regulation of organ remodelling [20–23]. However, when abnormal in structure and/or quantity and/or function, and/or location, chaperones can cause disease, the chaperonopathies [7,14], and numerous scientific reports showed their involvement in the pathogenesis and progression of various human neoplasms [15,19,24]. High tissue levels of Hsps are often associated with cancer progression and invasiveness, as shown by studies in which it was suggested that these proteins are augmented in some types of tumors with tendency to invade surrounding tissues and to spread to distant organs [19,25–27].

Hsp27 was initially characterized as a chaperone that facilitates the refolding of damaged proteins in response to heat shock. Further investigations revealed that Hsp27 also responds to oxidative and chemical stressors, mainly acting as an antioxidant and antiapoptotic agent. It was observed that an increase of Hsp27 levels is transiently induced at specific stages during development and cell differentiation and occurs concomitantly with the differentiation-associated decrease of cellular proliferation [28,29]. Other studies reported that Hsp27 is augmented in different types of tumors and its levels are directly associated with a more aggressive malignant behavior (cancer cell proliferation, invasiveness, and metastasis) and resistance to chemotherapy [30,31]. Furthermore, Hsp27 mediates endothelial cell mobility, improving angiogenesis [32].

The eukaryotic Hsp60 resides and works in the mitochondrial matrix where, together with its co-chaperonin Hsp10, drives the proper folding of proteins destined to the mitochondrial matrix. In addition to this intramitochondrial function, Hsp60 plays a role in other cellular processes beyond the mitochondrion, for instance in the cytosol, plasma-cell membrane, extracellular environment, and biological fluids [33]. Hsp60 seems to be directly or indirectly involved in carcinogenesis in different organs, since its levels change during the carcinogenetic steps [15,24]. Hsp60 levels are increased in various tumors such as colorectal cancer, liver and uterine cervical cancers and its levels are correlated with cancer progression, which makes this chaperonin a useful biomarker indicating poor prognosis [34,35].

There are many reports of a strong association of Hsp70 with cancer development. For instance, it promotes carcinogenesis by acting as survival factor owing to its tumor-associated expression and anti-apoptotic effects [36]. Hsp70 abundance gives the neoplasm greater invasiveness [37].

Hsp90 is also augmented in various cancers, apparently playing important roles in cancer biology by regulating tumor growth, invasion, metastasis, angiogenesis, and apoptosis, and induces neoangiogenesis by stabilizing vascular endothelial growth factor and nitric oxide syntheses [38–40].

In light of what is available in the literature in the field of Hsp and cancer, very briefly summarized in the preceding paragraphs, we decided to evaluate the tissue levels of the four molecular chaperones discussed above, simultaneously, in samples of thyroid follicular neoplasms, about which there is little information. We also observed the localization of these Hsp in tumor cells to evaluate their possible localization change.

Hsp27 levels did not show significant quantitative differences between the groups studied. This result is in contrast with the data present in the literature on other types of tumors, which indicates that the thyroid tumors deserve detailed analysis to elucidate the basis for this unique feature regarding Hsp27. However, even if we did not find a quantitative difference, we observed a nuclear localization that, according to the data in the literature, would be linked to the phosphorylation of the chaperone [41].

Conversely, we observed a higher immunopositivity of Hsp60, Hsp70, and Hsp90 in FC compared to FA and their adjacent parenchyma. These data are in agreement with what has been published in the literature on other types of tumors. The increase of Hsp60 and Hsp70 in FC suggest its implication in carcinogenesis and in the progression of this tumor. Hsp60 and Hsp70 levels in FC were higher compared to adjacent parenchyma levels. In normal cells, Hsp 60 is detected in the mitochondria while in tumoral cells it is abundant in the cytoplasm. These data are interesting because both Hsps could be considered tumor tissue markers. Likewise, the higher levels of Hsp90 might indicate its implication in the process of FC invasion of surrounding tissue. This could be attributed to the known stabilizing effects of Hsp90 on matrix metalloproteinases, which would favor tumor infiltration and invasion [42,43].

In conclusion, our immunohistochemical data suggest an involvement of Hsp60, Hsp70, and Hsp90 in the mechanisms of carcinogenesis of thyroid follicular carcinoma. The immunomorphological observation showed a change in cellular localization of the Hsps studied. This pattern is found in various carcinogenic processes [19,24]. It is necessary to continue these studies to clarify the molecular mechanisms underlying the increase in tissue levels of these chaperones in this human cancer. In this regard, determination of chaperone-gene expression levels and elucidation of post-transcriptional mechanisms that might be involved in augmenting the levels of the chaperones in thyroid tumors seem to be the most promising approaches toward finding points of attacks by anti-cancer agents.

Author Contributions: Conceptualization: C.C., F.C. and F.R.; Methodology: A.P., L.P., S.D., S.M.; Validation: D.C.; Investigation: A.P., G.G.; Resources: A.M.V., L.P., S.M., A.F.; Data Curation: F.C., F.R.; Writing–Original Draft Preparation: F.R., A.M.V.; Writing–Review & Editing, F.B., A.J.L.M. and E.C.deM.; Supervision: A.J.L.M. and E.C.deM.

Funding: A.J.L.M., and E.C.deM. were partially supported by IMET. This work was done under the agreement between IEMEST (Italy) and IMET (USA) (this is IMET contribution number IMET 19-016).

Conflicts of Interest: The authors declare no conflict of interest.

References

1. La Vecchia, C.; Malvezzi, M.; Bosetti, C.; Garavello, W.; Bertuccio, P.; Levi, F.; Negri, E. Thyroid cancer mortality and incidence: A global overview. *Int. J. Cancer* **2015**, *136*, 2187–2195. [CrossRef]
2. Kondo, T.; Ezzat, S.; Asa, S.L. Pathogenetic mechanisms in thyroid follicular-cell neoplasia. *Nat. Rev. Cancer* **2006**, *6*, 292–306. [CrossRef]
3. DeGroot, L.J. Morbidity and mortality in follicular thyroid cancer. *J. Clin. Endocrinol. Metab.* **1995**, *80*, 2946–2953.
4. McHenry, C.R.; Phitayakorn, R. Follicular Adenoma and Carcinoma of the Thyroid Gland. *Oncologist* **2011**, *16*, 585–593. [CrossRef]
5. Bartolazzi, A.; Gasbarri, A.; Papotti, M.; Bussolati, G.; Lucante, T.; Khan, A.; Inohara, H.; Marandino, F.; Orlandi, F.; Nardi, F.; et al. Application of an immunodiagnostic method for improving preoperative diagnosis of nodular thyroid lesions. *Lancet* **2001**, *357*, 1644–1650. [CrossRef]
6. Macario, A.J.L.; Conway de Macario, E. Chaperone proteins and chaperonopathies. In *Stress Physiology, Biochemistry, and Pathology*; Handbook of Stress; Fink, G., Ed.; Elsevier: Amsterdam, The Netherlands; Academic Press: Cambridge, MA, USA, 2019; Volume 3, pp. 135–152.
7. Macario, A.J.L.; Conway de Macario, E.; Cappello, F. *The Chaperonopathies. Diseases with Defective Molecular Chaperones*; Springer: Dordrecht, The Netherlands; Heidelberg, Germany; New York, NY, USA; London, UK, 2013.
8. Finka, A.; Sharma, S.K.; Goloubinoff, P. Multi-layered molecular mechanisms of polypeptide holding, unfolding and disaggregation by HSP70/HSP110 chaperones. *Front. Mol. Biosci.* **2015**, *2*, 29. [CrossRef] [PubMed]
9. Mogk, A.; Bukau, B.; Kampinga, H.H. Cellular Handling of Protein Aggregates by Disaggregation Machines. *Mol. Cell* **2018**, *69*, 214–226. [CrossRef] [PubMed]
10. Willison, K.R. The structure and evolution of eukaryotic chaperonin-containing TCP-1 and its mechanism that folds actin into a protein spring. *Biochem. J.* **2018**, *475*, 3009–3034. [CrossRef] [PubMed]
11. Adams, B.M.; Oster, M.E.; Hebert, D.N. Protein Quality Control in the Endoplasmic Reticulum. *Protein J.* **2019**, *38*, 317–329. [CrossRef]
12. Dahiya, V.; Buchner, J. Functional principles and regulation of molecular chaperones. *Insights Enzym. Mech. Funct. Exp. Comput. Methods* **2019**, *114*, 1–60.
13. Kampinga, H.H.; Hageman, J.; Vos, M.J.; Kubota, H.; Tanguay, R.M.; Bruford, E.A.; Cheetham, M.E.; Chen, B.; Hightower, L.E. Guidelines for the nomenclature of the human heat shock proteins. *Cell Stress Chaperones* **2009**, *14*, 105–111. [CrossRef]
14. Macario, A.J.L.; Conway de Macario, E. Sick Chaperones, Cellular Stress, and Disease. *N. Engl. J. Med.* **2005**, *353*, 1489–1501. [CrossRef] [PubMed]
15. Rappa, F.; Sciume, C.; Bello, M.L.; Bavisotto, C.C.; Gammazza, A.M.; Barone, R.; Campanella, C.; David, S.; Carini, F.; Zarcone, F.; et al. Comparative analysis of Hsp10 and Hsp90 expression in healthy mucosa and adenocarcinoma of the large bowel. *Anticancer Res.* **2014**, *34*, 4153–4159.
16. Chatterjee, S.; Burns, T.F. Targeting Heat Shock Proteins in Cancer: A Promising Therapeutic Approach. *Int. J. Mol. Sci.* **2017**, *18*, 1978. [CrossRef] [PubMed]

17. Mineva, I.; Gärtner, W.; Hauser, P.; Kainz, A.; Löffler, M.; Wolf, G.; Oberbauer, R.; Weissel, M.; Wagner, L. Differential expression of alphaB-crystallin and Hsp27-1 in anaplastic thyroid carcinomas because of tumor-specific alphaB-crystallin gene (CRYAB) silencing. *Cell Stress Chaperones* **2005**, *10*, 171–184. [CrossRef] [PubMed]
18. Mo, X.-M.; Li, L.; Zhu, P.; Dai, Y.-J.; Zhao, T.-T.; Liao, L.-Y.; Chen, G.G.; Liu, Z.-M. Up-regulation of Hsp27 by ERα/Sp1 facilitates proliferation and confers resistance to apoptosis in human papillary thyroid cancer cells. *Mol. Cell. Endocrinol.* **2016**, *431*, 71–87. [CrossRef]
19. Rappa, F.; Farina, F.; Zummo, G.; David, S.; Campanella, C.; Carini, F.; Tomasello, G.; Damiani, P.; Cappello, F.; Conway de Macario, E.; et al. HSP-molecular chaperones in cancer biogenesis and tumor therapy: An overview. *Anticancer Res.* **2012**, *32*, 5139–5150.
20. Walsh, D.; Grantham, J.; Zhu, X.O.; Lin, J.W.; Van Oosterum, M.; Taylor, R.; Edwards, M. The role of heat shock proteins in mammalian differentiation and development. *Environ. Med.* **1999**, *43*, 79–87.
21. Barna, J.; Csermely, P.; Vellai, T. Roles of heat shock factor 1 beyond the heat shock response. *Cell. Mol. Life Sci.* **2018**, *75*, 2897–2916. [CrossRef]
22. Park, A.-M.; Kanai, K.; Itoh, T.; Sato, T.; Tsukui, T.; Inagaki, Y.; Selman, M.; Matsushima, K.; Yoshie, O. Heat Shock Protein 27 Plays a Pivotal Role in Myofibroblast Differentiation and in the Development of Bleomycin-Induced Pulmonary Fibrosis. *PLoS ONE* **2016**, *11*, e0148998. [CrossRef]
23. Hance, M.W.; Dole, K.; Gopal, U.; Bohonowych, J.E.; Jezierska-Drutel, A.; Neumann, C.A.; Liu, H.; Garraway, I.P.; Isaacs, J.S. Secreted Hsp90 Is a Novel Regulator of the Epithelial to Mesenchymal Transition (EMT) in Prostate Cancer. *J. Boil. Chem.* **2012**, *287*, 37732–37744. [CrossRef]
24. Rappa, F.; Pitruzzella, A.; Marino Gammazza, A.; Barone, R.; Mocciaro, E.; Tomasello, G.; Carini, F.; Farina, F.; Zummo, G.; Conway de Macario, E.; et al. Quantitative patterns of Hsps in tubular adenoma compared with normal and tumor tissues reveal the value of Hsp10 and Hsp60 in early diagnosis of large bowel cancer. *Cell Stress Chaperones* **2016**, *21*, 927–933. [CrossRef]
25. Li, X.-S.; Xu, Q.; Fu, X.-Y.; Luo, W.-S. Heat Shock Protein 60 Overexpression Is Associated with the Progression and Prognosis in Gastric Cancer. *PLoS ONE* **2014**, *9*, e107507. [CrossRef]
26. Lianos, G.D.; Alexiou, G.A.; Mangano, A.; Mangano, A.; Rausei, S.; Boni, L.; Dionigi, G.; Roukos, D.H.; Dionigi, M.P.G. The role of heat shock proteins in cancer. *Cancer Lett.* **2015**, *360*, 114–118. [CrossRef]
27. Wu, J.; Liu, T.; Rios, Z.; Mei, Q.; Lin, X.; Cao, S. Heat Shock Proteins and Cancer. *Trends Pharm. Sci* **2017**, *38*, 226–256. [CrossRef]
28. Vidyasagar, A.; Wilson, N.A.; Djamali, A. Heat shock protein 27 (HSP27): Biomarker of disease and therapeutic target. *Fibrogenes. Tissue Repair* **2012**, *5*, 7. [CrossRef]
29. Concannon, C.G.; Gorman, A.; Samali, A. On the role of Hsp27 in regulating apoptosis. *Apoptosis* **2003**, *8*, 61–70. [CrossRef]
30. Zheng, G.; Zhang, Z.; Liu, H.; Xiong, Y.; Luo, L.; Jia, X.; Peng, C.; Zhang, Q.; Li, N.; Gu, Y.; et al. HSP27-Mediated Extracellular and Intracellular Signaling Pathways Synergistically Confer Chemoresistance in Squamous Cell Carcinoma of Tongue. *Clin. Cancer Res.* **2018**, *24*, 1163–1175. [CrossRef]
31. Sheng, B.; Qi, C.; Liu, B.; Lin, Y.; Fu, T.; Zeng, Q. Increased HSP27 correlates with malignant biological behavior of non-small cell lung cancer and predicts patient's survival. *Sci. Rep.* **2017**, *7*, 13807. [CrossRef]
32. Keezer, S.M.; Ivie, S.E.; Krutzsch, H.C.; Tandle, A.; Libutti, S.K.; Roberts, D.D. Angiogenesis inhibitors target the endothelial cell cytoskeleton through altered regulation of heat-shock protein 27 and cofilin. *Cancer Res.* **2003**, *63*, 6405–6412.
33. Cappello, F.; Marino Gammazza, A.; Palumbo Piccionello, A.; Campanella, C.; Pace, A.; Conway de Macario, E.; Macario, A.J.L. Hsp60 chaperonopathies and chaperonotherapy: Targets and agents. *Expert Opin. Ther. Targets* **2014**, *18*, 185–208. [CrossRef]
34. Martorana, G.; Belfiore, P.; Martorana, A.; Bucchieri, F.; Cappello, F.; Bellafiore, M.; Palma, A.; Marciano, V.; Farina, F.; Zummo, G. Expression of 60-kD Heat Shock Protein Increases during Carcinogenesis in the Uterine Exocervix. *Pathobiology* **2002**, *70*, 83–88.
35. Cappello, F.; Bellafiore, M.; Palma, A.; David, S.; Marcianò, V.; Bartolotta, T.; Sciumè, C.; Modica, G.; Farina, F.; Zummo, G.; et al. 60KDa chaperonin (HSP60) is over-expressed during colorectal carcinogenesis. *Eur. J. Histochem.* **2003**, *47*, 105–110. [CrossRef]
36. Rérole, A.-L.; Jego, G.; Garrido, C. Hsp70: Anti-apoptotic and Tumorigenic Protein. *Adv. Struct. Saf. Stud.* **2011**, *787*, 205–230.

37. Ciocca, D.R.; Calderwood, S.K. Heat-shock proteins in cancer: Diagnostic, prognostic, predictive, and treatment implications. *Cell Stress Chaperones* **2005**, *10*, 86–103. [CrossRef]
38. Burrows, F.; Zhang, H.; Kamal, A. Hsp90 Activation and Cell Cycle Regulation. *Cell Cycle* **2004**, *3*, 1530–1536. [CrossRef]
39. Sun, J.; Liao, J.K. Induction of angiogenesis by heat-shock protein 90 mediated by protein kinase Akt and endothelial nitric oxide syntethase. *Aterioscler. Thromb. Vasc. Biol.* **2004**, *24*, 2238–2244. [CrossRef]
40. Feron, O.; Pfosser, A.; Thalgott, M.; Büttner, K.; Brouet, A.; Boekstegers, P.; Kupatt, C. Liposomal Hsp90 cDNA induces neovascularization via nitric oxide in chronic ischemia. *Cardiovasc. Res.* **2005**, *65*, 728–736.
41. Bryantsev, A.L.; Chechenova, M.B.; Shelden, E.A. Recruitment of phosphorylated small heat shock protein Hsp27 to nuclear speckles without stress. *Exp. Cell Res.* **2007**, *313*, 195–209. [CrossRef]
42. Baker-Williams, A.J.; Hashmi, F.; Budzyński, M.A.; Woodford, M.R.; Gleicher, S.; Himanen, S.V.; Makedon, A.M.; Friedman, D.; Cortes, S.; Namek, S.; et al. Co-chaperones TIMP2 and AHA1 Competitively Regulate Extracellular HSP90:Client MMP2 Activity and Matrix Proteolysis. *Cell Rep.* **2019**, *28*, 1894–1906. [CrossRef]
43. Xiang, L.; Gilkes, D.M.; Chaturvedi, P.; Luo, W.; Hu, H.; Takano, N.; Liang, H.; Semenza, G.L. Ganetespib blocks HIF-1 activity and inhibits tumor growth, vascularization, stem cell maintenance, invasion, and metastasis in orthotopic mouse models of triple-negative breast cancer. *J. Mol. Med.* **2014**, *92*, 151–164. [CrossRef]

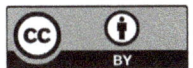

© 2019 by the authors. Licensee MDPI, Basel, Switzerland. This article is an open access article distributed under the terms and conditions of the Creative Commons Attribution (CC BY) license (http://creativecommons.org/licenses/by/4.0/).

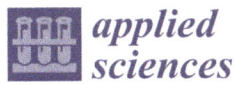

Article

Clinical and Functional Characterization of a Novel URAT1 Dysfunctional Variant in a Pediatric Patient with Renal Hypouricemia

Blanka Stiburkova [1,2,*], Jana Bohata [1,3], Iveta Minarikova [1], Andrea Mancikova [4], Jiri Vavra [4], Vladimír Krylov [4] and Zdenek Doležel [5]

1. Institute of Rheumatology, Na Slupi 4, 128 50 Prague, Czech Republic
2. Department of Pediatrics and Adolescent Medicine, First Faculty of Medicine, Charles University and General University Hospital in Prague, Ke Karlovu 2, 120 00 Prague, Czech Republic
3. Department of Rheumatology, First Faculty of Medicine, Charles University, Na Slupi 4, 128 50 Prague, Czech Republic
4. Department of Cell Biology, Faculty of Science, Charles University, Vinicna 7, 128 00 Prague, Czech Republic
5. Department of Pediatrics, University Hospital Brno, Medical Faculty of Masaryk University, Jihlavska 20, 625 00 Brno, Czech Republic
* Correspondence: stiburkova@revma.cz; Tel.: (+420)-234-075-319; Fax: (+420)-224-914-451

Received: 22 July 2019; Accepted: 20 August 2019; Published: 23 August 2019

Abstract: Renal hypouricemia (RHUC) is caused by an inherited defect in the main (reabsorptive) renal urate transporters, URAT1 and GLUT9. RHUC is characterized by decreased concentrations of serum uric acid and an increase in its excretion fraction. Patients suffer from hypouricemia, hyperuricosuria, urolithiasis, and even acute kidney injury. We report the clinical, biochemical, and genetic findings of a pediatric patient with hypouricemia. Sequencing analysis of the coding region of *SLC22A12* and *SLC2A9* and a functional study of a novel RHUC1 variant in the *Xenopus* expression system were performed. The proband showed persistent hypouricemia (67–70 μmol/L; ref. range 120–360 μmol/L) and hyperuricosuria (24–34%; ref. range 7.3 ± 1.3%). The sequencing analysis identified common non-synonymous allelic variants c.73G > A, c.844G > A, c.1049C > T in the *SLC2A9* gene and rare variants c.973C > T, c.1300C > T in the *SLC22A12* gene. Functional characterization of the novel RHUC associated c.973C > T (p. R325W) variant showed significantly decreased urate uptake, an irregular URAT1 signal on the plasma membrane, and reduced cytoplasmic staining. RHUC is an underdiagnosed disorder and unexplained hypouricemia warrants detailed metabolic and genetic investigations. A greater awareness of URAT1 and GLUT9 deficiency by primary care physicians, nephrologists, and urologists is crucial for identifying the disorder.

Keywords: *SLC22A12*; URAT1; hypouricemia; uric acid transporters; excretion fraction of uric acid

1. Introduction

Hypouricemia is defined as serum uric acid concentrations below 119 μmol/L (2 mg/dL). It is characterized by increased uric acid clearance or decreased uric acid production. Hypouricemia is a relatively rare condition, occurring in about 0.15–3.3% of the general population and 1.2–4% in hospitalized patients [1,2]. Malignancy is ranked first as a possible etiology of secondary hypouricemia, followed by diabetes mellitus, renal tubulopathies such as Fanconi syndrome, and medication. Excretion fraction of uric acid (EF-UA) is a key biochemical marker for a differential diagnosis of primary hypouricemia. Markedly elevated EF-UA suggests renal hypouricemia while lower or normal EF-UA suggests hereditary xanthinuria [3].

Renal hypouricemia (RHUC) is a heterogeneous hereditary disorder caused by a dysfunction of the main renal urate transporters, URAT1 and GLUT9. Characteristic biochemical markers include markedly decreased serum uric acid concentrations (S-UA) and elevated EF-UA. Clinical markers include exercise-induced acute renal failure, urolithiasis, and hematuria along with fatigue, nausea, vomiting, and diffuse abdominal discomfort. However, RHUC is also characterized by clinical variability, and only about 10% of all patients with a URAT1 defect have nephrolithiasis and/or acute kidney injury due to spasms of the renal artery. Currently there is no treatment for RHUC; however, allopurinol has been used to prevent recurrence of acute kidney injury episodes, and oral supplementation with antioxidants is recommended [4].

The role of URAT1 and the association of genetic variants of the *SLC22A12* gene with renal hypouricemia (RHUC type 1, OMIM no. 220150) were identified in 2002 [5], and to date, about 200 patients have been identified. The relationship between the GLUT9 transporter (gene *SLC2A9*) and renal hypouricemia (RHUC type 2, OMIM no. 612076) was reported in 2008 [6], and to date, about 15 patients have been identified. Homozygous or compound heterozygous loss-of-function mutations in the *SLC22A12* gene lead to a partial defect in absorption of uric acid, while variants in the *SLC2A9* are responsible for severe hypouricemia and hyperuricosuria (SUA < 10 µmol/L, EF-UA > 90%), which is often complicated by nephrolithiasis and acute kidney injury, such as that seen in RHUC1. Genetic variants in the *SLC22A12* gene are the primary cause of renal hypouricemia (>90%) with major variants reported in Asia region (Japanese and Korea, variant p.W258X with frequencies 2.3%) and in the Roma population (p.L415_G417del and p.T467M with frequencies of 1.9% and 5.6%, respectively) [7–10].

This case study expands our understanding of the molecular mechanisms of renal hypouricemia and confirms the distribution of dysfunctional URAT1 variants in non-Asian patients.

2. Materials and Methods

2.1. Patient

A three-year-old Caucasian girl was referred for an endocrine examination due to her small stature. The child's mother had been under long-term treatment for a psycho-affective disorder, which also included the pregnancy with her daughter; the father was healthy. The child was born during the 31st week of pregnancy, by C-section, due to premature discharge of amniotic fluid. Birth weight was 1330 g, and length was 37 cm. Oxygen therapy was necessary for 5 days but without the need for artificial pulmonary ventilation. During development, the child showed symptoms of psychomotor retardation. Therefore, developmental rehabilitation was initiated. Rehabilitation was carried out, however, family compliance was poor. The mother abandoned the family, and the girl was in alternating custody of her father and grandmother. On initial examination by an endocrinologist, the girl was 94.5 cm tall (−3.4 SD), had a body weight of 13.4 kg (−1.8 SD), and had only grown about 2.7 cm in the previous year. The father's body height was 163.5 cm, but the mother's height was unknown. The child's physical examination was without irregularities except for orbital hypertelorism. Her level psychomotor development corresponded approximately to that of a two-year-old child. Because hypouricemia (67–70 µmol/L) was repeatedly found during endocrine re-examinations, further analyses were carried out, mainly focused on purine metabolism disorders. High-performance liquid chromatography determination of hypoxanthine and xanthine in urine was performed on Waters Alliance 2695 [3].

2.2. Genetic Analysis

Genomic DNA was extracted from a blood sample using a QIAmp DNA Mini Kit (QiagenGmbH, Hilden, Germany). All coding exons and intron-exon boundaries of *SLC22A12* and *SLC2A9* were amplified from genomic DNA using polymerase chain reaction and subsequent purificated using a PCR DNA Fragments Extraction Kit (Geneaid, New Taipei City, Taiwan). DNA sequencing was performed on an automated 3130 Genetic Analyzer (Applied Biosystems Inc., Foster City, CA, USA). Primer sequences and PCR conditions used for amplification were described previously [11,12]. The reference genomic sequence was defined as version NC_000011.8, region 64,114,688..64126396, NM_144585.3 for *SLC22A12*; NM_020041.2, NP-064425.2, SNP source dbSNP 132 for *SLC2A9*.

2.3. Functional Analysis

A missense variant of URAT1, p.R325W, was tested for urate transport activity using in vitro expression analysis in *Xenopus* oocytes as previously described [11,13]. Subcellular localization was determined using immunocytochemical analysis. Immunodetection of URAT1 was performed on 3.5 μm paraffin sections using rabbit anti-SLC22A12 polyclonal antibody (Sigma, St. Louis, MO, USA). The paraffin sections were stained after heat-induced antigen retrieval (10 mM citrate buffer, pH 6.1, for 20 min at 97.0 °C in a water base) using standard blocking procedures. The primary antibody against URAT1 was diluted 1:25 in PBS and applied overnight at 4 °C. Detection of bound primary antibodies was achieved using Alexa Fluor 488-conjugated with anti-rabbit IgG (diluted 1:500; Abcam, Cambridge, Britain). For image acquisition, we used an Olympus BX53 fluorescent microscope (Olympus, Hamburg, Germany).

3. Results

3.1. Patient

The proband had persistent hyperuricemia (67–70 μmol/L; ref. range 120–360 μmol/L) and an increased EF-UA (24.3–34.2%; ref. range 7.3 ± 1.3%) with normal urinary excretion of hypoxanthine and xanthine, Table 1. No clinical or laboratory symptoms of renal disease were present in the patient. During follow-up, the patient was without episodes of acute kidney injury; her ultrasound exam showed no nephrolithiasis, and her creatinine clearance (estimated as eGF) was within the normal range. Supporting examinations to determine the cause of her small stature found normal serum levels of Thyroid Stimulating Hormone (TSH) and fT4, however, IGFBP-3 was low, and IGF-1 was well below the reference level. A growth hormone deficit was demonstrated with stimulation tests (clonidine test, hypoglycemia test). Brain magnetic resonance imaging found a markedly small hypophysis; the pituitary stalk was evaluated as normal. Cytogenetic analysis demonstrated a normal 46, XX karyotype. Growth hormone replacement therapy was initiated.

Table 1. Biochemical and genetic parameters of the proband and her father. [a] reference range for women and children; [b] reference range for men.

Table *Cont.*	Serum UA (μmol/L)	EF-UA (%)	Serum Creatinine (μmol/L)	Identified Variants in *SLC22A12*
Proband	67–70	24.3–34.2	32	c.973C > T (C/T); c.1300C > T (C/T)
Father of proband	205	N/A	62	c.1300C > T (C/T)
Reference range	120–360 [a] 120–420 [b]	7.3 ± 1.3 [a] 10.3 ± 4.2 [b]	50–110	-

3.2. Genetic Analysis

Sequencing analysis of *SLC2A9* revealed six intron variants (rs2240722, rs2240721, rs2240720, rs28592748, rs13115193 and rs61256984), three synonymous variants (rs13113918, rs10939650 and rs13125646) and three common non-synonymous allelic variants (rs2276961, p.G25R; rs16890979, p.V282I and rs2280205, p.P350L). A sequencing analysis of *SLC22A12* revealed one intron variant (rs11231837), four synonymous (rs3825016, rs11231825, rs1630320, and rs7932775), and two heterozygous rare non-synonymous allelic c.973C > T variants (p.R325W, rs150255373, Figure 1A,B), and a previously identified c.1300C > T variant (p.R434C, rs145200251) [14]. Segregation analysis was not fully performed because the child's family was not interested.

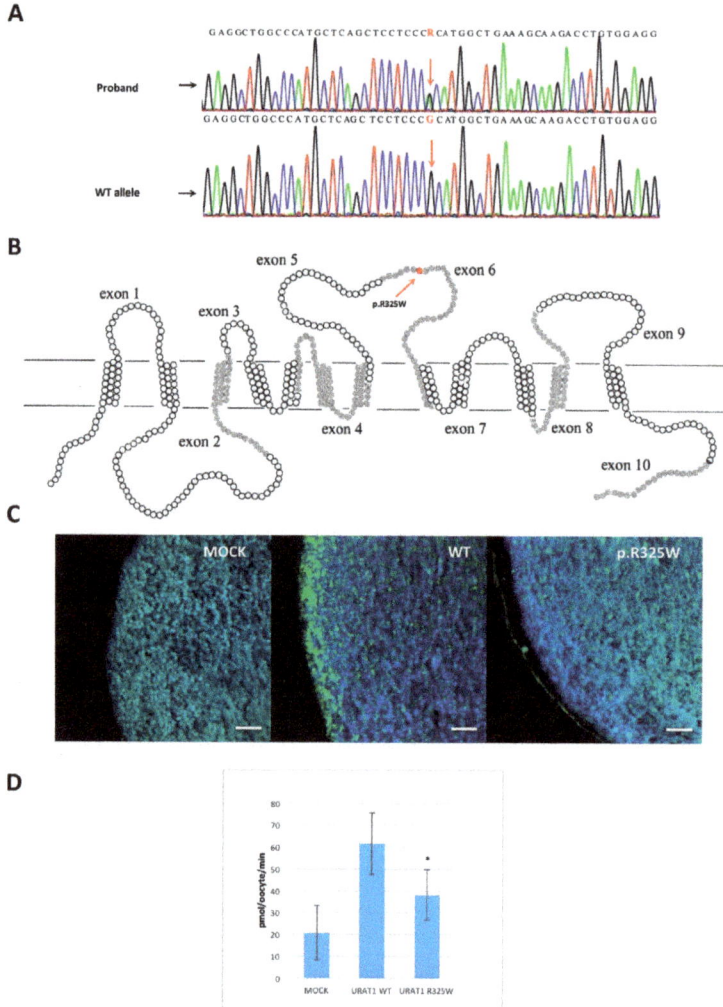

Figure 1. Illustration of allelic variant p.R325W in genetic, protein and functional context. (**A**) Electropherograms of partial sequences of exon 6 showing a heterozygous c.973C > T variant in the *SLC22A12* gene. (**B**) Position of identified allelic variant p.R325W in a URAT1 membrane topology model. (**C**) Immunohistochemical analysis of *Xenopus* oocytes injected with 50 ng of cRNA encoding the wt or p.R325W using anti-URAT1 polyclonal antibodies. The URAT1 signal is green, autofluorescent granules in the cytoplasm of oocytes are blue. Water-injected oocyte without any detectable URAT1 signal. Oocyte injected with wt cRNA exhibited a strong linear signal on the plasma membrane and a finely granular intracytoplasmic signal. The variant p.R325W was characterized by a weak discontinuous URAT1 signal on the plasma membrane, and reduced intracytoplasmic staining compared to the wt. Scale bar represents 50 µm. (**D**) Uric acid accumulation in *Xenopus* oocytes transfected with wt URAT1 and p.R325W URAT1 allelic variant after 30 min of incubation in [8-^{14}C] 600 µM uric acid/ND - 96 solution. The data was tested by One-way Analysis of variance (ANOVA). In comparison to wt URAT1, significantly lower UA accumulation (* $p < 0.05$) was detected in p.R325W URAT1 injected oocytes (n = 5; means ± SD). H$_2$O injected (mock) oocytes were used as a negative control.

3.3. Functional Analysis

Urate transport via the p.R325W variant was significantly decreased in comparison to the wild type (wt) (* $p < 0.05$), Figure 1C. This finding indicated that the above-mentioned URAT1 variant leads to reduced urate reabsorption at the apical membrane of proximal renal tubules leading to decreased serum urate levels. Oocytes expressing the wt exhibited strong continuous URAT1 immunostaining on the plasma membrane and dispersed finely granular staining in the cytoplasm. Oocytes expressing p.R325W showed a weak discontinuous URAT1 signal on the plasma membrane and intracytoplasmic staining was lower than in the wt, Figure 1D.

4. Discussion and Conclusions

Urate transport in the kidney is a complex process involving several transmembrane proteins that provide reabsorption (URAT1, GLUT9) and secretion (ABCG2). In genome-wide association studies, the *SLC2A9* gene is a well-established locus that is significantly associated with hyperuricemia while the *ABCG2* locus had the most significant association with gout susceptibility [15–17]. The dysfunctional variants in URAT1 and GLUT9 cause hereditary renal hypouricemia, and genetic analysis is needed to confirm the diagnosis and/or to identify the specific type of renal hypouricemia.

The *SLC22A12* gene is located on chromosome 11q13. Ten exons encode two transcript variants of the URAT1 transporter (332 and 553 amino acids), which are specifically expressed on the epithelial cells of the proximal tubules in the renal cortex [4]. At present, 52 variations in the *SLC22A12* coding region (40 missense/nonsense, two splicing, three regulatory, three small deletions, two small insertions, one gross deletion, and one complex rearrangement) have been described (HGMD Professional 2018.4, http://www.hgmd.cf.ac.uk). Thirty-six URAT1 variants are currently associated with the hypouricemia phenotype. Functional analysis confirmed in part of these variants impact on urate uptake ability and/or cytoplasmatic expression and localization [7,11,13,14]. However, not all URAT1 allelic variants have effect on decreasing of protein expression and/or function (p.R228E, R477H) [7,11].

The analysis of *SLC2A9* coding regions in our proband revealed three common non-synonymous variants: heterozygous rs2276961 (p.G25R, Caucasian MAF = 0.53), rs16890979 (p.V282I, Caucasian MAF = 0.21), and homozygous rs2280205 (p.P350L, Caucasian MAF = 0.48). These variants have not been previously reported in association with hypouricemia. Variant p.V282I was previously described relative to the hyperuricemia and gout phenotype [18]. Moreover, in our previous study, which used association analysis together with functional and immunohistochemical characterization of these variants identified in the adult population, we did not find any influence of these allelic variants on expression, subcellular localization, or urate uptake of GLUT9 transporters [19].

Our analysis of *SLC22A12* coding regions revealed two rare heterozygous non-synonymous variants: rs150255373 (p.R325W, Caucasian MAF = 0.001) and rs145200251 (p.R434C, Caucasian MAF unknown). Variant p.R434C was previously associated with renal hypouricemia 1 in a five-year-old Macedonian girl suffering from distal renal tubular acidosis and renal hypouricemia [14]. The patient had symptoms of dehydration, polyuria, and vomiting. The patient also had rickets and slow growth. There was evidence of hyperchloremic metabolic acidosis (pH 7.23, HCO_3 13.6 mmol/L, BE = 12.6 mmol/L), hypokalemia (3.0 mmol/L), hypophosphatemia (0.84 mmol/L), hypouricemia (73 μmol/L), and hyperuricosuria (EF-UA 24–31%). Bilateral nephrocalcinosis and a solitary cyst in the left kidney were discovered during an ultrasound examination. The patient was given alkali therapy; metabolic compensation was achieved, serum electrolytes normalized, and low molecular proteinuria resolved. Only the hypouricemia parameter persisted during the two-year observational period. The mother of this patient was a heterozygote for the same missense variant (S-UA 136 μmol/L, EF-UA 19%) and a history of renal colic and the passage of a single renal calculus. Functional studies of p.R434Cs were previously performed using transiently transfected HEK293 cells [14]. Plasma membrane expression levels of the p.R434C variant were low, intracellular localization was not strongly observed, and urate uptake showed a significant reduction of urate transport function ($P < 0.001$).

The structural model for URAT1 is mainly focused on the organization and alignment of residues within 12 transmembrane spanning domains. Variant p.R325W was localized within the putative extracellular loop. This variant has not yet been identified in the patients of those with renal hypouricemia, but the nature of this mutation strongly suggests that it is pathogenic; PolyPhen software (http://genetics.bwh.harvard.edu/pph/) suggested that the variant is possibly damaging (score 0.72). Moreover, another predictive software, SIFT (http://sift.jcvi.org/), suggests that this variant is deleterious (score 0). On the other hand, CADD (https://cadd.gs.washington.edu/), REVEL, and MetaLR predictive software indicate that the impact of the variant is likely to be tolerated or benign. In the middle stands Mutation Assessor (http://mutationassessor.org/r3/) which predicts a moderate functional impact. Evolutionary analysis of URAT1 paralogs, including six mammalian species, revealed conservation of p.R325W only between human and chimpanzee (Figure 2). Human and Simian monkeys possess high affinity and low capacity URAT1 transporter which diverged from the original low affinity, high capacity paralog (mouse, rat, horse and dog) 43 MYA [20]. Authors described four key amino acid substitutions in human URAT1 positions 25, 27, 365 and 414 as a crucial for the high to low affinity and low to high capacity shift. Similarly, as a variant p.R325W, all four amino acid residues are conserved between human and baboon, but not among other mammalian species. The functional characterization of p.R325W showed significantly decreased urate uptake and a weak, discontinuous URAT1 signal on the plasma membrane and reduced intracytoplasmic staining. The results suggested that p.R325W variant may not affect URAT1 function qualitatively (via alteration of its intrinsic transporter activity), but rather do so quantitatively (via decreasing its cellular protein level). Taken together, the data confirm the causality of the p.R325W variant relative to renal hypouricemia 1.

	p.R325W	p.R434C
Human	VLLSAMREELSMG	HEMGALRSALAVL
Chimpanzee	VLLSAMREELSMG	HEMGALRSALAVL
Horse	VLLSAMQEELSAS...	EWLWDLRSALAAL
Dog	VLLSAMQEELSAG....	YEMGALRSALAVL
Rat	VLRSAMQEEPNGN...	REMG I LRSSLAVL
Mouse	VLRSAMEEEPSRD,..	HGMGVLRSALAVL

Figure 2. Alignment of the p.R325W URAT1 amino acids in the studied allelic variants with chimpanzee, horse, dog, rat and mouse paralogs.

Detailed investigations of serum uric acid concentrations and excretion fractions of uric acid in patients with unexplained hypouricemia are needed. Many patients with RHUC may be asymptomatic; however, pediatric nephrologists know that RHUC can cause acute renal failure, especially after strenuous physical activity. Another risk of RHUC is the development of nephrolithiasis. Although renal hypouricemia is a rare hereditary disorder, the frequency of novel URAT1 associated variants shows that this condition is underdiagnosed. RHUC should be considered not only in patients from Japan or Asia. The phenotypic severity of RHUC1 is not correlated with results from functional characterizations of URAT1 variants. Functional studies regarding the impact of novel associated variants are necessary to determine their correlation with scores from prediction algorithms and to confirm causality.

Author Contributions: Conceptualization, B.S.; validation, B.S.; J.B. conducted sequencing analyses; I.M., A.M., J.V. and V.K. worked on experiments using *Xenopus* oocytes, and analyzed the data; Z.D. was responsible for clinical observations; data curation, B.S.; writing, B.S.; project administration, B.S.; funding acquisition, B.S.

Funding: Supported by the Ministry of Health of the Czech Republic: AZV 15-26693A, the project for conceptual development of research organization 00023728 (Institute of Rheumatology) and RVO VFN64165.

Conflicts of Interest: The authors declare no conflict of interest.

References

1. Son, C.N.; Kim, J.M.; Kim, S.H.; Cho, S.K.; Choi, C.B.; Sung, Y.K.; Kim, T.H.; Bae, S.C.; Yoo, D.H.; Jun, J.B. Prevalence and possible causes of hypouricemia at a tertiary care hospital. *Korean J. Intern. Med.* **2016**, *5*, 971–976. [CrossRef] [PubMed]
2. Bairaktari, E.T.; Kakafika, A.I.; Pritsivelis, N.; Hatzidimou, K.G.; Tsianos, E.V.; Seferiadis, K.I.; Elisaf, M.S. Hypouricemia in individuals admitted to an inpatient hospital-based facility. *Am. J. Kidney Dis.* **2003**, *41*, 1232–1255. [CrossRef]
3. Mraz, M.; Hurba, O.; Bartl, J.; Dolezel, Z.; Marinaki, A.; Fairbanks, L.; Stiburkova, B. Modern diagnostic approach to hereditary xanthinuria. *Urolithiasis* **2015**, *43*, 61–67. [CrossRef] [PubMed]
4. Bhasin, B.; Stiburkova, B.; De Castro-Pretelt, M.; Beck, N.; Bodurtha, J.N.; Atta, M.G. Hereditary renal hypouricemia: A new role for allopurinol? *Am. J. Med.* **2014**, *127*, e3–e4. [CrossRef] [PubMed]
5. Enomoto, A.; Kimura, H.; Chairoungdua, A.; Shigeta, Y.; Jutabha, P.; Cha, S.H.; Hosoyamada, M.; Takeda, T.; Sekine, T.; Igarashi, T.; et al. Molecular identification of a renal urate anion exchanger that regulates blood urate levels. *Nature* **2002**, *417*, 447–452. [CrossRef] [PubMed]
6. Matsuo, H.; Chiba, T.; Nagamori, S.; Nakayama, A.; Domoto, H.; Phetdee, K.; Wiriyasermkul, P.; Kikuchi, Y.; Oda, T.; Nishiyama, J.; et al. Mutations in glucose transporter 9 gene SLC2A9 cause renal hypouricemia. *Am. J. Hum. Genet.* **2008**, *83*, 744–751. [CrossRef] [PubMed]
7. Iwai, N.; Mino, Y.; Hosoyamada, M.; Tago, N.; Kokubo, Y.; Endou, H. A high prevalence of renal hypouricemia caused by inactive SLC22A12 in Japanese. *Kidney Int.* **2004**, *66*, 935–944. [CrossRef] [PubMed]
8. Lee, J.H.; Choi, H.J.; Lee, B.H.; Kang, H.K.; Chin, H.J.; Yoon, H.J.; Ha, I.S.; Kim, S.; Choi, Y.; Cheong, H.I. Prevalence of hypouricaemia and SLC22A12 mutations in healthy Korean subjects. *Nephrology* **2008**, *13*, 661–666. [CrossRef] [PubMed]
9. Gabrikova, D.; Bernasovska, J.; Sokolova, J.; Stiburkova, B. High frequency of SLC22A12 variants causing renal hypouricemia 1 in the Czech and Slovak Roma population; simple and rapid detection method by allele-specific polymerase chain reaction. *Urolithiasis* **2015**, *43*, 441–445. [CrossRef] [PubMed]
10. Stiburkova, B.; Gabrikova, D.; Čepek, P.; Šimek, P.; Kristian, P.; Cordoba-Lanus, E.; Claverie-Martin, F. Prevalence of URAT1 allelic variants in the Roma population. *Nucleosides Nucleotides Nucleic Acids* **2016**, *35*, 529–535. [CrossRef] [PubMed]
11. Stiburkova, B.; Sebesta, I.; Ichida, K.; Nakamura, M.; Hulkova, H.; Krylov, V.; Kryspinova, L.; Jahnova, H. Novel allelic variants and evidence for a prevalent mutation in URAT1 causing renal hypouricemia: Biochemical, genetics and functional analysis. *Eur. J. Hum. Genet.* **2013**, *21*, 1067–1073. [CrossRef] [PubMed]
12. Stiburkova, B.; Ichida, K.; Sebesta, I. Novel homozygous insertion in SLC2A9 gene caused renal hypouricemia. *Mol. Genet. Metab.* **2011**, *102*, 430–435. [CrossRef] [PubMed]
13. Mancikova, A.; Krylov, V.; Hurba, O.; Sebesta, I.; Nakamura, M.; Ichida, K.; Stiburkova, B. Functional analysis of novel allelic variants in URAT1 and GLUT9 causing renal hypouricemia type 1 and 2. *Clin. Exp. Nephrol.* **2016**, *20*, 578–584. [CrossRef] [PubMed]
14. Tasic, V.; Hynes, A.M.; Kitamura, K.; Cheong, H.I.; Lozanovski, V.J.; Gucev, Z.; Jutabha, P.; Anzai, N.; Sayer, J.A. Clinical and functional characterization of URAT1 variants. *PLoS ONE* **2011**, *6*, e28641. [CrossRef] [PubMed]
15. Köttgen, A.; Albrecht, E.; Teumer, A.; Vitart, V.; Krumsiek, J.; Hundertmark, C.; Pistis, G.; Ruggiero, D.; Seaghdha, M.C.O.; Haller, T.; et al. Genome-wide association analyses identify 18 new loci associated with serum urate concentrations. *Nat. Genet.* **2013**, *45*, 145–154. [CrossRef] [PubMed]
16. Nakayama, A.; Nakaoka, H.; Yamamoto, K.; Sakiyama, M.; Shaukat, A.; Toyoda, Y.; Okada, Y.; Kamatani, Y.; Nakamura, T.; Takada, T.; et al. GWAS of clinically defined gout and subtypes identifies multiple susceptibility loci that include urate transporter genes. *Ann. Rheum. Dis.* **2017**, *76*, 869–877. [CrossRef] [PubMed]
17. Stiburkova, B.; Pavelcova, K.; Zavada, J.; Petru, L.; Simek, P.; Cepek, P.; Pavlikova, M.; Matsuo, H.; Merriman, T.R.; Pavelka, K. Functional non-synonymous variants of ABCG2 and gout risk. *Rheumatology* **2017**, *56*, 1982–1992. [CrossRef] [PubMed]
18. Dehghan, A.; Köttgen, A.; Yang, Q.; Hwang, S.J.; Kao, W.H.L.; Rivadeneira, F.; Boerwinkle, E.; Levy, D.; Hofman, A.; Castor, B.; et al. Association of three genetic loci with uric acid concentration and risk of gout: A genome-wide association study. *Lancet* **2008**, *372*, 1953–1961. [CrossRef]

19. Hurba, O.; Mancikova, A.; Krylov, V.; Pavlikova, M.; Pavelka, K.; Stiburkova, B. Complex analysis of urate transporters SLC2A9, SLC22A12 and functional characterization of non-synonymous allelic variants of GLUT9 in the Czech population: No evidence of effect on hyperuricemia and gout. *PLoS ONE* **2014**, *9*, e107902. [CrossRef] [PubMed]
20. Tan, P.K.; Farrar, J.E.; Gaucher, E.A.; Miner, J.N. Coevolution of URAT1 and Uricase during Primate Evolution: Implications for Serum Urate Homeostasis and Gout. *Mol. Biol. Evol.* **2016**, *33*, 2193–2200. [CrossRef] [PubMed]

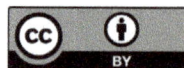

© 2019 by the authors. Licensee MDPI, Basel, Switzerland. This article is an open access article distributed under the terms and conditions of the Creative Commons Attribution (CC BY) license (http://creativecommons.org/licenses/by/4.0/).

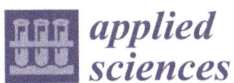

Article

Immunoexpression of Macroh2a in Uveal Melanoma

Lucia Salvatorelli [1],*, Lidia Puzzo [1], Giovanni Bartoloni [2], Stefano Palmucci [3], Antonio Longo [4], Andrea Russo [4], Michele Reibaldi [4], Manlio Vinciguerra [5], Giovanni Li Volti [6] and Rosario Caltabiano [1]

1. Department of Medical and Surgical Sciences and Advanced Technologies, G.F. Ingrassia, Azienda Ospedaliero-Universitaria "Policlinico-Vittorio Emanuele", Anatomic Pathology Section, School of Medicine, University of Catania, 95123 Catania, Italy
2. Pathology Department, University of Catania, 95123 Catania, Italy
3. Department of Medical Surgical Sciences and Advanced Technologies—Radiology I Unit, University Hospital "Policlinico-Vittorio Emanuele", 95123 Catania, Italy
4. Department of Ophthalmology, University of Catania, 95123 Catania, Italy
5. International Clinical Research Center, St. Anne's University Hospital, 65691 Brno, Czech Republic
6. Department of Biomedical and Biotechnological Sciences, University of Catania, 95123 Catania, Italy
* Correspondence: lucia.salvatorelli@unict.it; Tel.: +39-095-3782138

Received: 26 June 2019; Accepted: 6 August 2019; Published: 8 August 2019

Abstract: *MacroH2A* is a histone variant whose expression has been studied in several neoplasms, including cutaneous melanomas (CMs). In the literature, it has been demonstrated that *macroH2A.1* levels gradually decrease during CM progression, and a high expression of *macroH2A.1* in CM cells relates to a better prognosis. Although both uveal and cutaneous melanomas arise from melanocytes, uveal melanoma (UM) is biologically and genetically distinct from the more common cutaneous melanoma. Metastasis to the liver is a frequent occurrence in UM, and about 40%–50% of patients die of metastatic disease, even with early diagnosis, proper treatment, and close follow-up. We wanted to investigate macroH2A.1 immunohistochemical expression in UM. Our results demonstrated that mH2A.1 expression was higher in metastatic UM (21/23, 91.4%), while only 18/32 (56.3%). UMs without metastases showed mH2A.1 staining. These data could suggest a possible prognostic role for mH2A.1 and could form a basis for developing new pharmacological strategies for UM treatment.

Keywords: immunohistochemistry; macroH2A; prognostic factor; uveal melanoma; metastasis

1. Introduction

Uveal melanoma (UM) is the most frequent primitive intraocular neoplasm in middle age [1]: it occurs mainly in the choroid and ciliary bodies and less frequently in the iris, and some authors have suggested that these melanomas arise from previous benign nevi [2]. Histologically, three forms of UMs can be identified: (a) the spindle cell variant; (b) the epithelioid cell variant; and (c) the mixed cell variant, showing both epithelioid and spindle cells [3]. The prognosis of UM is poor because about 50% of patients will develop hepatic metastasis even 10–15 years after surgery [4]. Because of the strange behavior of this tumor, researchers have tried to determine what could be the mechanisms underlying the late development of liver metastases. Histone variants are chromatin components that replace replication-coupled histones in a fraction of nucleosomes and confer unique biological functions to chromatin [5]. MacroH2A (mH2A) is a histone variant whose expression has been studied in cutaneous melanomas (CMs). It has been shown that the loss of mH2A isoforms in cutaneous melanomas is correlated with increasing malignant phenotypes: this mechanism would seem to be mediated by the upregulation of CDK8, which inhibits the proliferation of melanoma cells. During CM progression, tumor cells show a low expression of mH2A, and conversely, high levels of mH2A expression correlate with a better prognosis [6,7].

In the present study, we studied the immunohistochemical expression of mH2A.1 in 55 primitive UMs, both with and without metastases, to understand whether expression may be correlated with a greater risk of metastasis in order to identify a marker able to predict the behavior of UM.

2. Materials and Methods

2.1. Patients and Tissue Samples

A retrospective study was performed on 55 primitive choroid and/or ciliary body melanomas after surgical treatment consisting of enucleation in cases not eligible for radiotherapy, such as plaque brachytherapy or proton beam radiotherapy [8], at the Eye Clinic, University of Catania, from October 2009 to October 2017.

No written informed consent was necessary because of the retrospective nature of the study.

The research protocols were conformed to the ethical guidelines of the Declaration of Helsinki.

The patients were 28 males and 27 females at an average age of 67 years (range 29–85). In particular, the patients with metastatic UM were 11 males and 12 females at an average age of 72 years (range 50–85): disease progression caused death in 13 of the 23 patients. The patients with nonmetastatic UM were 17 males and 15 females at an average age of 64 years (range 29–84) (Tables 1 and 2).

Table 1. Demographics, tumor parameters, disease-free time, follow-up, and macroH2A expression in primary uveal melanomas (UMs) without metastasis (n = 32).

Sex	Age (years)	Location	Thickness (mm)	Largest Diameter (mm)	Cell Type	Pathological T Stage	DFS (Months)	Follow-Up (Months)	MacroH2A			
									IS	ES	IRS	
F	29	Ch	14.2	16.2	Mc	pT2a	138	138	3	4	12	H
F	83	Ch/CB	14.84	16.8	Mc	pT2b	123	123	0	0	0	L
F	55	Ch	9.8	13.9	Sc	pT2a	122	122	0	0	0	L
F	30	Ch/CB	12.05	9.2	Sc	pT2b	122	122	2	1	2	L
M	74	Ch/CB	10.04	16.1	Sc	pT2b	121	121	3	4	12	H
M	64	Ch	7.7	11.5	Sc	pT1a	112	112	3	4	12	H
F	36	Ch	5.81	12.7	Sc	pT1a	109	109	3	1	3	L
F	59	Ch	8.4	16.7	Mc	pT2a	108	108	2	2	4	L
M	36	Ch	6.47	9.8	Mc	pT1a	108	108	0	0	0	L
M	84	Ch/CB	11.9	14.8	Mc	pT2b	106	106	0	0	0	L
F	67	Ch	10.42	13.02	Mc	pT3a	105	105	0	0	0	L
M	73	Ch	9.7	11.3	Mc	pT2a	102	102	0	0	0	L
F	45	Ch	13.7	10.2	Mc	pT2a	96	96	0	0	0	L
M	58	Ch	13.1	14.3	Mc	pT2a	96	96	2	1	2	L
M	63	Ch	3.3	11.7	Sc	pT2a	85	85	2	3	6	L
M	54	Ch	6.32	10	Sc	pT2a	83	83	3	4	12	H
F	84	Ch	11.7	17.4	Mc	pT3a	78	78	3	4	12	H
M	73	Ch	9.24	17.7	Ec	pT2a	72	72	2	1	2	L
M	83	Ch	10.62	9.4	Ec	pT3a	72	72	3	4	12	H
F	71	Ch	3.68	6.4	Ec	pT1a	71	71	0	0	0	L
M	55	Ch/CB	7.5	8.9	Ec	pT2b	61	61	3	4	12	H
M	52	Ch	9.2	12.1	Sc	pT2b	60	60	3	4	12	H
M	46	Ch	8.76	11.3	Sc	pT2a	54	54	0	0	0	L
F	76	Ch	8.02	10.7	Mc	pT1a	48	48	3	2	6	L
F	63	Ch	10.3	13.7	Mc	pT2a	42	42	0	0	0	L
F	41	Ch	5.85	10.3	Mc	pT1a	42	42	0	0	0	L
F	55	Ch	3.2	7.6	Mc	pT2a	24	24	2	4	8	L
F	74	Ch	8.6	10.2	Mc	pT4b	24	24	2	1	2	L
M	68	Ch/CB	10.1	10.1	Ec	pT1b	24	24	0	0	0	L
M	74	Ch/CB	14.45	17.5	Ec	pT4b	18	18	2	1	2	L
M	70	Ch/CB	16.27	20.8	Sc	pT4b	12	12	0	0	0	L
M	66	Ch	9.2	14.1	Mc	pT3a	12	12	1	1	1	L

Abbreviations: DFS, disease-free survival; Ch, choroid; CB, ciliary body; Mc, mixed cell; Sc, spindle cell; Ec, epithelioid cell.

Table 2. Demographics, tumor parameters, disease-free time, follow-up, and macroH2A expression in primary UMs with metastasis (n = 23).

Sex	Age (years)	Location	Thickness (mm)	Largest Diameter (mm)	Cell Type	Pathological T Stage	DFS (Months)	Follow-Up (Months)	MacroH2A			
									IS	ES	IRS	
F	58	Ch	6.04	17.8	Mc	pT2a	63	64 (†)	3	3	9	L
M	69	Ch	7.21	15.8	Mc	pT2a	54	81 (†)	3	4	12	H
F	75	Ch/CB	15.5	15.3	Mc	pT3b	44	62 (†)	3	4	12	H
F	50	Ch	7.36	15.6	Ec	pT2a	41	81	3	4	12	H
M	62	Ch	13.68	16	Mc	pT3a	38	51 (†)	3	4	12	H
F	51	Ch/CB	11.4	18.5	Mc	pT3b	38	61	3	4	12	H
M	71	Ch	13.14	17.1	Ec	pT3a	33	34 (†)	3	4	12	H
M	76	Ch/CB	11.6	6.5	Mc	pT1a	31	39	0	0	0	L
M	72	Ch	10.3	15.4	Mc	pT3b	27	35 (†)	3	4	12	H
F	85	Ch/CB	7.3	14.7	Sc	pT2d (EE)	26	49 (†)	3	4	12	H
M	73	Ch	5.73	11.7	Ec	pT2a	26	42 (†)	3	4	12	H
F	51	Ch	9.42	19	Mc	pT3a	25	39	1	1	1	L
F	74	Ch	5.7	12.1	Sc	pT2a	24	37 (†)	3	4	12	H
F	67	Ch	3.49	20	Mc	pT4a	24	31 (†)	3	4	12	H
M	74	Ch	11.35	10.5	Ec	pT3a	19	47	3	4	12	H
M	82	Ch	9.7	11	Ec	pT2a	19	42	3	4	12	H
F	72	Ch	6.7	15.2	Ec	pT2a	14	28 (†)	3	4	12	H
M	76	Ch	13.7	17.1	Mc	pT2a	14	70	3	4	12	H
M	79	Ch	13.91	16.1	Ec	pT3b	13	38	3	4	12	H
F	66	Ch/CB	8.95	12.5	Mc	pT2b	12	37 (†)	3	4	12	H
F	60	Ch	8.25	16.5	Ec	pT2a	11	37 (†)	3	4	12	H
F	57	Ch/CB	13.6	19	Ec	pT2b	6	55	3	4	12	H
M	72	Ch/CB	13.3	15.4	Mc	pT3b	0	51	3	4	12	H

Abbreviations: DFS, disease-free survival; Ch, choroid; CB, ciliary body; Mc, mixed cell; Sc, spindle cell; Ec, epithelioid cell; EE, extrascleral extension; (†) death.

The size and site of tumor onset were studied by ophthalmoscopy and A and B scan ultrasonography, while the study of metastases was performed by physical examination, hepatic ultrasound, and computerized tomography. The median follow-up period was 60 months (range 8–138 months). Forty melanomas were localized only in the choroid, while 15 involved both the choroid and the ciliary body: only in one case was an extrascleral extension found. As concerns histotypes, 15 cases were classified as epithelioid cells and 12 as spindle cells, and 28 cases were diagnosed as mixed type.

Based on the eighth TNM classification, 23 metastatic UMs were distributed as follows: pT1a (1 case, 4.3%), pT2a (9 cases, 39.1%), pT2b (2 cases, 8.7%), pT2d (1 case, 4.3%), pT3a (4 cases, 17.4%), pT3b (5 cases, 21.7%) and pT4a (1 case, 4.3%). TNM staging in 32 patients with metastatic UMs included pT1a (6 cases, 18.7%), pT1b (1 case, 3.1%), pT2a (12 cases, 37.5%), pT2b (6 cases, 18.7%), pT3a (4 cases, 12.5%), and pT4b (3 cases, 9.4%). We also tested mH2A in two cases of metastasis from uveal melanoma.

The cases were collected from the files of the Anatomic Pathology Department of Medical, Surgical, and Advanced Technologies, Gian Filippo Ingrassia, University of Catania. Some cases were excluded from the study for the following reasons: (1) if it was not possible to obtain sections from paraffin blocks for immunohistochemical staining, (2) the absence of representative tumor tissue, (3) the presence of exclusively necrotic material, and (4) preoperatively treated UMs.

Five sections were cut from each paraffin block. Briefly, the deparaffinized slides were pretreated with 10 mg/mL of ovalbumin in phosphate-buffered saline (PBS) followed by 0.2% biotin+ in PBS, each for 15 min at room temperature, and they were rinsed for 20 min with PBS (Bio-Optica, Milan, Italy) in order to reduce the usually seen nonspecific immunoreactivity due to endogenous biotin. Microwave pretreatment was performed to unmask antigenic sites. Then the slides were incubated overnight at 4 °C with rabbit polyclonal anti-macroH2A.1 antibody (ab37264; Abcam, Cambridge, UK) diluted 1:200 in PBS (Sigma, Milan, Italy). Sections were counterstained with hematoxylin, dehydrated, mounted (Zymed Laboratories, San Francisco, CA, USA), and observed with a light microscope (Carl Zeiss, Oberkochen, Germany).

The immunohistochemical expression of mH2A.1 was evaluated as positive if brown chromogen was observed in the nucleus. Normal skin was tested as a positive control, while the negative control was obtained through omission of the primary antibody.

Immunoreaction intensity and the percentage of stained cells were evaluated by light microscopy. Four levels (0–3) of the intensity of staining (IS) were identified: no evidence of immunoreactivity = 0, mild immunoreactivity = 1, intermediate immunoreactivity = 2, and intense immunoreactivity = 3, as described previously [9]. The extent score (ES), understood as the proportion of mH2A.1 immunopositive cells, included five levels: <5% (0), 5%–30% (+), 31%–50% (++), 51%–75% (+++), and >75% (++++). Counting was performed at 200× magnification. The intensity reactivity score (IRS) was obtained by multiplication of the intensity of staining (IS) and the percentage of positive cells: when the IRS was ≤6, mH2A.1 expression was considered to be "low" (L-IRS), while an IRS >6 was considered to be "high" expression (H-IRS).

The evaluation of immunohistochemical expression of mH2A was performed separately by three specialists in anatomic pathology (R.C., L.P., and L.S.), who were blind to the patient's identity, clinical data, and group identification.

2.2. Statistical Analysis

We compared the rate of high and low levels of mH2A.1 expression in melanoma of patients with and without metastasis using a chi-square test. The agreement among observations was assessed by Cohen's kappa coefficient.

We performed a univariate analysis based on a Cox proportional hazards regression model to test factors related to time free from metastasis. The parameters investigated were gender, age, melanoma location (choroid or ciliary body), temporal or nasal location, cell type (epithelioid, spindle cells, or mixed), echographic parameters (height, greatest diameter), and mH2A.1 expression (low and high).

Factors with a p-value <0.15 were included in the multivariate analysis.

We performed a survival analysis based on high and low mH2A.1 expression using the Kaplan–Meier test: survival rates were compared using a log-rank (Mantel–Cox) test, and p-values lower than 0.05 were considered to be statistically significant.

3. Results

3.1. Clinicopathological Characteristics of UMs

Comparing patients without metastasis and with metastasis, no significant difference was observed in median age, site (choroid or choroid/ciliary body), thickness, cell type, extrascleral extension, and pTNM: patients with metastatic melanoma showed a greater median largest diameter (15.6 mm vs 11.9 mm, $p = 0.007$) and higher median mH2A.1 expression (12 vs 2, $p < 0.001$). They also had lower median disease-free survival (25 months vs 81 months, $p < 0.001$) (Table 3).

Table 3. Medians (range) of demographics, tumor parameters, disease-free time, follow-up, and macroH2A expression in primary UMs without and with systemic metastasis.

	Sex m-f	Age (Years)	Location	Thickness	Largest Diameter	Cell Type	Extrascleral Extension	Pathological T Stage	DFS (Months)	Follow-Up (Months)	Macro H2A
All (n = 55)	28–27	67 (29–85)	Ch 40 Ch/CB 15	9.7 (3.2–16.3)	14.1 (6.4–20.8)	Ec: 15 Sc: 12 Mc: 28	No: 54 Yes: 1	pT1a: 7 pT1b:1 pT2a: 21 pT2b: 8 pT2d: 1 pT3a: 8 pT3b: 5 pT4a: 1 pT4b: 3	42 (0–138)	60 (8–138)	12 (0–12)
Metastasis-free (n = 32)	17–15	64 (29–84)	Ch24 Ch/CB 8	9.5 (3.2–16.3)	11.9 (6.4–20.8)	Ec: 6 Sc: 10 Mc: 16	No: 32	pT1a: 6 pT1b: 1 pT2a: 12 pT2b: 6 pT3a: 4 pT4b: 3	81 (12–138)	81 (8–138)	2 (0–12)
Metastasis (n = 23)	11–12	72 (50–85)	Ch 16 Ch/CB 7	9.7 (3.5–15.5)	15.6 (6.5–20)	Ec: 9 Sc: 2 Mc: 12	No: 22 Yes: 1	pT1a: 1 pT2a: 9 pT2b: 2 pT2d: 1 pT3a: 4 pT3b: 5 Pt4b: 1	25 (0–63)	42 13 deaths (28–81)	12 (0–12)
p (metastasis-free vs metastasis)	0.400 *	0.400 *	0.762 °	0.911 *	0.007 *	0.400 *	0.418°	0.560 *	<0.001 *	0.001 *	<0.001 *

* Kolmogorov–Smirnov test. ° Fisher's exact test. Abbreviations: Mc, mixed cell; Sc, spindle cell; Ec, epithelioid cell.

3.2. mH2A.1 Expression and Clinicopathological Features in UMs

Immunohistochemistry showed only mH2A.1 nuclear staining: no immunohistochemical expression of mH2A.1 was observed in non-neoplastic ocular tissue. Interobserver agreement was excellent (kappa = 0.943).

Considering the whole group ($n = 55$), the median mH2A.1 value was 12: H-IRS was observed in 28 (50.9%) melanomas and L-IRS in 27 (49.1%).

In 32 nonmetastatic primary UMs, mH2A.1 IS was intense/intermediate in 18 cases (56.3%) and mild in only one case (3.1%), while in 13 (40.6%) cases no immunoreactivity was observed (Figure 1). ES was >50% in 10 cases (31.3%) and 5%–30% in 9 cases (28.1%). Only 8/32 cases (25%) showed H-IRS, while 24 cases (75%) showed L-IRS (Table 1) (Fisher's exact test, $p < 0.001$, Table 4).

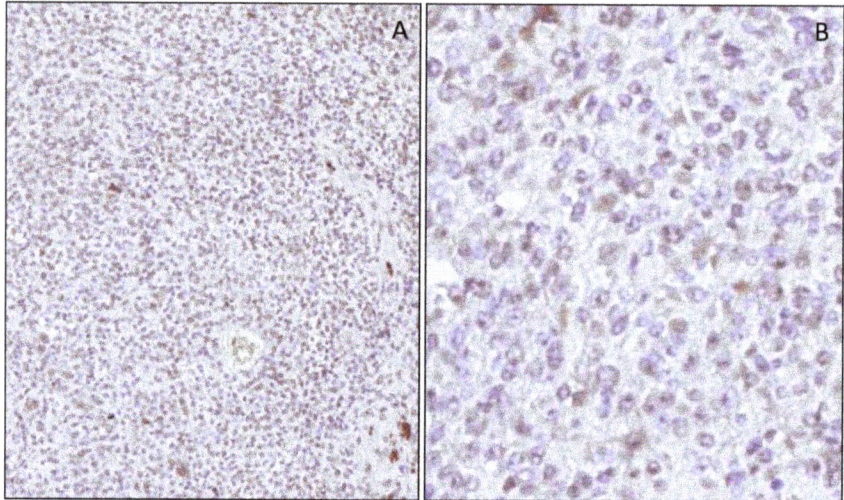

Figure 1. Immunohistochemical expression of mH2A.1 in nonmetastatic uveal melanomas. Melanoma cells showed weak staining for macroH2A.1 (low magnification in (**A**) and high magnification in (**B**)).

Table 4. Number of UMs (with and without metastasis) with low and high macroH2A.

mH2A	Metastasis ($n = 23$)	Metastasis-Free ($n = 32$)
Low	3 (13%) *	24 (75%)
High	20 (87%)	8 (25%)

Abbreviations: mH2A, macroH2A. p (Fisher's exact test). * $p < 0.0001$.

In 23 metastatic primary UMs, mH2A.1 IS was intense/intermediate in 21 cases (91.4%) and mild in 1 case (4.3%). Only 1 case (4.3%) showed an absence of immunoreactivity (Figure 2). ES was >75% in 20 cases (87%), 50%–75% in 1 case (4.3%), and 5%–30% in 1 case (4.3%). Here, 20/23 cases (87%) showed H-IRS, while only 3 cases (13%) had L-IRS (Table 2) (Fisher's exact test, $p < 0.001$, Table 4).

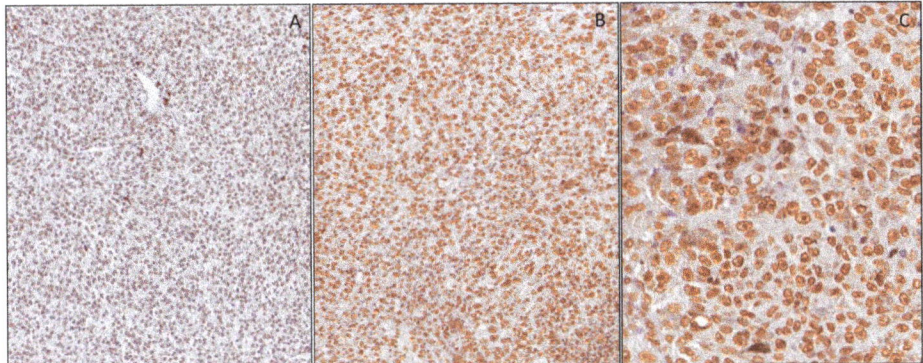

Figure 2. Immunohistochemical expression of mH2A.1 in metastatic uveal melanomas. Tumor cells revealed moderate (IS 2) immunoreactivity in (**A**). (**B**) and (**C**) show strong staining (IS 3), respectively, at low and high magnifications.

In two cases of metastasis from uveal melanoma, mH2A.1 showed diffuse and intense immunoreactivity with H-IRS (Figure 3).

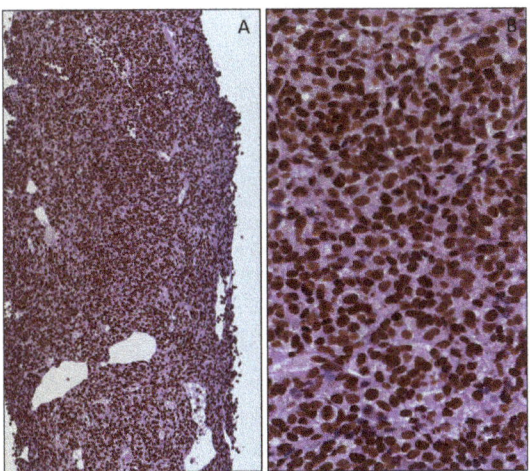

Figure 3. Immunohistochemical expression of mH2A.1 in metastases from uveal melanomas. Metastatic cells revealed diffuse (ES 4) and strong (IS 4) immunoreactivity, respectively, at low (**A**) and high magnifications (**B**).

Univariate analysis based on a Cox proportional hazards regression model revealed that factors related to the presence of metastasis were age ($p = 0.053$), greater tumor size ($p = 0.009$), pT (pathological Tumor) stage ($p = 0.016$), the epithelioid variant ($p = 0.011$), and mH2A.1 expression ($p < 0.001$). Factors significantly related to the presence of metastasis in the multivariate analysis were mH2A.1 expression ($p = 0.002$), greater tumor size ($p = 0.026$), and the epithelioid variant ($p = 0.019$).

Here, mH2A.1 expression was not related to histological type (Spearman's rho, $p = 0.173$). A Kaplan–Meier survival analysis showed that the estimated survival times free from metastasis were greater in patients with low mH2A.1 expression in UMs: mean values (SE (Standard error), with 95% CI (confidential interval)) were 110.3 (6.80) (CI: 97.0 to 123.7) in patients with low mH2A.1 expression and 56.7 (10.0) (CI: 37.2 to 76.2) in patients with high mH2A.1 expression ($p < 0.001$, log-rank (Mantel–Cox) test, Figure 4).

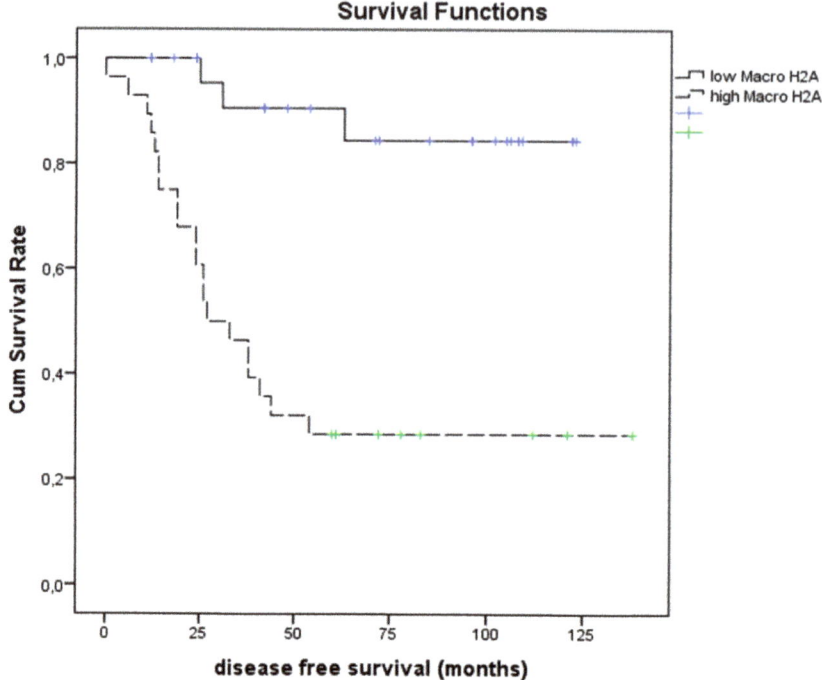

Figure 4. Kaplan–Meier test. Survival analyses (Kaplan–Meier) in patients with UMs with low and high macroH2A expression ($p < 0.001$, log-rank (Mantel–Cox) test).

4. Discussion

UM is an ambiguous neoplasia because regardless of the histological subtype and initial stage, it can metastasize to the liver, even after 10–15 years [4]. From the diagnosis of hepatic metastasis, death usually occurs within one year, and there is a lack of effective treatment. Asymptomatic patients with an early detection of metastasis seem to have an apparent benefit, while adjuvant therapies and screening do not seem to provide a significant survival benefit [10,11]. The prognosis of UM depends on multiple clinical data points: adult/senile age, male gender, large tumor, tumor thickness, ciliary body site, eye or skin melanocytosis, extraocular involvement at presentation, and advanced stage. Histopathological parameters (epithelioid cell variant, numerous mitoses, microvascular proliferation, microvascular loops and patterns, intratumoral lymphocytes, intratumoral macrophages, strong expression of IGF-1R (insulin-like growth factor-1 receptor) and HLA (Human Leucocyte Antigen) class I and II), cytogenetic factors (monosomy 3, chromosome 8q-gain or 8p-loss, chromosome 1p-loss, chromosome 6q-loss), and transcriptomic factors (gene expression profile class 2) [10,11] play a role as prognostic factors.

However, much remains to be understood to limit the onset of metastases or to identify effective treatments in metastatic patients.

Indeed, research is being focused on factors that can identify tumors with aggressive behavior and find new therapeutic targets. Our research group has tried to determine the unusual behavior of UM by testing different molecules and factors such as ADAM10, RKIP, pRKIP, ABCB5, and SPANX-C [9,12,13].

Recent studies have reported the inactivation of somatic mutations in gene-encoding BRCA-1-associated protein 1 (BAP1) in about 84% of metastasizing UMs [14]: the high frequency of BAP1 mutations in metastatic UMs encouraged us to search for new therapeutic strategies with the target molecule BAP1, which have deubiquitinase activity on histone H2A [15,16]. In different tumors, including skin melanoma, mH2A and its variants, which are widely distributed along chromatin [17–19], have been regarded as a potential prognostic marker [20,21].

Previously, Kapoor et al. [6] reported that the histone variant mH2A suppressed the tumor progression of malignant cutaneous melanoma and that the loss of mH2A isoforms was positively correlated with increasing malignant phenotypes of cutaneous melanoma cells in culture and human tissue samples. In addition, they suggested that the tumor-promoting function of mH2A loss was mediated, at least in part, through direct transcriptional upregulation of CDK8.

Lei et al. [7] showed that high expression of mH2A suppressed melanoma cell progression and arrested cells in the G2/M phase. Thus, we hypothesized that an alteration in mH2A expression could contribute to a change in the phenotype of UMs, promoting tumor progression. Therefore, mH2A would be the basis for this mechanism, whose final effect would be stabilizing the cell cycle, which is frequently observed in malignant neoplasms, in particular in tumor lesions with a low proliferative index. Furthermore, the arrest of the cell cycle would make the cell not very sensitive to chemotherapy, suggesting a further predictive role in the response to therapy. In the present study, we showed that an elevated increased expression of mH2A correlated with tumor progression: indeed, metastasizing UMs showed the highest expression of mH2A. This assay might prove that a high expression of histone protein correlates with an advanced tumor phase.

In this study, we saw that mH2A overexpression was a prognostic factor for the risk of metastasis. In our series of UMs, mH2A was strongly expressed in more than 75% of neoplastic cells, with a median IRS value of 12. In patients with H-IRS, we observed an increased incidence of metastasis after surgical treatment. These data were also confirmed by the high expression of mH2A in metastases, although this was limited to only two cases. Conversely, the cases with L-IRS showed a decreased risk of metastasis. In addition, a Kaplan–Meier survival analysis showed that patients with UMs and H-IRS had lower metastasis-free survival times.

In conclusion, our results highlight the important role played by mH2A in UM progression. The immunohistochemical expression of mH2A could be a suitable and easily detectable marker in the primary tumor, predicting the risk of UM metastasis and thus directing strategies for monitoring and therapy.

Author Contributions: Conceptualization, L.S. and R.C.; data curation, G.B., S.P., A.L., A.R., M.R., M.V., G.L.V., and R.C.; methodology, L.S., L.P., and R.C.; resources, R.C.; writing—original draft, L.S.; writing—review and editing, L.S. and R.C.

Funding: The project was funded by the intradepartmental research plan 2016/2018 of the Department of Medical, Surgical, and Advanced Technologies, University of Catania (funding number 5C722012114, 2018) and by the European Social Fund and European Regional Development Fund—Project MAGNET (No. CZ.02.1.01/0.0/0.0/15_003/0000492).

Acknowledgments: The authors would like to thank the Department "GF Ingrassia" of the University of Catania for financial support, and the Scientific Bureau of the University of Catania for language assistance.

Conflicts of Interest: The authors declare no conflicts of interest.

References

1. Pukrushpan, P.; Tulvatana, W.; Pittayapongpat, R. Congenitaluvealmalignantmelanoma. *J. AAPOS* **2014**, *18*, 199–201. [CrossRef] [PubMed]
2. Spagnolo, F.; Caltabiano, G.; Queirolo, P. Uveal melanoma. *Cancer Treat. Rev.* **2012**, *38*, 549–553. [CrossRef] [PubMed]
3. McLean, I.W.; Foster, W.D.; Zimmerman, L.E.; Gamel, J.W. Modifications of Callender's classification of uveal melanoma at the Armed Forces Institute of Pathology. *Am. J. Ophthalmol.* **1983**, *96*, 502–509. [CrossRef]
4. Willson, J.K.; Albert, D.M.; Moy, C.S. Collaborative Ocular Melanoma Study Group, Assessment of metastaticdisease status atdeath in 435 patients with large choroidal melanoma in the Collaborative Ocular Melanoma Study (COMS): COMS report no. 15. *Arch. Ophthalmol.* **2001**, *119*, 670–676. [CrossRef]
5. Cantariño, N.; Douet, J.; Buschbeck, M. MacroH2A–An epigeneticregulator of cancer. *Cancer Lett.* **2013**, *336*, 247–252. [CrossRef]

6. Kapoor, A.; Goldberg, M.S.; Cumberland, L.K.; Ratnakumar, K.; Segura, M.F.; Emanuel, P.O.; Menendez, S.; Vardabasso, C.; Leroy, G.; Vidal, C.I.; et al. The histonevariant macroH2A suppresses melanoma progressionthroughregulation of CDK8. *Nature* **2010**, *468*, 1105–1109. [CrossRef] [PubMed]
7. Lei, S.; Long, J.; Li, J. MacroH2A suppresses the proliferation of the B16 melanoma cell line. *Mol. Med. Rep.* **2014**, *10*, 1845–1850. [CrossRef]
8. Choudhary, M.M.; Triozzi, P.L.; Singh, A.D. Uveal melanoma: Evidence for adjuvanttherapy. *Int. Ophthalmol. Clin.* **2015**, *55*, 45–51. [CrossRef]
9. Caltabiano, R.; Puzzo, L.; Barresi, V.; Ieni, A.; Loreto, C.; Musumeci, G.; Castrogiovanni, P.; Ragusa, M.; Foti, P.; Russo, A.; et al. ADAM 10 expression in primaryuveal melanoma asprognosticfactor for risk of metastasis. *Pathol. Res. Pract.* **2016**, *212*, 980–987. [CrossRef]
10. Augsburger, J.J.; Corrêa, Z.M.; Trichopoulos, N. Surveillancetesting for metastasis from primaryuveal melanoma and effect on patientsurvival. *Am. J. Ophthalmol.* **2011**, *152*, 5–9. [CrossRef]
11. Kaliki, S.; Shields, C.L. Uveal melanoma: Relatively rare butdeadlycancer. *Eye* **2017**, *31*, 241–257. [CrossRef] [PubMed]
12. Caltabiano, R.; Puzzo, L.; Barresi, V.; Cardile, V.; Loreto, C.; Ragusa, M.; Russo, A.; Reibaldi, M.; Longo, A. Expression of RafKinaseInhibitorProtein (RKIP) is apredictor of uveal melanoma Metastasis. *Histol Histopathol.* **2014**, *29*, 1325–1334. [CrossRef] [PubMed]
13. Salvatorelli, L.; Puzzo, L.; Russo, A.; Reibaldi, M.; Longo, A.; Ragusa, M.; Aldo, C.; Rappazzo, G.; Caltabiano, R.; Salemi, M. Immunoexpression of SPANX-C in metastaticuveal melanoma. *Pathol. Res. Pract.* **2019**, *29*, 152431. [CrossRef] [PubMed]
14. Harbour, J.W.; Onken, M.D.; Roberson, E.D.; Duan, S.; Cao, L.; Worley, L.A.; Council, M.L.; Matatall, K.L.; Helms, C.; Bowcock, A.M.; et al. Frequentmutation of BAP1 in metastasizinguvealmelanomas. *Science* **2010**, *330*, 1410–1413. [CrossRef] [PubMed]
15. Scheuermann, J.C.; de Ayala Alonso, A.G.; Oktaba, K.; Ly-Hartig, N.; McGinty, R.K.; Fraterman, S. Histone H2A deubiquitinaseactivity of the Polycomb repressive complex PR-DUB. *Nature* **2010**, *465*, 243–247. [CrossRef] [PubMed]
16. Machida, Y.J.; Machida, Y.; Vashisht, A.A.; Wohlschlegel, J.A.; Dutta, A. The deubiquitinatingenzyme BAP1 regulatescellgrowth via interaction with HCF-1. *J. Biol. Chem.* **2009**, *284*, 34179–34188. [CrossRef] [PubMed]
17. Costanzi, C.; Pehrson, J.R. Histone macroH2A1 isconcentrated in the inactive X chromosome offemalemammals. *Nature* **1998**, *393*, 599–601. [CrossRef] [PubMed]
18. Zhang, R.; Poustovoitov, M.V.; Ye, X.; Santos, H.A.; Chen, W.; Daganzo, S.M.; Erzberger, J.P.; Dunbrack, R.L.; Adams, P.D.; Berger, J.M.; et al. Formation ofMacroH2A-containing senescence-associatedheterochromatin foci and senescencedriven by ASF1aand HIRA. *Dev. Cell.* **2005**, *8*, 19–30. [CrossRef]
19. Bernstein, E.; Muratore-Schroeder, T.L.; Diaz, R.L.; Chow, J.C.; Changolkar, L.N.; Shabanowitz, J.; Heard, E.; Pehrson, J.R.; Hunt, D.F.; Allis, C.D. A phosphorylated subpopulation of the histone variant macroH2A1 is excluded from the inactive X chromosome and enriched during mitosis. *Proc. Natl. Acad. Sci. USA* **2008**, *105*, 1533–1538. [CrossRef]
20. Lo Re, O.; Fusilli, C.; Rappa, F.; Van Haele, M.; Douet, J.; Pindjakova, J.; Pata, L.; Vinciguerra, M.; Mazza, T.; Buschbeck, M.; et al. Induction of cancercellstemness by depletion of macrohistone H2A1 in hepatocellular carcinoma. *Hepatology* **2018**, *67*, 636–650. [CrossRef]
21. Hua, S.; Kallen, C.B.; Dhar, R.; Baquero, M.T.; Mason, C.E.; Russell, B.A.; White, K.P.; Rimm, D.L.; Krausz, T.N.; Shah, P.K.; et al. Genomicanalysis of estrogencascaderevealshistonevariant H2A.Z associated with breastcancerprogression. *Mol. Syst. Biol.* **2008**, *4*, 188. [CrossRef] [PubMed]

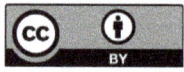

© 2019 by the authors. Licensee MDPI, Basel, Switzerland. This article is an open access article distributed under the terms and conditions of the Creative Commons Attribution (CC BY) license (http://creativecommons.org/licenses/by/4.0/).

Article

Immunohistochemical Expression of ABCB5 as a Potential Prognostic Factor in Uveal Melanoma

Giuseppe Broggi [1,*], Giuseppe Musumeci [2], Lidia Puzzo [1], Andrea Russo [3], Michele Reibaldi [3], Marco Ragusa [4], Antonio Longo [3] and Rosario Caltabiano [1]

1. Department G.F. Ingrassia, Section of Anatomic Pathology, University of Catania, 95123 Catania, Italy; lipuzzo@unict.it (L.P.); rosario.caltabiano@unict.it (R.C.)
2. Department of Bio-medical Sciences, Division of Anatomy and Histology, University of Catania, 95123 Catania, Italy; g.musumeci@unict.it
3. Department of Ophthalmology, University of Catania, 95123 Catania, Italy; clinica.oculistica@unict.it (A.R.); mreibaldi@libero.it (M.R.); antlongo@unict.it (A.L.)
4. Department of Bio-medical Sciences, Section of Molecular Biomedicine, University of Catania, 95123 Catania, Italy; mragusa@unict.it
* Correspondence: giuseppe.broggi@gmail.com; Tel.: +39-095-378-2022; Fax: +39-095-378-2023

Received: 24 December 2018; Accepted: 26 March 2019; Published: 29 March 2019

Abstract: Uveal melanoma represents the most common primary intraocular malignancy in adults; it may arise in any part of the uveal tract, with choroid and ciliary bodies being the most frequent sites of disease. In the present paper we studied ABCB5 expression levels in patients affected by uveal melanoma, both with and without metastasis, in order to evaluate if ABCB5 is associated with a higher risk of metastatic disease and can be used as a poor prognostic factor in uveal melanoma. The target population consisted of 23 patients affected by uveal melanoma with metastasis and 32 without metastatic disease. A high expression of ABCB5 was seen in patients with metastasis (14/23, 60.9%), compared to that observed in patients without metastasis (13/32, 40.6%). In conclusion, we found that ABCB5 expression levels were correlated with faster metastatic progression and poorer prognosis, indicating their role as a prognostic factor in uveal melanoma.

Keywords: ABCB5; uveal melanoma; prognosis; metastasis; immunohistochemistry

1. Introduction

Uveal melanoma (UM) is a rare neoplasm which, despite its rarity, represents the most common primary ocular malignancy in adults; it develops more frequently from melanocytes of the choroid but can also arise in other sites, such as ciliary bodies and iris [1]. UM has rarely been reported in pediatric ages, especially in advanced stages, with extraocular extension [2,3].

Several risk factors have been proposed in the pathogenesis of UM, including the presence of choroidal nevus, exposure to ultraviolet radiation, clear phototypes, ocular melanocytosis and extraocular conditions such as cutaneous dysplastic nevus syndrome, nevus of Ota and type 1 neurofibromatosis [4].

Clinically, although UM may remain silent and be accidentally detected by routine ophthalmic screening, a retinal detachment, causing visual disturbances like photopsia, is the most common presenting symptom of the disease; intraocular infections, vitreous bleeding and secondary glaucoma are frequent complications characterizing the natural history of the neoplasm [5].

Histologically, three distinct histotypes of UM have been identified: epithelioid cells, spindle cells and mixed cell type; a greater proportion of epithelioid cells has traditionally been associated with poorer prognosis [6].

It has been demonstrated on the basis of cytogenetic studies that monosomy 3 is the most common chromosomal aberration in UMs and correlates with lower survival rates; other cytogenetic alterations including loss of 1p, 6q and gain of 6p and 8q have been also associated with UM [7].

The biological history of the neoplasm has been characterized in almost 50% of cases by hematogenous dissemination, with the onset of secondary disease localizations, especially at the liver. Despite the improvements in therapeutic strategies, no significant increase in survival has been obtained and liver metastases are expected within 10–15 years after the diagnosis in about half of patients [8].

ATP-binding cassette sub-family B member 5 (ABCB5) is a human transmembrane P-glycoprotein that plays an active role in transmembrane transport of several substances including chemotherapeutic drugs; therefore, it is physiologically involved in the development of chemoresistance of cancer cells [9–11]. An overexpression of ABCB5 has been found in tumor stem cells, of which it is therefore a full-fledged marker of several malignancies such as hepatocellular carcinoma, breast cancer, cutaneous melanoma and Merkel cell carcinoma [12–14]. Furthermore, ABCB5 has been shown to be correlated with tumor growth and invasion [15,16].

Regarding cutaneous melanoma, ABCB5-positive malignant melanoma-initiating cells (MMICs) are believed to be involved both in the onset and in the progression of disease and ABCB5 has also been found to play a crucial role in promoting distant metastasis through the activation of the NF-kB signaling pathway [17].

In the present study, we retrospectively investigated ABCB5 expression in primary uveal melanoma in patients both with non-metastatic and metastatic disease and we evaluated its potential role as a prognostic marker and predictive factor of metastatic potential of the neoplastic cells.

2. Materials and Methods

A retrospective analysis of clinical data and histologic specimens of all cases of uveal melanoma treated by enucleation at the Eye Clinic of the University of Catania, during the eight years until to October 2017, was performed. Tumors not suitable for radiotherapy, such as plaque brachytherapy or proton beam radiotherapy were subjected to enucleation. Formalin-fixed and paraffin-embedded tissue specimens were obtained from the surgical pathology archive at the Section of Anatomic Pathology, Department G.F. Ingrassia, University of Catania. Cases in which paraffin blocks containing the tumor could not be used to obtain additional slides for immunohistochemical evaluation, representative tumor tissue was not present, the tumor was totally necrotic or had been treated previously, were excluded from the study. At least five sections were obtained from paraffin-embedded tissue specimens. Because of the retrospective nature of the study, no written informed consent from patients was obtained. The research protocols were approved by the Local Medical Ethics Committee (University of Catania) and conformed to the ethical guidelines of the Declaration of Helsinki. 23 UMs with metastasis and 32 UMs without metastasis were part of the study. The following clinical data were collected: tumor size and location, evaluated through ophthalmoscopy and A and B scan ultrasonography, and presence of metastasis, investigated with standard methods such as physical examination, liver ultrasound and total body computed tomography. The A-scan ultrasound refers to a mono-dimensional amplitude modulation scan, mainly used in common sight disorders because it provides important data on the axial length of the eye; the other major use of the A-scan is to determine the size and ultrasound characteristics of intraocular masses. B-scan ultrasound is a two-dimensional, cross-section brightness scan, that, when used in conjunction with A-scan imaging, allows direct visualization of the lesion, including anatomic location, shape, borders, and size, thereby ensuring a more detailed preoperative diagnosis. All histological sections were evaluated by two pathologists (GB and RC) in order to get the most objective assessment possible.

2.1. Immunohistochemistry

Sections were processed as previously described [18,19]. Briefly, the slides were dewaxed in xylene, hydrated using graded ethanols and incubated for 30 min in 0.3% H_2O_2/methanol to quench endogenous peroxidase activity, then rinsed for 20 min with phosphate-buffered saline (PBS; Bio-Optica, Milan, Italy). The sections were heated (5 min × 3) in capped polypropylene slide-holders with citrate buffer (10 mM citric acid, 0.05% Tween 20, pH 6.0; Bio-Optica, Milan, Italy), using a microwave oven (750 W) to unmask antigenic sites. To reduce the commonly seen non-specific immunoreactivity due to endogenous biotin, sections were pretreated with 10 mg/mL of ovalbumin in PBS followed by 0.2% biotin in PBS, each for 15 min at room temperature. Then, the sections were incubated for 18 h at 4 °C with mouse monoclonal anti-ABCB5 antibody (ab140667; Abcam, Cambridge, UK), diluted 1:100 in PBS (Sigma, Milan, Italy). The secondary biotinylated anti-mouse antibody was applied for 30 min at room temperature, followed by the avidin–biotin–peroxidase complex (Vector Laboratories, Burlingame, CA, USA) for a further 30 min at room temperature. The immunoreaction was visualized by incubating the sections for 4 min in a 0.1% 3,3'-diaminobenzidine (DAB) and 0.02% hydrogen peroxide solution (DAB substrate kit, Vector Laboratories, CA, USA). The sections were lightly counterstained with Mayer's hematoxylin (Histolab Products AB, Göteborg, Sweden) mounted in GVA mountant (Zymed Laboratories, San Francisco, CA, USA) and observed with a Zeiss Axioplan light microscope (Carl Zeiss, Oberkochen, Germany).

2.2. Evaluation of Immunohistochemistry

Immunostained histologic sections were separately evaluated by two pathologists (GB and RC), with no information on clinical data. Immunohistochemical positive ABCB5 staining was defined as the presence of brown chromogen detection in the cell membrane. Liver cancer and breast cancer tissues (Figure 1a) were used as positive controls to test the validity of the antibody reaction. Negative controls, involving benign prostatic tissue, were included (Figure 1b).

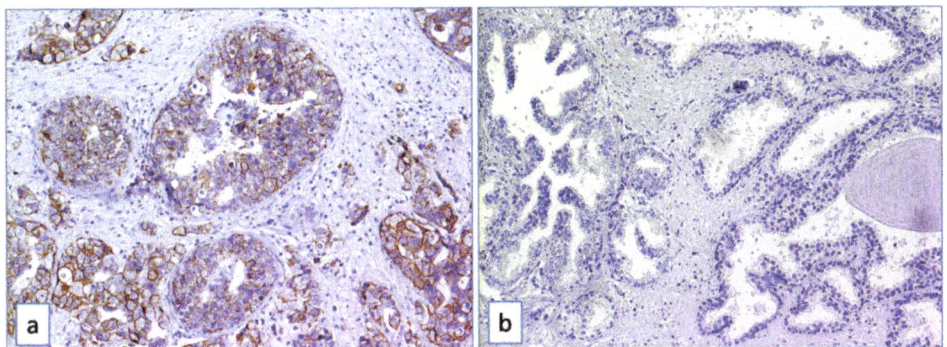

Figure 1. (**a**) ABCB5 staining on breast cancer tissue used as positive control (Immunoperoxidase stain; original magnification 150×); (**b**) absence of expression of ABCB5 in benign prostatic tissue used as negative control (Immunoperoxidase stain; original magnification 150×).

Stain intensity and proportion of immunopositive cells were assessed by light microscopy, as previously described [18]. Intensity of staining (IS) was graded on a scale of 0–3, according to the following assessment: no detectable staining = 0, weak staining = 1, moderate staining = 2, strong staining = 3. The percentage of ABCB5 immunopositive cells (Extent Score, ES) was scored in five categories: <5% (0); 5–30% (+); 31–50% (++); 51–75% (+++), and >75% (++++). Counting was performed at 200× magnification. Staining intensity was multiplied by the percentage of positive cells to obtain the intensity reactivity score (IRS); IRS < 6 was considered as low expression (L-IRS), IRS > 6 was considered as high expression (H-IRS).

2.3. Statistical Analysis

Non parametric comparison of the rate of high and low levels of ABC5 expression in melanoma of patients with and without metastasis was performed by chi-square test. Agreement among observers was tested by Cohen K.

Univariate and multivariate analysis were based on a Cox proportional hazards regression model (time free from metastasis as outcome); this model included gender, age, melanoma location (choroid or ciliary body), temporal or nasal location, cells type (epithelioid, spindle cells or mixed), echographic parameters (height, greatest diameter), ABCB5 expression (low and high). All predictors that had a p-value < 0.15 (cut off) in the univariate analysis were included in the multivariate analysis. Survival analysis according to ABC5 expression levels (high and low) was performed by Kaplan-Meyer test; survival rates were compared by log-rank (Mantel-Cox) test. p-values < 0.05 were considered as statistically significant.

3. Results

3.1. Clinico-Pathological Characteristic of Uveal Melanomas

The study was conducted on of 55 patients, 28 of whom were males and 27 women; median age was 67 years (range 29–85). 40 melanomas were localized only in the choroid, while 15 affected both choroid and ciliary body; extrascleral involvement was present and histologically confirmed in only one case. Regarding the histotypes, 15 cases were classified as epithelioid cells, 12 as spindle cells, while 28 cases were diagnosed as mixed type UM with both epithelioid and spindle cells. Considering the "TNM classification of malignant tumours", pathological T stage was: pT1a in 7 patients, pT1b in 1 patient, pT2a in 21 patients, pT2b in 8 patients, pT2d in 1 patient, pT3a in 8 patients, pT3b in 5 patients, pT4a in 1 patient and pT4b in 3 patients. Liver metastasis were present in 23 patients. Median follow-up period was 60 months (range 12–138 months).

Out of 32 patients without metastatic disease, 17 were males and 15 females; the median age was 64 years (range 29–84). Considering 23 patients with metastatic localization of primary UM, 11 were males and 12 females; median age was 72 (range 50–85). 13 of 23 patients died during the follow-up period for disease progression (Tables 1 and 2).

Comparing patients without metastasis and those with metastasis, no significant difference was seen in median age, location of the melanoma (choroid or choroid/ciliary body), tumor thickness, cell type, extrascleral extension, pathological pT stage; patients who developed metastasis had melanoma with greater median largest diameter (15.6 mm vs 11.9 mm, $p = 0.007$), and higher median ABCB5 expression (9 vs 3, $p = 0.030$); they had lower median disease free survival (25 months vs 81 months, $p < 0.001$). (Table 3)

Table 1. Demographics, tumor parameters, disease free time, follow-up and ABCB5 expression in primary uveal melanoma without metastasis ($n = 32$).

Sex	Age (Yrs)	Location	Thickness (mm)	Largest Diameter (mm)	Cell Type	Pathological T Stage	DFS (Months)	Follow-up (Months)	ABCB5 IS	ABCB5 ES	ABCB5 IRS	
F	29	Ch	14.2	16.2	mixed	pT2a	138	138	0	0	0	L
F	83	Ch/CB	14.84	16.8	mixed	pT2b	123	123	2	3	6	H
F	55	Ch	9.8	13.9	spindle	pT2a	122	122	1	3	3	L
F	30	Ch/CB	12.05	9.2	spindle	pT2b	122	122	0	0	0	L
M	74	Ch/CB	10.04	16.1	spindle	pT2b	121	121	2	3	6	H
M	64	Ch	7.7	11.5	spindle	pT1a	112	112	1	2	2	L
F	36	Ch	5.81	12.7	spindle	pT1a	109	109	2	3	2	L
F	59	Ch	8.4	16.7	mixed	pT2a	108	108	1	1	6	H
F	36	Ch	6.47	9.8	mixed	pT1a	108	108	1	1	1	L
M	84	Ch/CB	11.9	14.8	mixed	pT2b	106	106	2	2	4	L
F	67	Ch	10.42	13.02	mixed	pT3a	105	105	3	3	9	H
M	73	Ch	9.7	11.3	mixed	pT2a	102	102	0	0	0	L
F	45	Ch	13.7	10.2	mixed	pT2a	96	96	2	3	6	H
M	58	Ch	13.1	14.3	mixed	pT2a	96	96	2	3	6	H
M	63	Ch	3.3	11.7	spindle	pT2a	85	85	1	2	2	L
M	54	Ch	6.32	10	spindle	pT2a	83	83	3	3	9	H
M	84	Ch	11.7	17.4	mixed	pT3a	78	78	3	3	9	H
F	73	Ch	9.24	17.7	epith	pT2a	72	72	2	2	4	L
M	83	Ch	10.62	9.4	epith	pT3a	72	72	2	1	2	L
F	71	Ch	3.68	6.4	epith	pT1a	71	71	1	2	2	L
M	55	Ch/CB	7.5	8.9	epith	pT2b	61	61	0	0	0	L
M	52	Ch	9.2	12.1	spindle	pT2b	60	60	1	1	1	L
M	46	Ch	8.76	11.3	spindle	pT2a	54	54	3	3	9	H
F	76	Ch	8.02	10.7	mixed	pT1a	48	48	0	0	0	L
F	63	Ch	10.3	13.7	mixed	pT2a	42	42	0	2	6	H
F	41	Ch	5.85	10.3	mixed	pT1a	42	42	1	2	2	L
F	55	Ch	3.2	7.6	mixed	pT2a	42	42	0	0	0	L
F	74	Ch	8.6	10.2	mixed	pT4b	24	24	1	1	1	L
M	68	Ch/CB	10.1	10.1	epith	pT1b	24	24	2	3	6	H
M	74	Ch/CB	14.45	17.5	epith	pT4b	24	24	3	3	9	H
M	70	Ch/CB	16.27	20.8	spindle	pT4b	18	18	2	3	6	H
M	66	Ch	9.2	14.1	mixed	pT3a	12	12	0	0	0	L
							12	12	1	3	3	L
									2	3	6	H

Abbreviations: DFS, disease free survival; ABCB5, ATP-binding cassette sub-family B member 5; Ch, choroid; CB, ciliary body; epith, epithelioid.

Table 2. Demographics, tumor parameters, disease free time, follow-up and ABCB5 expression in primary uveal melanoma with metastasis (n = 23).

Sex	Age (Yrs)	Location	Thickness (mm)	Largest Diameter (mm)	Cell Type	Pathological T Stage	DFS (Months)	Follow-up (Months)	ABCB5 IS	ABCB5 ES	ABCB5 IRS	
F	58	Ch	6.04	17.8	mixed	pT2a	63	64 (†)	1	4	0	L
M	69	Ch	7.21	15.8	mixed	pT2a	54	81 (†)	0	0	0	L
F	75	Ch/CB	15.5	15.3	mixed	pT3b	44	62 (†)	2	2	6	H
F	50	Ch	7.36	15.6	epith	pT2a	41	81	3	3	9	H
M	62	Ch	13.68	16	mixed	pT3a	38	51 (†)	1	2	2	L
F	51	Ch/CB	11.4	18.5	mixed	pT3b	38	61	1	1	1	L
M	71	Ch	13.14	17.1	epith	pT3a	33	34 (†)	2	3	2	L
M	76	Ch/CB	11.6	6.5	mixed	pT1a	31	39	2	3	6	H
M	72	Ch	10.3	15.4	mixed	pT3b	27	35 (†)	1	2	2	L
F	85	Ch/CB	7.3	14.7	spindle	pT2d (EE)	26	49 (†)	1	2	2	L
M	73	Ch	5.73	11.7	epith	pT2a	26	42 (†)	3	3	9	H
F	51	Ch	9.42	19	mixed	pT3a	25	39	3	3	9	H
F	74	Ch	5.7	12.1	spindle	pT2a	24	37 (†)	3	3	9	H
F	67	Ch	3.49	20	mixed	pT4a	24	31 (†)	1	2	2	L
M	74	Ch	11.35	10.5	epith	pT3a	19	47	3	3	9	H
M	82	Ch	9.7	11	epith	pT2a	19	42	3	3	9	H
F	72	Ch	6.7	15.2	epith	pT2a	14	28 (†)	2	3	12	H
M	76	Ch	13.7	17.1	mixed	pT2a	14	70	3	3	9	H
M	79	Ch	13.91	16.1	epith	pT3b	13	38	1	2	2	L
F	66	Ch/CB	8.95	12.5	mixed	pT2b	12	37 (†)	3	4	12	H
F	60	Ch	8.25	16.5	epith	pT2a	11	37 (†)	3	3	9	H
F	57	Ch/CB	13.6	19	epith	pT2b	6	55	2	2	12	H
M	72	Ch/CB	13.3	15.4	mixed	pT3b	0	51	3	4	12	H

Abbreviations: DFS, disease free survival; ABCB5, ATP-binding cassette sub-family B member 5; Ch, choroid; CB, ciliary body; epith, epithelioid; EE, extrascleral extension; (†) death.

Table 3. Median (range) of demographics, tumour parameters, disease free time, follow-up, ABCB5 expression in primary uveal melanoma without and with systemic metastasis.

	Sex (m-f)	Age (yrs)	Location	Thickness	Largest diameter	Cell type	Extrascleral extension	Pathological T stage	DFS (months)	Follow-up (months)	ABCB5
All (n=55)	28-27	67 (29-85)	Ch 40 Ch/CB 15	9.7 (3.2-16.3)	14.1 (6.4-20.8)	Epith: 15 Spindle: 12 Mixed: 28	No: 54 Yes: 1	pT1a: 7 pT1b: 1 pT2a: 21 pT2b: 8 pT2d: 1 pT3a: 8 pT3b: 5 pT4a: 1 pT4b: 3	42 (0-138)	60 (8-138)	4 (0-12)
Metastasis free (n=32)	17-15	64 (29-84)	Ch 24 Ch/CB 8	9.5 (3.2-16.3)	11.9 (6.4-20.8)	Epith: 6 Spindle: 10 Mixed: 16	No: 32	pT1a: 6 pT1b: 1 pT2a: 12 pT2b: 6 pT3a: 4 pT4b: 3	81 (12-138)	81 (8-138)	3 (0-9)
Metastasis (n=23)	11-12	72 (50-85)	Ch 16 Ch/CB 7	9.7 (3.5-15.5)	15.6 (6.5-20)	Epith: 9 Spindle: 2 Mixed: 12	No: 22 Yes: 1	pT1a: 1 pT2a: 9 pT2b: 2 pT2d: 1 pT3a: 4 pT3b: 5 pT4a: 1	25 (0-63)	42 13 death (28-81)	9 (0-12)
p (metastasis free vs metastasis)	0.400*	0.400*	0.762°	0.911*	0.007*	0.400*	0.418°	0.560*	<0.001*	0.001*	0.030*

Abbreviations: DFS, disease free survival; ABCB5, ATP-binding cassette sub-family B member 5; Ch, choroid; CB, ciliary body; epith, epithelioid

- * Kolmogorov-Smirnov test
- ° Fisher's exact test

3.2. Correlations between ABCB5 Expression and Clinico-Pathological Factors in Uveal Melanomas

In the whole group (n = 55) the median ABCB5 value was 4. ABCB5 expression was high in 27 (49.1%) melanomas (Figure 2), and low in 28 (50.9%) melanomas (Figure 3).

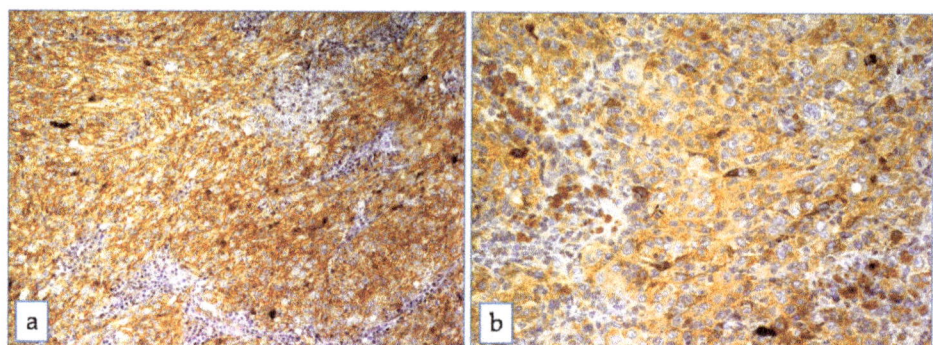

Figure 2. ABCB5 in uveal melanoma. Strong and diffuse cytoplasmic positivity in mixed cell type uveal melanoma at medium (**a**) and high magnification (**b**) (Immunoperoxidase stain; original magnification 100× (**a**) and 200× (**b**)).

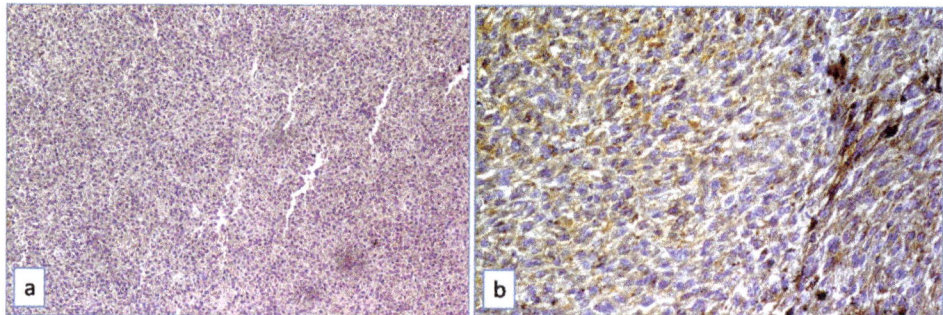

Figure 3. ABCB5 in uveal melanoma. Mild and heterogeneous cytoplasmic positivity in mixed cell type uveal melanoma at medium (**a**) and high magnification (**b**) (Immunoperoxidase stain; original magnification 100× (**a**) and 200× (**b**)).

In 32 primary uveal melanomas without metastasis, ABCB5 IS was strong/moderate in 14 cases (43.7%) and weak in 10 cases (31.3%). 8 cases (25%) were totally negative; ES was >50% in 14 cases (43.7%), variable between 5–30% in 10 cases (31.3%). Only 13/32 cases (40.6%) showed H-IRS, while the remaining 19 cases showed L-IRS (59.4%) (Fisher's exact test, p = 0.026, Table 4). In 23 primary uveal melanomas with metastasis, ABCB5 IS was strong/moderate in 15 cases (65.2%) and weak in 7 cases (30.5%). Only 1 case (4.3%) was completely negative. ES was >75% in 3 cases (13.1%), >50% in 11 cases (47.8%), 30–50% in 7 cases (30.5%), <30% in 1 case (4.3%); lack of expression of ABCB5 was observed in only 1 case (4.3%). 14/23 cases (60.9%) showed H-IRS, while only 9 cases (39.1%) had L-IRS (Fisher's exact test, p = 0.026, Table 4).

Table 4. Number of uveal melanoma (with and without metastasis) with low and high ABCB5.

	Metastasis (n=23)	Metastasis free (n=32)
Low	10 (43.5%) *	18 (56.3%)
High	13 (56.5%)	14 (43.8%)

Abbreviations: ABCB5, ATP-binding cassette sub-family B member 5. p (Fisher's exact test). * $p = 0.026$

Factors related to the presence of metastasis at univariate analysis on a Cox proportional hazards regression model were: age ($p = 0.053$), tumor greater diameter ($p = 0.009$), pT stage ($p = 0.016$), epithelioid cell type ($p = 0.011$) and ABCB5 expression ($p = 0.047$); at multivariate analysis tumor greater diameter ($p = 0.010$), ABCB5 expression ($p = 0.003$) and epithelioid cell type ($p = 0.026$) were significant.

No correlation was found between the histological type and ABCB5 expression (Spearman's rho $p = 0.334$).

Figure 4 shows the results of Kaplan-Meier survival analyses in patients with uveal melanomas with low and high ABCB5 expression. The estimated survival times free from metastasis (SE, with 95% CI) were respectively: 101.1 (10.0) (CI: 81.6 to 120.7) and 64.4(10.5) (CI: 43.9 to 85.0).

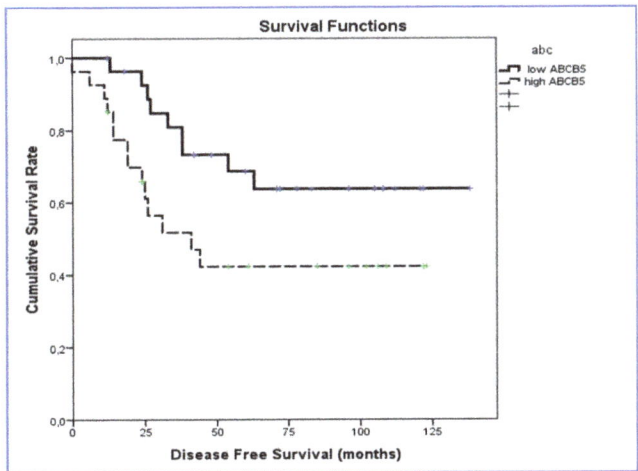

Figure 4. Kaplan–Meier survival analyses in patients with uveal melanomas with low and high ABCB5 expression. The log-rank test showed a significant difference ($p = 0.039$) between the two groups in ABCB5 expression.

The log-rank test showed a significant difference ($p = 0.039$) between the two groups in ABCB5 expression.

4. Discussion

UM is a rare neoplasm with an "indolent" but slowly progressive biological behavior, characterized by the onset of liver metastasis within 10–15 years after diagnosis in about 50% of patients and a high rate of mortality [8]. Although in the last years several improvements have been recorded in the conservative management of UM with the aim of preserving the visual function [20], recurrence of disease and metastasis are still frequent events in the natural history of this neoplasm. Therefore, the study of molecular alterations in UM is currently of great scientific interest aiming at identifying possible biological factors capable of predicting a more aggressive biological behavior of the disease.

Histopathological factor of poor prognosis such as epithelioid cell type, tumor size, mitotic index, tumor infiltrating lymphocytes (TILs), extrascleral invasion, vascular pattern and necrosis, and clinical risk factor (male sex and older age of the patient) are not very accurate in identifying a high-risk prognostic category of patients.

Cytogenetic studies demonstrated that patients with disomy 3 have a lower risk of developing metastasis; instead, the loss of heterozygosis of chromosome 3 was associated with a high rate of metastatic disease and poorer prognosis in UM: in particular, Prescher et al. [21] evaluated 30 patients with UM in association with monosomy 3 and 24 patients with disomy 3, and reported that 50% of patients with monosomy 3 showed metastasis within 3 years, whereas no metastatic disease was noted in those with disomy 3. In recent years, inactivating mutations of BRCA1 associated protein-1 (BAP-1), confirmed by lower nuclear immunohistochemical expression, have been found and reported in literature as poor prognostic factors [22,23]; moreover, high levels of expression of nestin, a member of the intermediate filament protein family, seem to correlate with metastatic progression and reduced survival rate in UM [24]. We previously evaluated the expression of ADAM10, RKIP and pRKIP [19,25], demonstrating their role as negative prognostic markers: in particular, regarding ADAM10 expression, high levels were found in 11/13 patients with metastatic UM and in only 15/39 patients without metastasis, and the difference was statistically significant [19].

As previously said, ABCB5 is a marker of cancer stem cells and is implicated in the tumorigenesis and tumor growth of several neoplasms, such as cutaneous melanoma, breast cancer and hepatocellular carcinoma [9–16]. Particularly, Wang et al. [17] found that in vitro ABCB5-negative melanoma cell sub-population displayed a reduction in cell migration and invasion compared to the ABCB5-positive one; this finding was also confirmed at the transwell assays: lentivirus-mediated knockdown of ABCB5 in two different melanoma cell cultures induced a decline of cell migration and invasion. NF-kB signaling pathway has been discovered to be involved in this process: ABCB5 activates the NF-kB pathway by inhibiting p65 ubiquitination to enhance p65 protein stability, resulting in an accumulation of p65 in ABCB5-positive MMICs [17]. Among the traditional NF-kB targeting genes, MMP9 is involved in tumor cells invasion and metastasis [26]: an overexpression of MMP9, induced by ABCB5, seems to be one of the most important steps in the stimulation of metastatic potential of cutaneous melanoma [17]. In this paper, we first tested ABCB5 as prognostic factor in UM and observed that higher immunohistochemical levels of ABCB5 correlated to higher risk of metastasis. In our study, the median value of ABCB5 was 4 (moderate staining in more than 75% of neoplastic cells, or severe staining in more than 50% of neoplastic cells). Higher risk of metastasis was observed in UMs with higher expression of ABCB5 and lower metastatic risk in UMs with lower expression of the antibody. According to Kaplan-Meier survival analyses, lower survival times free from metastasis were seen in patients with UM and high expression of ABCB5.

In conclusion, we suggest using ABCB5 as an easily detectable prognostic marker in primary UMs and advocate its use as a predictor of the risk of liver metastasis and as guide for monitoring and treatment. In fact, ABCB5 levels expressed in UM biopsies could be a useful guide towards better treatment between enucleation and more conservative method.

The weakness of the present study was to evaluate only the morphological evidence based on immunohistochemistry, to investigate the expression of ABCB5 as a potential prognostic factor in uveal melanoma. Further studies are needed to confirm our morphological data with other relevant and sensitive techniques, such as quantitative RT-PCR, ELISA (or similar), and/or western blot.

Author Contributions: Conceptualization, G.B. and R.C.; Data curation, A.R., M.R. and A.L.; Investigation, M.R.; Methodology, G.M., L.P. and R.C.; Software, G.M.; Writing—original draft, G.B.; Writing—review& editing, G.B. and R.C.

Funding: This research received no external funding.

Conflicts of Interest: The authors declare no conflict of interest.

References

1. Mahendraraj, K.; Lau, C.S.; Lee, I.; Chamberlain, R.S. Trends in incidence, survival, and management of uveal melanoma: A population-based study of 7516 patients from the surveillance, epidemiology, and end results database (1973–2012). *Clin. Ophthalmol.* **2016**, *10*, 2113–2119. [CrossRef] [PubMed]
2. Pukrushpan, P.; Tulvatana, W.; Pittayapongpat, R. Congenital uveal malignant melanoma. *J. Am. Assoc. Pediatr. Ophthalmol. Strabismus* **2014**, *18*, 199–201. [CrossRef] [PubMed]
3. Gray, M.E.; Shaikh, A.H.; Corrêa, Z.M.; Augsburger, J.J. Primary uveal melanoma in a 4-year-old black child. *J. Am. Assoc. Pediatr. Ophthalmol. Strabismus* **2013**, *17*, 551–553. [CrossRef] [PubMed]
4. Krantz, B.A.; Dave, N.; Komatsubara, K.M.; Marr, B.P.; Carvajal, R.D. Uveal melanoma: Epidemiology, etiology, and treatment of primary disease. *Clin. Ophthalmol.* **2017**, *11*, 279–289. [CrossRef] [PubMed]
5. Eskelin, S.; Kivelä, T. Mode of presentation and time to treatment of uveal melanoma in Finland. *Br. J. Ophthalmol.* **2002**, *86*, 333–338. [CrossRef] [PubMed]
6. Griewank, K.G.; van de Nes, J.; Schilling, B.; Moll, I.; Sucker, A.; Kakavand, H.; Haydu, L.E.; Asher, M.; Zimmer, L.; Hillen, U.; et al. Genetic and clinico-pathologic analysis of metastatic uveal melanoma. *Mod. Pathol.* **2014**, *27*, 175–183. [CrossRef]
7. Jovanovic, P.; Mihajlovic, M.; Djordjevic-Jocic, J.; Vlajkovic, S.; Cekic, S.; Stefanovic, V. Ocular melanoma: An overview of the current status. *Int. J. Clin. Exp. Pathol.* **2013**, *6*, 1230–1244.
8. Chattopadhyay, C.; Kim, D.W.; Gombos, D.S.; Oba, J.; Qin, Y.; Williams, M.D.; Esmaeli, B.; Grimm, E.A.; Wargo, J.A.; Woodman, S.E.; et al. Uveal melanoma: From diagnosis to treatment and the science in between. *Cancer* **2016**, *122*, 2299–2312. [CrossRef]
9. Frank, N.Y.; Margaryan, A.; Huang, Y.; Schatton, T.; Waaga-Gasser, A.M.; Gasser, M.; Sayegh, M.H.; Sadee, W.; Frank, M.H. ABCB5-mediated doxorubicin transport chemoresistance in human malignant melanoma. *Cancer Res.* **2005**, *65*, 4320–4333. [CrossRef]
10. Cheung, S.T.; Cheung, P.F.; Cheng, C.K.; Wong, N.C.; Fan, S.T. Granulin-epithelin precursor and ATP-dependent binding cassette (ABC)B5 regulate liver cancer cell chemoresistance. *Gastroenterology* **2011**, *140*, 344–355. [CrossRef]
11. Wilson, B.J.; Schatton, T.; Zhan, Q.; Gasser, M.; Ma, J.; Saab, K.R.; Schanche, R.; Waaga-Gasser, A.M.; Gold, J.S.; Huang, Q.; et al. ABCB5 identifies a therapy-refractory tumor cell population in colorectal cancer patients. *Cancer Res.* **2011**, *71*, 5307–5316. [CrossRef]
12. Kleffel, S.; Lee, N.; Lezcano, C.; Wilson, B.J.; Sobolewski, K.; Saab, K.R.; Mueller, H.; Zhan, Q.; Posch, C.; Elco, C.P.; et al. ABCB5-targeted chemoresistance reversal inhibits merkel cell carcinoma growth. *J. Invest Dermatol.* **2016**, *136*, 838–846. [CrossRef]
13. Wilson, B.J.; Saab, K.R.; Ma, J.; Schatton, T.; Pütz, P.; Zhan, Q.; Murphy, G.F.; Gasser, M.; Waaga-Gasser, A.M.; Frank, N.Y.; et al. ABCB5 maintains melanoma-initiating cells through a proinflammatory cytokine signaling circuit. *Cancer Res.* **2014**, *74*, 4196–4207. [CrossRef] [PubMed]
14. Cheung, P.F.; Cheung, T.T.; Yip, C.W.; Ng, L.W.; Fung, S.W.; Lo, C.M.; Fan, S.T.; Cheung, S.T. Hepatic cancer stem cell marker granulin-epithelin precursor and β-catenin expression associate with recurrence in hepatocellular carcinoma. *Oncotarget* **2016**, *7*, 21644–21657. [CrossRef]
15. Yao, J.; Yao, X.; Tian, T.; Fu, X.; Wang, W.; Li, S.; Shi, T.; Suo, A.; Ruan, Z.; Guo, H.; et al. ABCB5-ZEB1 axis promotes invasion and metastasis in breast cancer cells. *Oncol. Res.* **2017**, *25*, 305–316. [CrossRef]
16. Guo, Q.; Grimmig, T.; Gonzalez, G.; Giobbie-Hurder, A.; Berg, G.; Carr, N.; Wilson, B.J.; Banerjee, P.; Ma, J.; Gold, J.S.; et al. ATP-binding cassette member B5 (ABCB5) promotes tumor cell invasiveness in human colorectal cancer. *J. Biol. Chem.* **2018**, *293*, 11166–11178. [CrossRef]
17. Wang, S.; Tang, L.; Lin, J.; Shen, Z.; Yao, Y.; Wang, W.; Tao, S.; Gu, C.; Ma, J.; Xie, Y.; et al. ABCB5 promotes melanoma metastasis through enhancing NF-κB p65 protein stability. *Biochem. Biophys. Res. Commun.* **2017**, *492*, 18–26. [CrossRef] [PubMed]
18. Leonardi, R.; Loreto, C.; Talic, N.; Caltabiano, R.; Musumeci, G. Immunolocalization of lubricin in the rat periodontal ligament during experimental tooth movement. *Acta Histochem.* **2012**, *114*, 700–704. [CrossRef] [PubMed]
19. Caltabiano, R.; Puzzo, L.; Barresi, V.; Ieni, A.; Loreto, C.; Musumeci, G.; Castrogiovanni, P.; Ragusa, M.; Foti, P.; Russo, A.; et al. ADAM 10 expression in primaryuveal melanoma asprognostic factor for risk of metastasis. *Pathol. Res. Pract.* **2016**, *212*, 980–987. [CrossRef]

20. Pereira, P.R.; Odashiro, A.N.; Lim, L.A.; Miyamoto, C.; Blanco, P.L.; Odashiro, M.; Maloney, S.; de Souza, D.F.; Burnier, M.N., Jr. Current and emerging treatment options for uveal melanoma. *Clin. Ophthalmol.* **2013**, *7*, 1669–1682. [CrossRef] [PubMed]
21. Prescher, G.; Bornfeld, N.; Hirche, H.; Horsthemke, B.; Jöckel, K.H.; Becher, R. Prognostic implications of monosomy 3 in uveal melanoma. *Lancet* **1996**, *347*, 1222–1225. [PubMed]
22. Harbour, J.W.; Onken, M.D.; Roberson, E.D.; Duan, S.; Cao, L.; Worley, L.A.; Council, M.L.; Matatall, K.A.; Helms, C.; Bowcock, A.M. Frequent mutation of BAP1 in metastasizing uveal melanomas. *Science* **2010**, *330*, 1410–1413. [CrossRef] [PubMed]
23. Szalai, E.; Wells, J.R.; Ward, L.; Grossniklaus, H.E. Uveal melanoma nuclear BRCA1-associated protein-1 immunoreactivity is an indicator of metastasis. *Ophthalmology* **2018**, *125*, 203–209. [CrossRef]
24. Djirackor, L.; Shakir, D.; Kalirai, H.; Petrovski, G.; Coupland, S.E. Nestin expression in primary and metastatic uveal melanoma—Possible biomarker for high risk uveal melanoma. *Acta Ophthalmol.* **2018**, *96*, 503–509. [CrossRef] [PubMed]
25. Caltabiano, R.; Puzzo, L.; Barresi, V.; Cardile, V.; Loreto, C.; Ragusa, M.; Russo, A.; Reibaldi, M.; Longo, A. Expression of raf kinase inhibitor protein (RKIP) is a predictor of uveal melanoma metastasis. *Histol. Histopathol.* **2014**, *29*, 1325–1334. [PubMed]
26. Kessenbrock, K.; Plaks, V.; Werb, Z. Matrix metalloproteinases: Regulators of the tumor microenvironment. *Cell* **2010**, *141*, 52–67. [CrossRef] [PubMed]

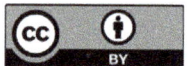

© 2019 by the authors. Licensee MDPI, Basel, Switzerland. This article is an open access article distributed under the terms and conditions of the Creative Commons Attribution (CC BY) license (http://creativecommons.org/licenses/by/4.0/).

 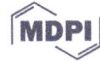

Article

Adapted Moderate Training Exercise Decreases the Expression of Ngal in the Rat Kidney: An Immunohistochemical Study

Michelino Di Rosa [1,†], Paola Castrogiovanni [1,†], Francesca Maria Trovato [2], Lorenzo Malatino [2], Silvia Ravalli [1], Rosa Imbesi [1], Marta Anna Szychlinska [1,‡] and Giuseppe Musumeci [1,*,‡]

1. Department of Biomedical and Biotechnological Sciences, Human Anatomy and Histology Section, School of Medicine, University of Catania, 95100 Catania, Italy; mdirosa@unict.it (M.D.R.); pacastro@unict.it (P.C.); silviaravalli@gmail.com (S.R.); roimbesi@unict.it (R.I.); marta.sz@hotmail.it (M.A.S.)
2. Department of Clinical and Experimental Medicine, School of Medicine, University of Catania, 95100 Catania, Italy; trovatofrancesca@gmail.com (F.M.T.); Malatino@unict.it (L.M.)
* Correspondence: g.musumeci@unict.it; Tel.: +39-095-3782043
† co-first authorship.
‡ co-last authorship.

Received: 1 February 2019; Accepted: 8 March 2019; Published: 13 March 2019

Abstract: Neutrophil gelatinase-associated lipocalin (NGAL) is a biomarker of several injuries and is upregulated in inflammatory conditions. Vitamin D was shown to have anti-inflammatory effects and to increase after physical activity. This work aimed to assess, through immunohistochemistry, the effects of an adapted moderate training exercise (AMTE) on the expression of NGAL and vitamin D receptor (VDR) in the kidney and heart of rats. Sixteen rats were distributed into two groups: the sedentary control group and the experimental group, subjected to AMTE on the treadmill for 12 weeks. The results showed the basal expression of NGAL and VDR in both the heart and the kidney in sedentary rats; no differences in the expression of both NGAL and VDR in the heart; and a decreased NGAL and an increased VDR expression in the kidney of rats subjected to AMTE. These results suggest a possible protective role of AMTE on NGAL-associated injuries in the kidney, probably through the vitamin D signaling pathway. Our results represent an interesting preliminary data that may open new horizons in the management of NGAL-associated kidney injuries. However, further studies are needed to confirm these results and to comprehend the specific interaction between NGAL and VDR pathways in the kidney.

Keywords: training exercise; NGAL; VDR; kidney; heart; immunohistochemistry

1. Introduction

The adapted moderate training exercise (AMTE), corresponding to the adapted nonexhaustive aerobic physical activity is an exciting approach, is increasingly considered by the scientific community to prevent metabolic disabling diseases and increase physical well-being. Data from the literature show that moderate physical activity can reduce inflammation and improve general physical function in humans [1–9] and animals [10,11]. In a rat model, aerobic interval exercise protocol was shown to prevent the development of diabetic nephropathy and to affect the metabolism of certain minerals [12]. Moreover, aerobic training in association with L-arginine supplementation also demonstrated to ameliorate kidney and liver damage in myocardial infarction rats, via antioxidant mechanisms [13]. The expression of many cytokines and adipokines associated with metabolic syndrome has also been investigated in obese women, after aerobic training protocol, with positive results [14]. In recent literature, authors described that AMTE has beneficial effects on the preservation of articular cartilage and muscle tissues, confirming its protective role on the musculoskeletal system as well [15–18].

Neutrophil gelatinase-associated lipocalin (NGAL) is a small protein of the lipocalin superfamily, also known as lipocalin-2 [19]. It is physiologically and basally present at low levels in many tissues including heart, kidney, liver, uterus, bone marrow, lung, adipose tissue, and macrophages [20–22]. Its upregulation follows the activation of the NF-kB pathway [23]. NGAL was shown to play a pivotal role as a modulator of the innate immune system in inflammation [24–26]. Of note, the complex NGAL-MMP-9 extends the proteolytic activity of the latter by inhibiting its degradation [27], which leads to several pathophysiological conditions [28]. In human diseases, several studies have shown that NGAL increases significantly and rapidly in case of renal cell damage, suggesting that NGAL is a biomarker of various forms of kidney injuries [29,30]. NGAL upregulation could also be a biomarker in patients who suffer from heart failure [31] or in those who undergo cardiac surgery [32]. NGAL is upregulated in several other inflammatory states, like chronic obstructive pulmonary disorder and bowel inflammatory condition [33]. Strenuous exercise, causing oxidative stress and reactive oxygen species (ROSs) production, can induce changes in NGAL concentration as well [34–36]. Bongers et al. reported that prolonged endurance exercise in healthy adults could induce an increase in NGAL urinary concentration [34]. Increased NGAL urinary levels have also been found in endurance cycling athletes [35]. These findings were validated by Lippi et al., who demonstrated increased acute expression of serum NGAL in long distance running athletes (strenuous exercise) [36]. The expression of NGAL has also been investigated in physically active individuals, after short-term maximal exercise, but no differences in its expression have been reported [37,38]. However, the expression of NGAL in association with an AMTE protocol has never been investigated.

Another, recently emerging important compound positively associated with physical activity is represented by vitamin D. It is a fat-soluble molecule able to exert antioxidant functions, responsible for the body's mineral homeostasis. This vitamin can be taken exogenously with food or endogenously produced by the skin during the exposure to sunlight. After synthesis, vitamin D is inactive. The liver operates the conversion from the inactive form to 25-hydroxyvitamin D or calcidiol by hydroxylation at carbon 25. The latter is then collected in the adipose tissue as a reserve. To become active, 25-hydroxyvitamin D needs the participation of kidneys and 1-hydroxylase enzyme to be converted into 1,25-dihydroxyvitamin D, known as calcitriol [39]. The body cells respond to vitamin D in its active form through its receptor called vitamin D receptor (VDR) [40]. Vitamin D can regulate important mechanisms of immunity and inflammation and to modulate cardiovascular and musculoskeletal systems [41]. Indeed, it was shown that calcitriol suppresses NF-κB activity in a VDR-dependent manner. VDR binds IKKβ, and this interaction is enhanced by calcitriol. Thus, VDR overexpression downregulates IKKβ-induced NF-κB activity [42]. Its deficiency represents a risk factor for the onset of metabolic syndrome, but it also determines an increase in oxidative stress. Several studies indicate that physical activity promotes an increase in vitamin D level, despite sun exposure [43–46]. Indeed, it has been evidenced that the vitamin D receptor (VDR) increases during exercise [47,48]. These findings would suggest that physical activity exerts its positive effects also through the vitamin D pathway. Summing up, (i) physical activity is shown to increase the circulating levels of vitamin D [43–46]; (ii) vitamin D is also shown to exert its anti-inflammatory effects through the NKκB inhibition [49]; and (iii) NGAL is shown to be upregulated by induction of the NF-kB pathway [50,51]. The question remains: Does AMTE have any effect on NGAL expression? If so, does the VDR expression change as well? The goal of the present research was to answer these questions and to evaluate the expression of NGAL and VDR in kidneys and hearts of rats subjected to AMTE for 12 weeks.

2. Materials and Methods

2.1. Breeding and Housing of Animals

Sixteen 3-month-old healthy male Wistar Outbred Rats (Charles River Laboratories, Milan, Italy) with an average body weight of 300 ± 20 g were housed in polycarbonate cages (cage dimensions: 10.25″ W × 18.75″ D × 8″ H) at controlled temperature (20–23 °C) and humidity during the entire experimentation at the "Center for Advanced Preclinical In Vivo Research (CAPIR)". The animals had free access to food and water and lived a photoperiod of 12 h light/dark. The day after the last training (the experiment lasted 12 weeks), the rats were sacrificed by an intravenous lethal injection of anesthetic overdose using a mixture of Zoletil 100 (Virbac, Milan, Italy) at a dose of 80 mg/kg and DEXDOMITOR (Virbac, Milan, Italy) at a dose of 50 mg/kg. After the sacrifice, kidney and heart were explanted and histological and immunohistochemical analyses were performed. All procedures conformed to the guidelines of the Institutional Animal Care and Use Committee (I.A.C.U.C.) of the University of Catania (Protocol n. 2112015-PR of the 14.01.2015, Italian Ministry of Health). The experiments were performed accordingly with the European Community Council Directive (86/609/EEC) and the Italian Animal Protection Law (116/1992).

2.2. Experimental Design

Sixteen 3-month-old healthy male Wistar Rats were randomly divided into two groups, with 8 rats per group:

- Group 1: sedentary rats.
- Group 2: rats undergoing AMTE on treadmill.

Group 2 rats performed moderate exercise on the treadmill (2Biological instrument, Varese, Italy), for 12 weeks, five days a week, for 20/30 min daily. The treadmill was set with an inclination of 2° (between 2 and 6 degrees) and speed of 10/30 m/minute (type of exercise: interval training, between mild and moderate intensity). Physical activity was executed by the method previously described [52,53]. Briefly, a minimal electric shock (0.2 mA) forced the rat to walk on the treadmill. The shock serves to stimulate the rat to walk and to instruct it. Usually, the rat learns this activity in the first 2 min of the exercise. This type of exercise is used to stimulate the muscles, joints, and bones in the work of flexion–extension of the limbs. During the exercise, the possible suffering of the animals was evaluated. The rats that exceeded five electric shocks (0.2 mA) without learning the work to be done on the treadmill, have been discarded from the experiment. On the day following the last training (after 12 weeks of the experiment) the animals were humanely sacrificed by a lethal intravenous injection of anesthetic overdose, and kidney/heart samples were explanted and fixed for the histological and immunohistochemical analysis.

2.3. Histology

Kidney and heart samples were fixed in 10% neutral buffered formalin (Bio-Optica, Milan, Italy). Embedding in paraffin followed overnight washing, as previously described [54]. The samples were placed in the cassettes after wax infiltration. A rotary manual microtome (Leica RM2235, Milan, Italy) was used to cut the paraffin blocks into tissue samples (4–5 μm) which were then mounted on silane-coated slides (Menzel-Gläser, Braunschweig, Germany) and stored at room temperature. Histological analysis and examination of structural alterations were possible by dewaxing the sections in xylene, hydrating them by graded ethanol, and then staining with hematoxylin and eosin.

A Zeiss Axioplan light microscope (Carl Zeiss, Oberkochen, Germany) and a digital camera (AxioCam MRc5, Carl Zeiss, Oberkochen, Germany) were used to examine slides.

2.4. Immunohistochemistry

Kidney and heart samples were processed for immunohistochemical evaluation as formerly discussed [55]. Thoroughly, the slides were dewaxed in xylene, hydrated by graded ethanol, incubated for 30 min in 0.3% hydroperoxyl (H_2O_2)/methanol to block endogenous peroxidase activity, and then rinsed in phosphate-buffered saline (PBS; Bio-Optica, Milan, Italy) for 20 min. The antigenic sites were unmasked by storing the slides in capped polypropylene slide holders with citrate buffer (10 mM citric acid, 0.05% Tween 20, pH 6.0; Bio-Optica, Milan, Italy) and heated for 5 min for three times inside a microwave oven (750 W, LG Electronics Italia S.p.A., Milan, Italy). Nonspecific binding of the antibodies was prevented by the applying of a blocking buffer with 5% bovine serum albumin (BSA, Sigma, Milan, Italy) in PBS for one h in a moist chamber, and then the primary antibodies were applied. The sections of tissue were then incubated overnight at 4 °C with the following antibodies; rat monoclonal anti-vitamin D receptor (ab115495; Abcam, Cambridge, UK) diluted 1/100 in PBS (Bio-Optica, Milan, Italy) and rabbit monoclonal anti-NGAL [EPR5084] (ab125075; Abcam, Cambridge, UK), diluted 1/100 in PBS (Bio-Optica, Milan, Italy). The slides were then covered with a biotinylated antibody (horseradish peroxidase (HRP)-conjugated anti-rat and anti-rabbit were used as secondary antibodies), and the peroxidase-labeled streptavidin allowed the detection of the immune complexes (labeled streptavidin-biotin (LSAB) + System-HRP, K0690, Dako, Glostrup, Denmark), after incubation for 10 min at room temperature. The immunoreaction was perceived by incubating the sections for 2 min in a 0.1% 3,3′-diaminobenzidine, 0.02% hydrogen peroxide solution (DAB substrate Chromogen System; Dako, Denmark). The slides were mildly counterstained with Mayer's Hematoxylin (Histolab Products AB, Goteborg, Sweden) and mounted in GVA mount (Zymed, Laboratories Inc., San Francisco, CA, USA).

2.5. Computerised Densitometric Measurements and Image Analysis

Image analysis software (AxioVision Release 4.8.2-SP2 Software, Carl Zeiss Microscopy GmbH, Jena, Germany) was used to quantify the grade of staining of positive anti-vitamin D receptor and anti-NGAL antibodies immunolabeling. It also calculated the densitometric count (Log2 densitometric count-pixel2) of the immunostained area in seven fields, the area of which was about 150,000 μm^2, randomly selected from slides. Digital micrographs were taken using the Zeiss Axioplan light microscope (Carl Zeiss, Oberkochen, Germany), using a lens with a magnification of ×20, i.e., total magnification 200) fitted with a digital camera (AxioCam MRc5, Carl Zeiss, Oberkochen, Germany). Evaluations were performed by three blinded investigators (two anatomical morphologists and one histologist). The values were accepted as correct if they did not show statistically significant difference [56]. Every single interpretation of the results was discussed in favor of a standard agreement, in case of disputes [53].

2.6. Statistical Analysis

GraphPad Instat® Biostatistics version 3.0 software (GraphPad Software, Inc., La Jolla, CA, USA) and IBM SPSS Statistics (version 20, IBM Corporation, Somers, Armonk, NY, USA) were used as instruments of statistical evaluations. An unpaired *t*-test was used to compare two groups. *p*-values of less than 0.05 were considered statistically significant (* $p < 0.05$; ** $p < 0.01$; *** $p < 0.001$; **** $p < 0.0001$ and ns not significant) as previously described [57]. The data were presented as the mean ± SD.

3. Results

3.1. Histology

Hematoxylin & eosin staining made possible to inspect morphological alterations in the kidney and heart tissue of the experimental groups. No damages in the histological structure of kidney and heart tissue were appreciated (data not shown).

3.2. Immunohistochemistry (IHC) Observations and Statistical Analysis

3.2.1. NGAL-Kidney

NGAL immunostaining was mainly detected in the cytoplasm of cells in the medulla of kidney samples of both Groups, 1 and 2, involving collecting ducts and loops of Henle (Figure 1A,C). In the cortex, the NGAL immunostaining was found at the different degree in groups, involving both distal and proximal convoluted tubules; glomeruli were rarely and slightly immunostained (Figure 1B,D). The intensity of NGAL immunostaining (Log2 densitometric count-pixel2) was lower in Group 2

(16.60 ± 1.71) when compared to sedentary control group (Group 1) (17.87 ± 0.59) (*p* = 0.0028), as reported in graph (Figure 1E).

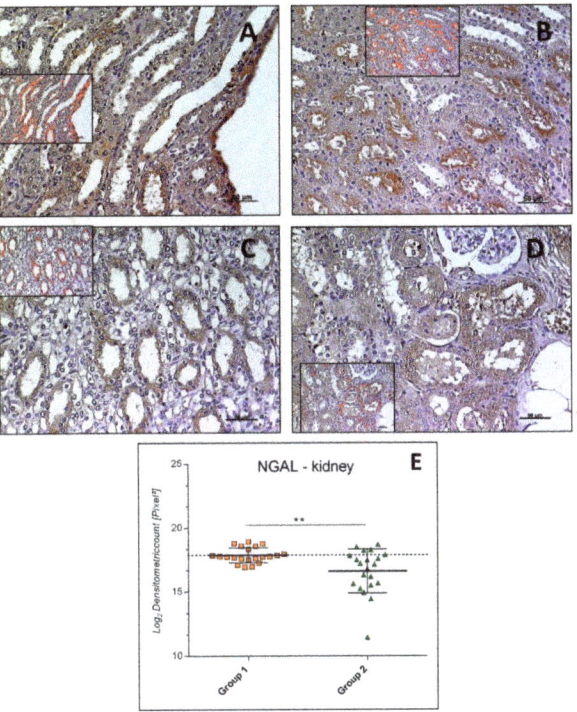

Figure 1. Kidney neutrophil gelatinase-associated lipocalin (NGAL) immunohistochemistry in Group 1 (**A**,**B**) and in Group 2 (**C**,**D**). NGAL immunostaining in kidney tissue and image analysis by software in which the red color indicates the immunolabeling (inserts). NGAL immunostaining was mainly detected in the medulla of kidney samples (**A**,**C**) and in the cortex where it was at a different degree in groups (**B**,**D**); glomeruli were rarely and slightly immunostained. (**E**) Graph showing the intensity of NGAL immunostaining (Log$_2$ Densitometric count pixel^2) with statistical analysis. For details, see the text. (**A**–**D**): scale bars: 50 µm. The data are presented as mean ± SD.

3.2.2. VDR-Kidney

VDR immunostaining was highlighted both in cytoplasm and nucleus of cells in kidney samples of both Groups, 1 and 2. It had different expression levels in the collecting ducts and loops of Henle of the medulla (Figure 2A,C) and the distal and proximal convoluted tubules of the cortex (Figure 2B,D) about different groups. Glomeruli were rarely VDR immunostained. The intensity of VDR immunostaining (Log2 densitometric count-pixel2) was much higher in Group 2 (18.15 ± 0.71) when compared to Group 1 (15.11 ± 2.09) ($p < 0.0001$), as reported in the graph (Figure 2E).

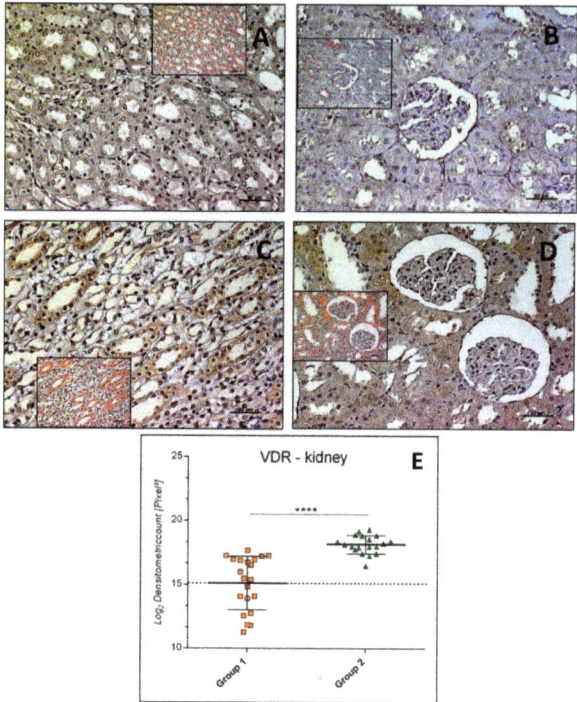

Figure 2. Kidney vitamin D receptor (VDR) immunohistochemistry in Group 1 (**A,B**) and in Group 2 (**C,D**). VDR immunostaining in kidney tissue and image analysis by software in which the red color indicates the immunolabeling (inserts). VDR immunostaining had different expression levels in the medulla (**A,C**) and in the cortex (**B,D**) in groups; glomeruli were rarely VDR immunostained. (**E**) Graph showing the intensity of VDR immunostaining (Log_2 Densitometric count pixel^2) with statistical analysis. For details, see the text. (**A–D**): scale bars: 50 µm. The data are presented as mean ± SD.

3.2.3. NGAL-Heart

NGAL immunostaining was mainly detected in the cardiomyocytes cytoplasm of both Groups, 1 and 2 (Figure 3A,B). The intensity of NGAL immunostaining (Log2 densitometric count-pixel2) was almost equal in Group 2 (19.56 ± 0.79) if compared to Group 1 (sedentary) (19.48 ± 0.89), and the difference between means was not significant (p = 0.7655, ns), as reported in the graph (Figure 3C).

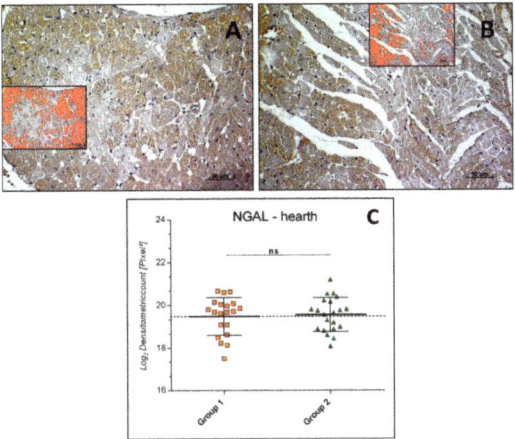

Figure 3. Heart NGAL immunohistochemistry in Group 1 (**A**) and Group 2 (**B**). NGAL immunostaining in heart tissue and image analysis by software in which the red color indicates the immunolabeling (inserts). NGAL immunostaining detected in the cytoplasm of cardiomyocytes, at similar levels of expression in the groups. (**C**) Graph showing the intensity of NGAL immunostaining (Log_2 Densitometric count pixel^2) with statistical analysis. For details, see the text. (**A**,**B**): scale bars: 50 μm. The data are presented as mean ± SD.

3.2.4. VDR-Heart

In heart samples, VDR immunostaining was detected mainly in the cytoplasm of cardiomyocytes of both Groups 1 and 2 (Figure 4A,B), and rarely in nuclei. The intensity of VDR immunostaining (Log_2 densitometric count-pixel2) was similar both in Group 2 (19.11 ± 0.79) and Group 1 (sedentary) (18.81 ± 0.67) and the difference between means was not significant ($p = 0.1847$, ns), as reported in the graph (Figure 4C).

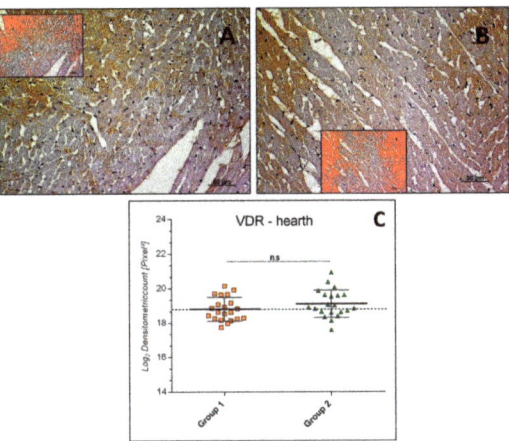

Figure 4. Heart VDR immunohistochemistry in Group 1 (**A**) and in Group 2 (**B**). VDR immunostaining in heart tissue and image analysis by software in which the red color indicates the immunolabeling (inserts). VDR immunostaining was found to have similar degrees of expression in the groups, mainly in the cardiomyocytes cytoplasm and rarely in nuclei. (**C**) Graph showing the intensity of VDR immunostaining (Log_2 Densitometric count pixel^2) with statistical analysis. For details, see the text. (**A**,**B**): scale bars: 50 μm. The data are presented as mean ± SD.

4. Discussion

The presented research aimed to assess if AMTE may exert a protective role on body homeostasis, through vitamin D and NGAL pathways. Our results, as expected, showed the augmented expression of VDR in kidneys of rats subjected to AMTE, in comparison to the sedentary controls. These results may hint an increased release of vitamin D in the circulation after physical activity, confirming findings from literature [43–46]. Makanae et al. demonstrated that indeed intramuscular VDR expression could be effectively promoted by physical activity [47]. Another work suggests that rats performing swimming activity experienced increases in vitamin D level in the serum and, consequently, a greater expression of its receptors in the pancreas, adipose tissue, and muscle [48]. In the present study, the authors did not evaluate the circulating levels of vitamin D in the serum of rats undergoing AMTE protocol; this represents a limitation of the study. Nevertheless, curiously, in our results, the expression of VDR in the heart of active rats did not change significantly when compared to the sedentary controls. A reason for that could be hypothesized by the fact that the circulating vitamin D is converted in its active form in the kidney and, then, determines the increased local expression of its receptor at this level, but does not determine its increase in other organs. Nevertheless, further long-term studies should be done to clarify this aspect. Vitamin D was shown to inhibit the NF-kB pathway [24,25]. Thus, since the promoter region of NGAL contains a consensus-binding site for NF-κB [58,59] and VDR was shown to inhibit the activation of NF-κB, it is conceivable that increased levels of circulating vitamin D indirectly inhibit the NGAL expression (Figure 5). In our work, we observed the basal expression of NGAL both in hearts and kidneys of sedentary rats, suggesting that sedentary lifestyle may represent a condition in which it is easier to develop NGAL-involved pathophysiological states. We also assisted to a significant reduction in the detection of NGAL in kidneys inactive rats, as expected, but curiously, not in their hearts. These data suggest that, regarding the crosslink between VDR and NGAL pathways, AMTE did not have any effects on heart tissue, but only on the kidney one. Moreover, a significant and inversely proportional expression of both proteins in kidneys, but not in hearts, of active rats, when compared to the sedentary controls, further confirms the involvement of VDR in the NGAL downregulation. This reasonably happened through the NF-κB inhibition. However, these preliminary findings certainly need further studies to confirm the crosslink between these two pathways. Albeit above reported scientific data highlight that physical activity may increase NGAL levels, they refer to strenuous anaerobic exercise. In our experimental design, we preferred to use AMTE, since this type of exercise is more inclined to induce an adaptive response by the body and our results were different from those reported concerning the strenuous anaerobic exercise. These findings have intriguing clinical implications related to physical activity in humans, emphasizing the beneficial effects of AMTE, but not strenuous exercise, particularly in obese people, given that obesity is associated with inflammation [60]. The limitations of our study refer to the nondosing of NGAL in organic liquids such as urine and blood, which could strengthen immunohistochemical data on tissue; this will lead us to further future studies to deepen the topic of our research.

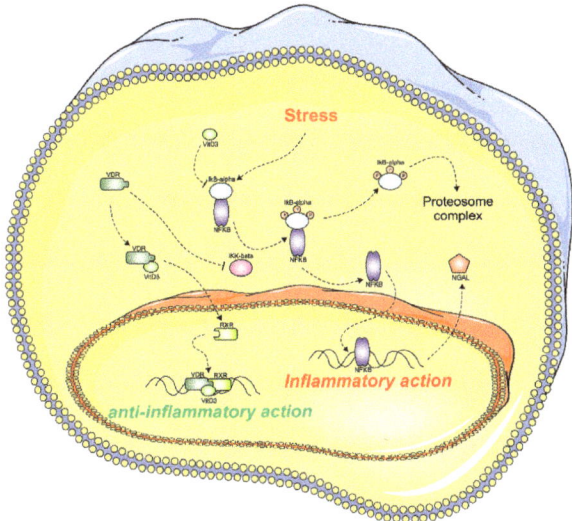

Figure 5. The possible VDR action on kidney cells. The hypothetical mechanism involved during the stress condition in kidney cells. The deprivation of vitamin D3 and stress condition determines the NKkB activation, which results in NGAL upregulation and inflammation. On the contrary, the increased levels of vitamin D3 may determine the inhibition of NFkB pathway, which indirectly may block NGAL synthesis, exerting its anti-inflammatory effect. This figure was drawn using the software CorelDraw (Version, Company, City, US State Abbr., Country and Year) and the vector image bank of Servier Medical Art (http://smart.servier.com/). Servier Medical Art by Servier is licensed under a Creative Commons Attribution 3.0 Unported License (https://creativecommons.org/licenses/by/3.0/).

5. Conclusions

In the present study, once again in agreement with the current literature, we provide experimental evidence supporting the concept that physical activity improves metabolic homeostasis, leading to physical wellness. We can also confirm the positive effects of physical activity-dependent vitamin D mobilization/synthesis, counteracted by NGAL behavior in the kidney. We believe that the present morphological study, although it has some limitations, can give an interesting contribution in basic research to better understand the role of molecule biomarkers for kidney injuries, such as NGAL, and, consequently, adopt strategies that can improve and maintain the state of health of the individual. However, additional investigations should be realized to confirm our preliminary morphological data.

Author Contributions: All authors contributed equally to the design of the study as well as results interpretation and concluding concepts. Conceptualization and Methodology, Writing—Original Draft, P.C.; Data Curation, Formal Analysis, Investigation, and Visualization: M.D.R.; Investigation: S.R. and F.M.T.; Resources: R.I. and L.M.; Methodology, Writing—Original Draft, and Investigation: M.A.S.; Conceptualization, Methodology, Writing—Review & Editing, and Project Administration: G.M. All authors approved the final submitted version.

Funding: This research gained the support of the University Research Project Grant (Triennial Research Plan 2016–2018), Department of Biomedical and Biotechnological Sciences (BIOMETEC), University of Catania, Italy.

Acknowledgments: The authors would like to express their gratitude to Iain Halliday for his valuable work of correction of the paper.

Conflicts of Interest: The authors declare no conflicts of interest.

References

1. Roubenoff, R. Physical activity, inflammation, and muscle loss. *Nutr. Rev.* **2007**, *65*, S208–S212. [CrossRef] [PubMed]

2. Castrogiovanni, P.; Imbesi, R. Oxidative stress and skeletal muscle in exercise. *Ital. J. Anat. Embryol.* **2012**, *117*, 107–117. [PubMed]
3. Ward-Ritacco, C.L.; Adrian, A.L.; Johnson, M.A.; Rogers, L.Q.; Evans, E.M. Adiposity, physical activity, and muscle quality are independently related to physical function performance in middle-aged postmenopausal women. *Menopause* **2014**, *21*, 1114–1121. [CrossRef] [PubMed]
4. Musumeci, G.; Loreto, C.; Imbesi, R.; Trovato, F.M.; Di Giunta, A.; Lombardo, C.; Castorina, S.; Castrogiovanni, P. Advantages of exercise in rehabilitation, treatment and prevention of altered morphological features in knee osteoarthritis. A narrative review. *Histol. Histopathol.* **2014**, *29*, 707–719. [CrossRef]
5. Moreira, L.D.; Oliveira, M.L.; Lirani-Galvão, A.P.; Marin-Mio, R.V.; Santos, R.N.; Lazaretti-Castro, M. Physical exercise and osteoporosis: Effects of different types of exercises on bone and physical function of postmenopausal women. *Arq. Bras. Endocrinol. Metabol.* **2014**, *58*, 514–522. [CrossRef]
6. Beiter, T.; Hoene, M.; Prenzler, F.; Mooren, F.C.; Steinacker, J.M.; Weigert, C.; Nieß, A.M.; Munz, B. Exercise, skeletal muscle and inflammation: ARE-binding proteins as key regulators in inflammatory and adaptive networks. *Exerc. Immunol. Rev.* **2015**, *21*, 42–57.
7. Castrogiovanni, P.; Trovato, F.M.; Szychlinska, M.A.; Nsir, H.; Imbesi, R.; Musumeci, G. The importance of physical activity in osteoporosis. From the molecular pathways to the clinical evidence. *Histol. Histopathol.* **2016**, *31*, 1183–1194. [CrossRef]
8. Du, Z.; Li, Y.; Li, J.; Zhou, C.; Li, F.; Yang, X. Physical activity can improve cognition in patients with Alzheimer's disease: A systematic review and meta-analysis of randomized controlled trials. *Clin. Interv. Aging* **2018**, *13*, 1593–1603. [CrossRef]
9. Musumeci, G.; Castrogiovanni, P.; Coleman, R.; Szychlinska, M.A.; Salvatorelli, L.; Parenti, R.; Magro, G.; Imbesi, R. Somitogenesis: From somite to skeletal muscle. *Acta Histochem.* **2015**, *117*, 313–328. [CrossRef]
10. Musumeci, G.; Trovato, F.M.; Imbesi, R.; Castrogiovanni, P. Effects of dietary extra-virgin olive oil on oxidative stress resulting from exhaustive exercise in rat skeletal muscle: A morphological study. *Acta Histochem.* **2014**, *116*, 61–69. [CrossRef]
11. Coqueiro, R.D.S.; Soares, T.J.; Pereira, R.; Correia, T.M.L.; Coqueiro, D.S.O.; Oliveira, M.V.; Marques, L.M.; de Sá, C.K.C.; de Magalhães, A.C.M. Therapeutic and preventive effects of exercise on cardiometabolic parameters in aging and obese rats. *Clin. Nutr. ESPEN* **2019**, *29*, 203–212. [CrossRef]
12. Martínez, R.; Kapravelou, G.; López-Chaves, C.; Cáceres, E.; Coll-Risco, I.; Sánchez-González, C.; Llopis, J.; Arrebola, F.; Galisteo, M.; Aranda, P.; et al. Aerobic interval exercise improves renal functionality and affects mineral metabolism in obese Zucker rats. *Am. J. Physiol. Renal. Physiol.* **2019**, *316*, F90–F100. [CrossRef]
13. Ranjbar, K.; Nazem, F.; Sabrinezhad, R.; Nazari, A. Aerobic training and L-arginine supplement attenuates myocardial infarction-induced kidney and liver injury in rats via reduced oxidative stress. *Indian Heart J.* **2018**, *70*, 538–543. [CrossRef]
14. Choi, K.M.; Kim, T.N.; Yoo, H.J.; Lee, K.W.; Cho, G.J.; Hwang, T.G.; Baik, S.H.; Choi, D.S.; Kim, S.M. Effect of exercise training on A-FABP, lipocalin-2 and RBP4 levels in obese women. *Clin. Endocrinol.* **2009**, *70*, 569–574. [CrossRef]
15. Musumeci, G.; Aiello, F.C.; Szychlinska, M.A.; Di Rosa, M.; Castrogiovanni, P.; Mobasheri, A. Osteoarthritis in the XXIst century: Risk factors and behaviours that influence disease onset and progression. *Int. J. Mol. Sci.* **2015**, *16*, 6093–6112. [CrossRef]
16. Musumeci, G. Sarcopenia and Exercise "The State of the Art". *J. Funct. Morphol. Kinesiol.* **2017**, *2*, 40. [CrossRef]
17. Musumeci, G. The Use of Vibration as Physical Exercise and Therapy. *J. Funct. Morphol. Kinesiol.* **2017**, *2*, 17. [CrossRef]
18. Castrogiovanni, P.; Di Giunta, A.; Guglielmino, C.; Roggio, F.; Romeo, D.; Fidone, F.; Imbesi, R.; Loreto, C.; Castorina, S.; Musumeci, G. The Effects of Exercise and Kinesio Tape on Physical Limitations in Patients with Knee Osteoarthritis. *J. Funct. Morphol. Kinesiol.* **2016**, *1*, 355–368. [CrossRef]
19. Kjeldsen, L.; Bainton, D.F.; Sengelov, H.; Borregaard, N. Identification of neutrophil gelatinase-associated lipocalin as a novel matrix protein of specific granules in human neutrophils. *Blood* **1994**, *83*, 799–807.
20. Xu, S.Y.; Carlson, M.; Engstrom, A.; Garcia, R.; Peterson, C.G.; Venge, P. Purification and characterization of a human neutrophil lipocalin (HNL) from the secondary granules of human neutrophils. *Scand. J. Clin. Lab. Investig.* **1994**, *54*, 365–376. [CrossRef]

21. Sivalingam, Z.; Larsen, S.B.; Grove, E.L.; Hvas, A.M.; Kristensen, S.D.; Magnusson, N.E. Neutrophil gelatinase-associated lipocalin as a risk marker in cardiovascular disease. *Clin. Chem. Lab. Med.* **2017**, *56*, 5–18. [CrossRef] [PubMed]
22. Flo, T.H.; Smith, K.D.; Sato, S.; Rodriguez, D.J.; Holmes, M.A.; Strong, R.K.; Akira, S.; Aderem, A. Lipocalin 2 mediates an innate immune response to bacterial infection by sequestrating iron. *Nature* **2004**, *432*, 917–921. [CrossRef]
23. Li, S.H.; Hawthorne, V.S.; Neal, C.L.; Sanghera, S.; Xu, J.; Yang, J.; Guo, H.; Steeg, P.S.; Yu, D. Upregulation of neutrophil gelatinase-associated lipocalin by ErbB2 through nuclear factor-kappaB activation. *Cancer Res.* **2009**, *69*, 9163–9168. [CrossRef]
24. Goetz, D.H.; Holmes, M.A.; Borregaard, N.; Bluhm, M.E.; Raymond, K.N.; Strong, R.K. The neutrophil lipocalin NGAL is a bacteriostatic agent that interferes with siderophore-mediated iron acquisition. *Mol. Cell.* **2002**, *10*, 1033–1043. [CrossRef]
25. Nasioudis, D.; Witkin, S.S. Neutrophil gelatinase-associated lipocalin and innate immune responses to bacterial infections. *Med. Microbiol. Immunol.* **2015**, *204*, 471–479. [CrossRef] [PubMed]
26. Lisowska-Myjak, B.; Skarżyńska, E.; Wilczyńska, P.; Jakimiuk, A. Correlation between the concentrations of lactoferrin and neutrophil gelatinase-associated lipocalin in meconium. *Biometals* **2018**, *31*, 123–129. [CrossRef] [PubMed]
27. Yan, L.; Borregaard, N.; Kjeldsen, L.; Moses, M.A. The high molecular weight urinary matrix metalloproteinase (MMP) activity is a complex of gelatinase B/MMP-9 and neutrophil gelatinase-associated lipocalin (NGAL). Modulation of MMP-9 activity by NGAL. *J. Biol. Chem.* **2001**, *276*, 37258–37265. [CrossRef]
28. Hemdahl, A.L.; Gabrielsen, A.; Zhu, C.; Eriksson, P.; Hedin, U.; Kastrup, J.; Thorén, P.; Hansson, G.K. Expression of neutrophil gelatinase-associated lipocalin in atherosclerosis and myocardial infarction. *Arterioscler. Thromb. Vasc. Biol.* **2006**, *26*, 136–142. [CrossRef]
29. Mishra, J.; Mori, K.; Ma, Q.; Kelly, C.; Yang, J.; Mitsnefes, M.; Barasch, J.; Devarajan, P. Amelioration of ischemic acute renal injury by neutrophil gelatinase-associated lipocalin. *J. Am. Soc. Nephrol.* **2004**, *15*, 3073–3082. [CrossRef]
30. Mishra, J.; Dent, C.; Tarabishi, R.; Mitsnefes, M.M.; Ma, Q.; Kelly, C.; Ruff, S.M.; Zahedi, K.; Shao, M.; Bean, J.; et al. Neutrophil gelatinase-associated lipocalin (NGAL) as a biomarker for acute renal injury after cardiac surgery. *Lancet* **2005**, *365*, 1231–1238. [CrossRef]
31. Yndestad, A.; Landro, L.; Ueland, T.; Dahl, C.P.; Flo, T.H.; Vinge, L.E.; Espevik, T.; Frøland, S.S.; Husberg, C.; Christensen, G.; et al. Increased systemic and myocardial expression of neutrophil gelatinase-associated lipocalin in clinical and experimental heart failure. *Eur. Heart. J.* **2009**, *30*, 1229–1236. [CrossRef] [PubMed]
32. Haase-Fielitz, A.; Bellomo, R.; Devarajan, P.; Bennett, M.; Story, D.; Matalanis, G.; Frei, U.; Dragun, D.; Haase, M. The predictive performance of plasma neutrophil gelatinase-associated lipocalin (NGAL) increases with grade of acute kidney injury. *Nephrol. Dial. Transplant.* **2009**, *24*, 3349–3354. [CrossRef] [PubMed]
33. Nymo, S.H.; Hartford, M.; Ueland, T.; Yndestad, A.; Lorentzen, E.; Truvé, K.; Karlsson, T.; Ravn-Fischer, A.; Aukrust, P.; Caidahl, K. Serum neutrophil gelatinase-associated lipocalin (NGAL) concentration is independently associated with mortality in patients with acute coronary syndrome. *Int. J. Cardiol.* **2018**, *262*, 79–84. [CrossRef] [PubMed]
34. Bongers, C.C.W.G.; Alsady, M.; Nijenhuis, T.; Hartman, Y.A.W.; Eijsvogels, T.M.H.; Deen, P.M.T.; Hopman, M.T.E. Impact of acute versus repetitive moderate intensity endurance exercise on kidney injury markers. *Physiol. Rep.* **2017**, *5*. [CrossRef] [PubMed]
35. Machado, J.C.Q.; Volpe, C.M.O.; Vasconcellos, L.S.; Nogueira-Machado, J.A. Quantification of NGAL in Urine of Endurance Cycling Athletes. *J. Phys. Act. Health* **2018**, *15*, 679–682. [CrossRef] [PubMed]
36. Lippi, G.; Sanchis-Gomar, F.; Salvagno, G.L.; Aloe, R.; Schena, F.; Guidi, G.C. Variation of serum and urinary neutrophil gelatinase associated lipocalin (NGAL) after strenuous physical exercise. *Clin. Chem. Lab. Med.* **2012**, *50*, 1585–1589. [CrossRef] [PubMed]
37. Kanda, K.; Sugama, K.; Sakuma, J.; Kawakami, Y.; Suzuki, K. Evaluation of serum leaking enzymes and investigation into new biomarkers for exercise-induced muscle damage. *Exerc. Immunol. Rev.* **2014**, *20*, 39–54.
38. Wołyniec, W.; Ratkowski, W.; Urbański, R.; Bartoszewicz, M.; Siluk, D.; Wołyniec, Z.; Kasprowicz, K.; Zorena, K.; Renke, M. Urinary Kidney Injury Molecule-1 but Not Urinary Neutrophil Gelatinase Associated Lipocalin Is Increased after Short Maximal Exercise. *Nephron* **2018**, *138*, 29–34. [CrossRef]

39. Nair, R.; Maseeh, A. Vitamin D: The "sunshine" vitamin. *J. Pharmacol. Pharmacother.* **2012**, *3*, 118–126.
40. Pike, J.W.; Meyer, M.B. The vitamin D receptor: New paradigms for the regulation of gene expression by 1,25-dihydroxyvitamin D3. *Rheum. Dis. Clin. N. Am.* **2012**, *38*, 13–27. [CrossRef]
41. Lombardi, G.; Corsetti, R.; Lanteri, P.; Grasso, D.; Vianello, E.; Marazzi, M.G.; Graziani, R.; Colombini, A.; Galliera, E.; Corsi-Romanelli, M.M.; et al. Reciprocal regulation of calcium-/phosphate-regulating hormones in cyclists during the Giro d'Italia 3-week stage race. *Scand. J. Med. Sci. Sports* **2014**, *24*, 779–787. [CrossRef]
42. Cohen-Lahav, M.; Shany, S.; Tobvin, D.; Chaimovitz, C.; Douvdevani, A. Vitamin D decreases NFkappaB activity by increasing IkappaBalpha levels. *Nephrol. Dial. Transplant.* **2006**, *21*, 889–897. [CrossRef]
43. Scott, D.; Ebeling, P.R.; Sanders, K.M.; Aitken, D.; Winzenberg, T.; Jones, G. Vitamin D and physical activity status: Associations with five-year changes in body composition and muscle function in community-dwelling older adults. *J. Clin. Endocrinol. Metab.* **2015**, *100*, 670–678. [CrossRef]
44. Gerdhem, P.; Ringsberg, K.A.M.; Obrant, K.J.; Akesson, K. Association between 25-hydroxy vitamin D levels, physical activity, muscle strength and fractures in the prospective population-based OPRA study of elderly women. *Osteoporos. Int.* **2005**, *16*, 1425–1431. [CrossRef]
45. Scott, D.; Blizzard, L.; Fell, J.; Ding, C.; Winzenberg, T.; Jones, G. A prospective study of the associations between 25-hydroxyvitamin D, sarcopenia progression, and physical activity in older adults. *Clin. Endocrinol. (Oxf.)* **2010**, *73*, 581–587. [CrossRef]
46. Bell, N.H.; Godsen, R.N.; Henry, D.P.; Shary, J.; Epstein, S. The effects of muscle-building exercise on vitamin D and mineral metabolism. *J. Bone Miner. Res.* **1988**, *3*, 369–373. [CrossRef]
47. Makanae, Y.; Ogasawara, R.; Sato, K.; Takamura, Y.; Matsutani, K.; Kido, K.; Shiozawa, N.; Nakazato, K.; Fujita, S. Acute bout of resistance exercise increases vitamin D receptor protein expression in rat skeletal muscle. *Exp. Physiol.* **2015**, *100*, 1168–1176. [CrossRef]
48. Aly, Y.E.; Abdou, A.S.; Rashad, M.M.; Nassef, M.M. Effect of exercise on serum vitamin D and tissue vitamin D receptors in experimentally induced type 2 Diabetes Mellitus. *J. Adv. Res.* **2016**, *7*, 671–679. [CrossRef]
49. Chen, Y.; Zhang, J.; Ge, X.; Du, J.; Deb, D.K.; Li, Y.C. Vitamin D receptor inhibits nuclear factor κB activation by interacting with IκB kinase β protein. *J. Biol. Chem.* **2013**, *288*, 19450–19458. [CrossRef]
50. Bu, D.X.; Hemdahl, A.L.; Gabrielsen, A.; Fuxe, J.; Zhu, C.; Eriksson, P.; Yan, Z.Q. Induction of neutrophil gelatinase-associated lipocalin in vascular injury via activation of nuclear factor-kappaB. *Am. J. Pathol.* **2006**, *169*, 2245–2253. [CrossRef]
51. Husi, H.; Human, C. Molecular determinants of acute kidney injury. *J. Inj. Violence Res.* **2015**, *7*, 75–86. [CrossRef] [PubMed]
52. Musumeci, G.; Trovato, F.M.; Pichler, K.; Weinberg, A.M.; Loreto, C.; Castrogiovanni, P. Extra-virgin olive oil diet and mild physical activity prevent cartilage degeneration in an osteoarthritis model: An in vivo and in vitro study on lubricin expression. *J. Nutr. Biochem.* **2013**, *24*, 2064–2075. [CrossRef] [PubMed]
53. Musumeci, G.; Castrogiovanni, P.; Trovato, F.M.; Imbesi, R.; Giunta, S.; Szychlinska, M.A.; Loreto, C.; Castorina, S.; Mobasheri, A. Physical activity ameliorates cartilage degeneration in a rat model of aging: A study on lubricin expression. *Scand. J. Med. Sci. Sports* **2015**, *25*, e222–e230. [CrossRef] [PubMed]
54. Trovato, F.M.; Imbesi, R.; Conway, N.; Castrogiovanni, P. Morphological and functional aspects of human skeletal muscle. *J. Funct. Morphol. Kinesiol.* **2016**, *1*, 289–302. [CrossRef]
55. Leonardi, R.; Rusu, M.C.; Loreto, F.; Loreto, C.; Musumeci, G. Immunolocalization and expression of lubricin in the bilaminar zone of the human temporomandibular joint disc. *Acta Histochem.* **2012**, *114*, 1–5. [CrossRef] [PubMed]
56. Musumeci, G.; Magro, G.; Cardile, V.; Coco, M.; Marzagalli, R.; Castrogiovanni, P.; Imbesi, R.; Graziano, A.C.; Barone, F.; Di Rosa, M.; et al. Characterization of matrix metalloproteinase-2 and -9, ADAM-10 and N-cadherin expression in human glioblastoma multiforme. *Cell Tissue Res.* **2015**, *362*, 45–60. [CrossRef] [PubMed]
57. Musumeci, G.; Mobasheri, A.; Trovato, F.M.; Szychlinska, M.A.; Graziano, A.C.; Lo Furno, D.; Avola, R.; Mangano, S.; Giuffrida, R.; Cardile, V. Biosynthesis of collagen I, II, RUNX2 and lubricin at different time points of chondrogenic differentiation in a 3D in vitro model of human mesenchymal stem cells derived from adipose tissue. *Acta Histochem.* **2014**, *116*, 1407–1417. [CrossRef]
58. Cowland, J.B.; Sørensen, O.E.; Sehested, M.; Borregaard, N. Neutrophil gelatinase-associated lipocalin is up-regulated in human epithelial cells by IL-1 beta, but not by TNF-alpha. *J. Immunol.* **2003**, *171*, 6630–6639. [CrossRef]

59. Fuchs, O. Transcription factor NF-κB inhibitors as single therapeutic agents or in combination with classical chemotherapeutic agents for the treatment of hematologic malignancies. *Curr. Mol. Pharmacol.* **2010**, *3*, 98–122. [CrossRef]
60. Deng, T.; Lyon, C.J.; Bergin, S.; Caligiuri, M.A.; Hsueh, W.A. Obesity, Inflammation, and Cancer. *Annu. Rev. Pathol.* **2016**, *11*, 421–449. [CrossRef]

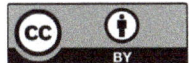

© 2019 by the authors. Licensee MDPI, Basel, Switzerland. This article is an open access article distributed under the terms and conditions of the Creative Commons Attribution (CC BY) license (http://creativecommons.org/licenses/by/4.0/).

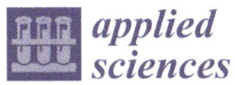

Review

Immunohistochemical Expression of Wilms' Tumor 1 Protein in Human Tissues: From Ontogenesis to Neoplastic Tissues

Lucia Salvatorelli [1,*], Giovanna Calabrese [2], Rosalba Parenti [2], Giada Maria Vecchio [1], Lidia Puzzo [1], Rosario Caltabiano [1], Giuseppe Musumeci [3] and Gaetano Magro [1]

1. Department of Medical and Surgical Sciences and Advanced Technologies, G.F. Ingrassia, Azienda Ospedaliero-Universitaria "Policlinico-Vittorio Emanuele", Anatomic Pathology Section, School of Medicine, University of Catania, 95123 Catania, Italy; giadamariavecchio@gmail.com (G.M.V.); lipuzzo@unict.it (L.P.); rosario.caltabiano@unict.it (R.C.); g.magro@unict.it (G.M.)
2. Department of Biomedical and Biotechnological Sciences, Physiology Section, University of Catania, 95123 Catania, Italy; giovanna.calabrese@unict.it (G.C.); parenti@unict.it (R.P.)
3. Department of Biomedical and Biotechnological Sciences, Human Anatomy and Histology Section, School of Medicine, University of Catania, 95123 Catania, Italy; g.musumeci@unict.it
* Correspondence: lucia.salvatorelli@unict.it; Tel.: +39-095-3702138; Fax: +39-095-3782023

Received: 4 October 2019; Accepted: 10 December 2019; Published: 19 December 2019

Abstract: The human Wilms' tumor gene (WT1) was originally isolated in a Wilms' tumor of the kidney as a tumor suppressor gene. Numerous isoforms of WT1, by combination of alternative translational start sites, alternative RNA splicing and RNA editing, have been well documented. During human ontogenesis, according to the antibodies used, *anti-C* or *N-terminus* WT1 protein, nuclear expression can be frequently obtained in numerous tissues, including metanephric and mesonephric glomeruli, and mesothelial and sub-mesothelial cells, while cytoplasmic staining is usually found in developing smooth and skeletal cells, myocardium, glial cells, neuroblasts, adrenal cortical cells and the endothelial cells of blood vessels. WT1 has been originally described as a tumor suppressor gene in renal Wilms' tumor, but more recent studies emphasized its potential oncogenic role in several neoplasia with a variable immunostaining pattern that can be exclusively nuclear, cytoplasmic or both, according to the antibodies used (*anti-C* or *N-terminus* WT1 protein). With the present review we focus on the immunohistochemical expression of WT1 in some tumors, emphasizing its potential diagnostic role and usefulness in differential diagnosis. In addition, we analyze the WT1 protein expression profile in human embryonal/fetal tissues in order to suggest a possible role in the development of organs and tissues and to establish whether expression in some tumors replicates that observed during the development of tissues from which these tumors arise.

Keywords: immunohistochemistry; WT1; human embryonal/fetal tissues; neoplastic tissue; differential diagnosis

---

1. Introduction

The human Wilms' tumor gene (WT1), first isolated as a tumor suppressor gene and involved in the development of Wilms' tumor of the kidney [1], was among the principal tumor suppressor genes to be cloned [2]. The WT1 gene maps to chromosomal band 11p13, and encodes a transcription factor of the zinc finger type family, containing four zinc finger motifs at the *C-terminus* and a proline/glutamine-rich DNA-binding domain at the *N-terminus*. It spans approximatively 50 kb of genomic sequence and comprises 10 exons that produce a 3 kb mRNA [3,4].

Numerous isoforms, developing from a combination of alternative translational start sites, alternative RNA splicing, and RNA editing, have been well-documented [5–8]. The most studied are the exon 5 variants and the KST (lysine–threonine–serine) isoforms, and, in some cases, these can have specific functions. Although WT1 was originally discovered as a tumor suppressor gene involved in the pathogenesis of renal Wilms' tumor, subsequent studies emphasized its potential oncogenic role in hematologic malignancies [9] and in different malignant solid tumors [10], including lung cancer [11], colorectal cancer [12], pancreatic cancer [13], breast cancer [14], desmoid tumors [15], ovarian cancer [16,17], brain tumors [18,19] and soft tissue sarcomas [20]. This hypothesis is supported by several functional studies showing that WT1 inhibition, by using antisense oligonucleotides, reduces cell proliferation, migration and endothelial tube formation [21]. WT1 could play an important role in angiogenesis, the onset of metastases and the inhibition of the immune response. In fact the endothelial cells, haematopoietic progenitor and myeloid-derived suppressor cells express high levels of WT1 inducing the control of the expression of CD31 and CD117. Therefore, the inactivation of WT1 in the aforementioned cells can reduce angiogenesis, the development of metastases and promote the immune response [22].

Although the first function defined for WT1 was that of a transcriptional regulator, in the last 10 years several studies have emerged indicating its function as an activator, a repressor or a coactivator [23,24]. Nevertheless, it is known that the role of WT1 is more complicated than once believed, and it could be involved in at least two distinct cellular processes: transcription control and RNA metabolism. All these roles of WT1 are supported by alternative splicing of the WT1 RNA to generate two main isoforms that differ by the insertion of three amino acids, KTS (lysine–threonine–serine), inside the zinc finger region of the protein [25–27]. In this regard, several studies have demonstrated that the isoform of WT1 that lacks the KTS insertion, –KTS WT1, binds to DNA with higher affinity and functions as a transcriptional regulator. On the other hand, the form having the KTS insertion, +KTS WT1, plays a role in mRNA splicing rather than transcriptional control [28,29]. Larsson et al. found the first correlation between the WT1 protein and RNA metabolism, showing that the +KTS WT1 isoform colocalized specially with splicing factors within nuclear speckles. In the last few years it has been demonstrated that a considerable amount of transcription and/or splicing factors shuttle to the cytoplasm, acquiring a new function. The cytoplasmic role attributed to shuttling proteins is predominantly the nucleocytoplasmic transport of mRNA or RNA. Niksic et al. [27], emphasized not only that WT1 is a shuttling protein, but also that a substantial part of endogenous WT1 protein is located in the cytoplasm. Furthermore, they showed that both WT1 isoforms shuttle between the nucleus and the cytoplasm [30].

WT1 is not only differentially spliced, but in turn alters the splicing and function of other genes, such as the vascular endothelial growth factor (VEGF), through the activation of Serine/arginine-rich, protein-specific splicing factor kinase (SRPK1), and indirectly Serine/arginine-rich splicing factor 1 (Srsf1). Comparing healthy tissues with neoplastic tissues, there is a greater expression of Wt1, Srpk1, Srsf1 and the pro-angiogenic VEGF isoforms. WT1 inhibition regulates negatively the expression of Srpk1 and Srsf1 in endothelial cells, inducing the development of the antiangiogenic VEGF isoform, associated with apoptotic cell death [31,32].

In the past many authors believed that WT1 immunohistochemical expression, using antibodies directed against the *C-terminal* portion of the protein [33,34], was exclusively limited to the nucleus, and that the occasional cytoplasmic staining obtained in some tumors was the result of an artifact (non-specific staining). The variability of staining with anti-WT1 *C-terminus* antibodies could be due to the use of different clones of the same antibody. Subsequently, with the advent of newly available antibodies against the *N-terminal* portion of WT1 (clone WT6F-H2), it has been demonstrated that WT1 expression can be found in the nucleus or in the cytoplasm, or concurrently in both the nucleus and cytoplasm [35–42].

During human ontogenesis, according to the antibodies used, *anti-C* or *N-terminus* WT1 protein, [36,39–47], nuclear expression can be frequently obtained in metanephric and mesonephric glomeruli, primary sex cords, gonadic stroma and mesothelial and sub-mesothelial cells, while cytoplasmic staining is usually found in developing skeletal muscles, myocardium, radial glia of the spinal cord and cerebral cortex, sympathetic neuroblasts, adrenal cortical cells and the endothelial cells of blood vessels [33,34,37,38,48–52]. With regard to neoplastic tissues, WT1 protein has been found in several tumors with variable immunostaining patterns, i.e., exclusively nuclear, cytoplasmic or both, according to the antibodies used (*anti-C* or *N-terminus* WT1 protein) [35,36,39–47]. The variable nuclear and cytoplasmic WT1 staining may be explained by assuming that the expression of this transcription factor in some neoplastic tissues (Wilms tumor, ovarian, mesothelial neoplasms, Sertoli cell tumor and rhabdomyosarcoma) mirrors its normal developmental regulation [37,38,41]. In addition, our research group have recently demonstrated that WT1 shows an oncofetal expression pattern, being abundantly detected in developing and neoplastic skeletal muscle tissues, while its expression is down-regulated in adult normal skeletal muscle tissues [41,46].

The present review focuses on the immunohistochemical expression of WT1 in some common and less common tumors (Table S1), emphasizing its potential diagnostic role and usefulness in differential diagnosis. In addition, we analyze WT1 protein expression profiles during human ontogenesis to provide suggestions about its role in the development of organs and tissues, and to establish if its expression in some tumors replicates that observed during the development of tissues from which these tumors arise.

2. WT1 Immunohistochemical Expression in Human Embryonal/Fetal and Neoplastic Tissues

2.1. WT1 Immunohistochemical Expression in Human Embryonal/Fetal Tissues

From gestational weeks 7 to 24, WT1 expression has been found in several tissues, in a nuclear or a cytoplasmic localization. WT1 nuclear staining can be observed in different structures of metanephros and mesonephros [37,51,52], including glomeruli and sub-capsular blastema of nephrogenic zone (Figure 1). WT1 expression in round, undifferentiated mesenchymal cells (blastematous component) undergoing epithelial differentiation is a model of controlled epithelial–mesenchymal transition resulting in nephrogenesis [53–56]. WT1 is expressed in mesothelial cells (excoelomic epithelium) that are found above both ovaries and testes, in the developing sex cords and in the gonadal mesenchyme (Figure 1). In the later phases of development, nuclear staining is manteined in the secondary sex cords of both testes and ovaries, while it gradually disappears from their surrounding mesenchyme, to be restricted to epithelial cells surrounding the oocytes [51]. Between the seventh and the tenth week of gestational age, WT1 nuclear expression can be found in the mesothelial cells of serosal surfaces covering the abdominal and pelvic visceral organs (uterus and ovaries, bladder, stomach, small and large intestine, pancreas) pleura and peritoneum. Notably, a conspicuous amount of mesenchymal sub-mesothelial cells along mesothelial cells displays WT1 nuclear expression [37].

During human developmental phases (from 8 to 28 wGA) small clusters of neuroblasts are located in the paravertebral regions, in the cortex of adrenal glands and within the muscle wall of the developing stomach and small/large intestine. WT1 cytoplasmic expression in neuroblasts is strong and diffuse during the different phases of development, while no nuclear immunoreactivity can be demonstrated. These cells gradually differentiate into ganglion cells, at first as immature ganglion cells and finally as mature ganglion cells. In immature ganglion cells, unlike neuroblasts, WT1 cytoplasmic immunoexpression is weak/focal and sometimes absent, while ganglion cells of adult sympathetic ganglia, adrenal glands and myoenteric nervous plexuses, are completely negative. Similar to the adult adrenal medulla and paraganglia, extra- and intra-adrenal differentiating chromaffin cells are not WT1 stained. The expression of WT1 is strongly localized in the cytoplasm of radial glia cells of both the developing spinal cord and cerebral cortex along the entire thickness of the neural tube. WT1 expression in the undifferentiated radial glial cells seems to support the theory that it is necessary to maintain cells in an undifferentiated state [30,57–59].

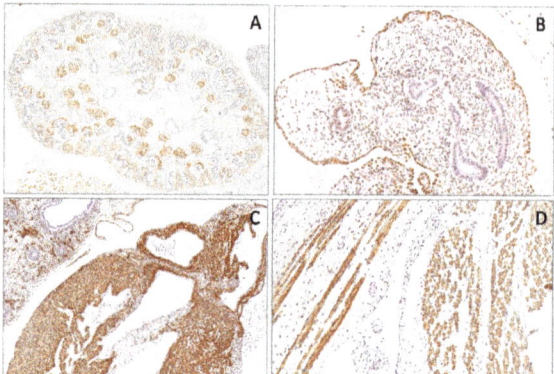

Figure 1. Nuclear expression of the Wilms' tumor gene (WT1) (*N-terminus*) in human metanephros (**A**), in gonadic stromal cells (**B**) and in the mesothelial cells covering the surface of the ovary (**B**) of the fetus of 11 weeks of gestational age. Cytoplasmic expression of WT1 (*N-terminus*) in myocardium (**C**) and in the skeletal cells (**D**) in a fetus of 22 weeks of gestational age.

During the early phases of development (from 6 wGA) embryonic myoblasts forming myotomes exhibit strong cytoplasmic staining for WT1. Moreover, in both primary and secondary myotubes of the developing muscles, WT1 is strongly and diffusely expressed in the cytoplasm of these cells. From 20 wGA, WT1 cytoplasmic expression becomes more heterogeneous, ranging from focally strong to weak or absent within the same muscle fiber (mosaic-type expression) (Figure 1). WT1 nuclear immunoreactivity is lacking in skeletal muscle during all phases of myogenesis [41]. Several studies have shown that WT1 is crucial for heart development [60,61], and it may also be involved in the proliferation of cardiac myocytes. In addition, WT1 plays a key role in the conversion of epicardial cells to mesenchymal cells. This is demonstrated by strong WT1 cytoplasmic expression in cardiomyocytes of both atria and ventricles during the different phases of heart development, as in somatic skeletal muscle cells. In addition, WT1 is expressed in the cytoplasm of the endothelial cells of blood vessels (aorta, arteries, veins, capillaries) in all developing tissues (Figure 1) [62]. These findings are also maintained in the endothelial cells of both adult tissues and benign and malignant tumors. In developing human lungs, from 8 to 14 wGA, WT1 nuclear staining is limited to the mesothelial cells of visceral pleura, with a weak cytoplasmic expression in some mesenchymal cells surrounding branching epithelial structures. Between 7 and 14 wGA, WT1 staining is missing in the human fetal epidermis, except for an intense cytoplasmic expression in the progenitor cells of the developing dermis [41].

WT1 is expressed in the myoenteric plexus of the developing gastroenteric system [38], while a weak cytoplasmic staining is observed in the cells of the muscularis propria, especially of the small intestine [52]. A strong WT1 nuclear staining is found in the mesothelial cells of serosal surfaces covering the stomach, small and large intestine, pancreas and liver [52].

2.2. Wilms' Tumor

Wilms' tumor is a malignant embryonal neoplasm, also known as a nephroblastoma of pediatric age, resulting from a disturbance of the differentiation of nephrogenic blastematous cells, which replicates various stages of the developing kidneys [53,54,63,64]. Microscopically, Wilms' tumor is typically composed of three components: blastematous, mesenchymal (stromal) and epithelial [65–67]. Most Wilms' tumors show all three components, but their proportions vary widely. Some tumors are biphasic, while others are monophasic. The blastematous component is extremely cellular and composed of small round-to-oval cells with scanty cytoplasm, dark nuclei and frequent mitotic figures, arranged in diffuse, nodular, cord-like (serpentine), or basaloid (with peripheral palisading) patterns. The stromal component is composed of spindle-shaped cells set in a myxoid stroma.

In most tumors, stromal differentiation, including smooth and skeletal muscle, bone and chondroid tissues, adipocytic tissue, or more rarely, neuroglia and mature ganglion cells, may be observed. Skeletal muscle in various stages of differentiation, including rhabdomyoblasts, represents the most common heterologous component [68,69]. The epithelial component is composed of tubules, papillary and glomerular-like structures, which are closely reminiscent of normal nephrogenesis.

There is not a single marker or panel of immunostains that is diagnostic of Wilms' tumor, but the immunohistochemical profile depends on the different tumor components examined. WT1 is certainly the most sensitive and specific marker for the diagnosis of Wilms' tumor, with positivity in more than 90% of cases (Figure 2). It is expressed in the nuclei of primitive blastemal cells using antibodies directed both to the *C-terminal* or *N-terminal* portions of the protein, while it is absent in the differentiated epithelial and stromal elements. When a Wilms' tumor is composed predominantly/exclusively of the blastematous component, it may be diagnostically challenging, especially when pathologists are dealing with small biopsies, and the differential diagnosis includes other small, round cell tumors (differential diagnosis with other small, round blue cell tumors-PNETs/Ewing sarcoma, neuroblastomas, rhabdomyosarcomas, clear cell sarcomas, synovial sarcomas and lymphomas). In this context, the demonstration of WT1 nuclear expression with antibodies directed against the *C-terminal* portion of the protein (clone WT1C19) is helpful in confirming the diagnosis.

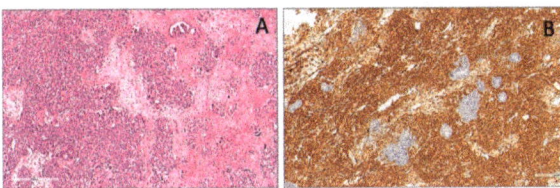

Figure 2. Wilms' tumor showing blastematous, epithelial and stromal components (**A**). Blastematous component showing diffuse and strong nuclear WT1 (*N-terminus*) expression (**B**).

2.3. Malignant Mesothelialioma

Malignant mesothelioma is a primary tumor of serosal membranes, including pleura, peritoneum, pericardium and tunica vaginalis of the testis. The majority of these tumors arise from pleura followed by peritoneum, and are related to asbestos exposure. Histologically, mesotheliomas are classified in three forms: epithelioid, sarcomatoid, or mixed (biphasic). The majority of these tumors are predominantly epithelioid, with tumor cells forming papillae, pseudoacini or solid epithelial nests [70]. These tumor cells show abundant and acidophilic cytoplasm with round nuclei and occasionally prominent nucleoli. Early forms can be difficult to distinguish from reactive mesothelial hyperplasia. Infiltration of deep tissues, obvious cytologic atypia, prominent cell groupings and necrosis favor the diagnosis of malignant mesothelioma [71]. Sarcomatoid mesothelioma [72] is composed of spindle cells with oval nuclei, scant amphophilic cytoplasm and occasionally prominent nucleoli, arranged in a fascicular pattern, sometimes with a fibrosarcoma-like appearance.

Epithelioid mesotheliomas may show a wide variety of morphologies, which can mimic numerous metastatic carcinomas, especially adenocarcinoma of the lung. The correct diagnosis of mesothelioma is usually achieved by the application of a panel of immunohistochemistry, including WT1 antibodies. Early studies on WT1 expression in mesotheliomas were published in 2000, reporting a positivity of 45–75% of the cases using a polyclonal antibody [73,74]. With the advent of new, commercially-available antibodies (6F-H2), a higher percentage of expression has been reported. Currently, WT1 is considered a highly sensitive and relatively specific marker for distinguishing mesothelioma from lung adenocarcinoma [75]. However, in daily diagnostic practice, WT1 must be used in combination with other, usually positive, markers for mesothelioma (calretinin, Keratin5/6).

In mesotheliomas, WT1 protein expression is restricted to the nucleus (Figure 3), even if it can be focally observed in the cytoplasm of the cells of sarcomatoid mesotheliomas [74–78]. As normal/

hyperplastic mesothelial cells lining pleura show nuclear staining for WT1 [37], this marker is not helpful in distinguishing benign from malignant lesions. Nuclear WT1 expression in mesothelioma is not surprising if we consider that a similar expression has been documented in embryonal/fetal mesothelial cells covering cavities. The diagnosis of mesothelioma continues to rely on a multimodal approach that incorporates clinical features, gross, microscopic and immunohistochemical features [79].

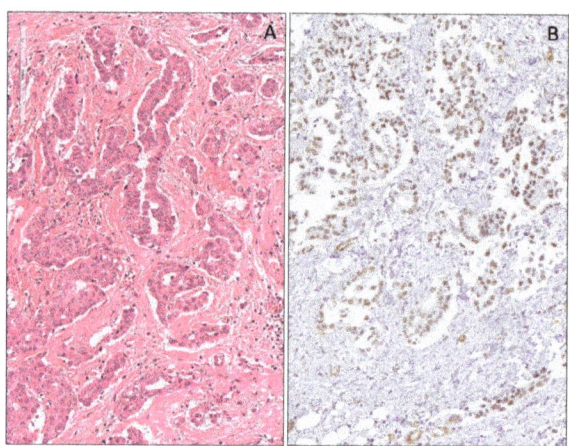

Figure 3. Epithelioid mesothelioma of the pleura (**A**). Diffuse nuclear expression of WT1 (*N-terminus*) in the neoplastic cells of mesothelioma (**B**).

2.4. WT1 Expression in Epithelial Tumors of Ovary

Epithelial tumors are the most common ovarian tumors, comprising about 60% of all ovarian tumors. Serous tumors constitute approximately 30% of all ovarian tumors. About half of the cases are benign, approximately 35% are malignant and the remaining cases are classified as borderline. They usually show positive staining for CK7, and they do not stain for CK20 or CDX-2. Parenti et al. [37] reported WT1 nuclear expression in mesothelial cells lining the fetal ovaries, thus it is not surprising if the tumors that originate from the epithelium covering the ovary express WT1. In fact, several studies show that the WT1 nuclear expression in serous ovarian tumors is around 90–95%, and that this marker is also helpful in differentiating ovarian serous carcinoma from endometrial serous carcinoma, which has a similar microscopic appearance, but is less likely to stain for WT1 [16,80–89]. WT1 shows a different expression in the different histological subtypes of ovarian carcinomas. Serous ovarian carcinomas that originate in the fallopian tubes, in the peritoneum and in the ovarian cortical inclusion cysts, are always WT1 positive. Recent studies demonstrated not only the diagnostic utility, but also the possible prognostic role of WT1. High grade serous ovarian carcinomas positive to WT1 have a better prognosis, especially when the neoplastic cells co-express WT1 and the estrogen receptor [90]. Mucinous and clear-cell carcinomas are negative, according to Waldstrøm and Grove [89], Goldstein et al. [80] and Hashi et al. [82]. In contrast, another study carried out by Shimizu et al. [16] demonstrated the immunohistochemical expression of WT1 in both mucinous and clear-cell carcinomas, with a higher expression in serous carcinomas than in clear-cell carcinomas, while not a significantly higher expression than mucinous carcinomas. It is likely that these conflicting results may be due to the use of different primary antibodies. Indeed, Shimizu et al. [16], used the C19 clone, whereas in other studies the 6F-H2 clone was the antibody used against WT1.

Numerous reports show that WT1 is not expressed in endometrioid carcinomas [82,86,87], with only a few studies showing focal WT1 positivity [81,83,84]. Recently, immunohistochemical studies indicated a significant difference in WT1 expression between highly-differentiated, endometrioid carcinomas, compared with tumors of lower grade [89]. As suggested by Gilks [88], low-grade

Appl. Sci. 2020, *10*, 40

endometrioid carcinomas differ from high-grade endometrioid carcinomas in biological behavior and gene expression profile, and this theory may explain the different expression of WT1.

2.5. WT1 Expression in Granulosa Cell Tumor

Granulosa cell tumors are sex cord–stromal ovarian neoplasms showing differentiation toward follicular granulosa cells. The two types of granulosa cell tumors are known as adult and juvenile types. Macroscopically, adult granulosa cell tumors appear as unilateral, usually solid or solid-cystic masses, with an area of hemorrhage or necrosis following torsion. In the adult type granulosa cell tumors, the tumor cells resemble normal granulosa cells. They are small and round, cuboidal, or spindle shaped, with pale cytoplasm and ill-defined cell borders. The nuclei are round or oval, with fine chromatin and a single small nucleolus. An important diagnostic feature is the presence of longitudinal folds or grooves in the nuclei with a 'coffee-bean' appearance [91]. Occasionally, mitotic figures, nuclear pleomorphism and bizarre nuclei are seen, but do not appear to affect the prognosis adversely [92–94]. The tumor cells are rarely extensively (>50% of cells) luteinized with abundant eosinophilic cytoplasm, well-defined cell borders and central nuclei resembling the luteinized granulosa cells of the corpus luteum. Cells are arranged in different patterns, including diffuse, trabecular, micro-follicular, macro-follicular, insular and pseudopapillary. Macroscopically juvenile granulosa cell tumors are solid-cystic masses, rarely exclusively solid. They are variably composed of a double component, granulosa and theca component. The former shows polygonal cells with abundant cytoplasm, from eosinophilic to vacuolated, and clear and hyperchromatic nuclei without grooves. The second is composed of oval- to spindle-shaped cells with pale cytoplasm. Several growth patterns are observed, from solid to follicular or pseudo-papillary. In the atypical forms, brisk mitotic activity is seen. Bizarre nuclei may occur. WT1 is a marker that has not been widely studied in granulosa cell tumors. It is expressed in 65% to 88% of adult granulosa cell tumors (Figure 4) [95–98]. Although several different non-sex cord-stromal tumors can express WT1 [99], most of them are not in the differential diagnosis of ovarian sex cord-stromal tumors, and tumors that are in the differential diagnosis are typically negative or limited for WT1 expression.

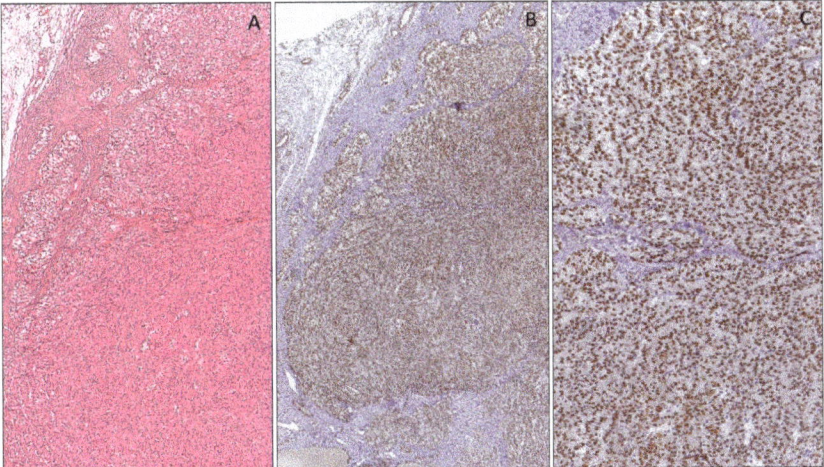

Figure 4. Ovarian granulosa cell tumor, adult type (**A**). Nuclear WT1 (*N-terminus*) expression in neoplastic cells at low (**B**) and high (**C**) magnification.

2.6. WT1 Expression in Sertoli Cell Tumors

Sertoli cell tumors are composed of Sertoli cells with rare Leydig cells. They are typically a solid mass with a tan to yellow cut surface. The tumor cells are cuboidal or columnar with pale cytoplasm, and less frequently, deeply eosinophilic or vacuolated. The nuclei are round–oval in shape and uniform with inconspicuous nucleoli. Atypical and bizarre nuclei are rarely observed. Mitotic activity is variable, but not > 5/10 HPF. The lesion is well limited by the surrounding ovarian parenchyma.

The cells are typically arranged in a diffuse or nodular pattern, but they can be observed as a mixture of different patterns (tubules, cord or trabeculae, sheets, pseudo-papillae and more rarely, retiform, islands or spindly patterns). The main differential diagnoses are the Sertoli–Leydig cell tumor, endometrioid carcinoma, carcinoid tumor and female adnexa tumor.

Several studies have investigated the expression of WT1 in Sertoli cell tumors in order to identify new diagnostic markers. Zhao et al. [99] suggested including WT1 protein (6F-H2 antibody) in the immunohistochemical panel, together with inhibin, to distinguish Sertoli cell tumors from endometrioid and neuroendocrine tumors. In addition, the authors stated that the diagnostic utility of WT1 in Sertoli cell tumors is similar to inhibin, and better than that of calretinin [99]. Another study evaluated WT1 expression in ovarian stroma and its tumors. The results showed that ovarian stromal cells, ovarian fibroma, cellular fibroma, fibrothecoma and ovarian leiomyoma expressed WT1, whereas non-gynecologic smooth muscle tumors and other spindle cell tumors were usually negative for WT1. These findings suggest that WT1 may be used as an immunohistochemical marker for spindle cell tumors derived from the ovary and uterus, including Sertoli cell tumors (Figure 5). WT1, SF-1 and inhibin are the most informative sex cord-stromal markers to be used for the distinction of non-sex cord-stromal tumors; however, the usefulness of immunohistochemistry for the diagnosis of fibroma/fibrothecoma is limited [100].

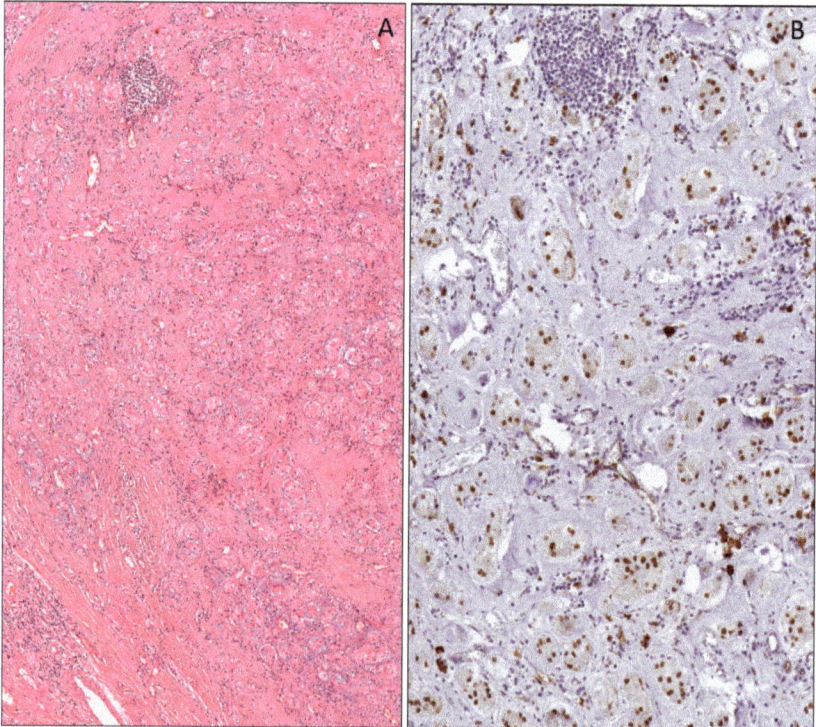

Figure 5. Sertoli cell tumor (**A**). Neoplastic cells showing nuclear WT1 (*N-terminus*) expression (**B**).

2.7. WT1 Expression in Breast Carcinoma

Several studies have demonstrated WT1 expression in breast carcinomas, with low expression in adjacent normal breast tissues. Nasomyon et al. [101], confirmed WT1 protein expression by using Western blotting. These results suggested that WT1 (17AA+) might be a crucial isoform in cancer progression and development, and might work together with WT1 (17AA−) as a protein partner. In the same study, the authors showed that WT1 plays an oncogenic role in ERα and HER2 protein regulation.

In addition, they observed that ER-α and HER2 proteins were highly expressed in breast cancer, but expressed at low levels in adjacent normal breast tissues, while WT1 (17AA+) was strongly expressed in breast cancer and slightly in adjacent normal breast tissues. The result of WT1 (17AA+) mRNA expression was confirmed at the protein level.

Several studies focused on immunohistochemical nuclear expression of WT1 in breast cancer, predominantly in the mucinous histotype [43,102–104], while it is occasionally co-expressed in non-mucinous carcinoma components of mixed mucinous carcinoma [102]. In addition, WT1 expression was observed, not only in mucinous carcinoma, but also in associated solid papillary carcinoma. A good correlation of WT1 immunohistochemical expression between solid papillary carcinoma and associated mucinous carcinomas does exist, indicating that the former could be the precursor of the latter [105]. With the advent of immunotherapy in malignancies, expression of WT1in mucinous breast carcinomas provides a molecular target in these relatively indolent breast tumors [102]. Conflicting results are reported regarding WT1 expression and the prognosis of breast carcinoma. A study demonstrated that WT1 expression in breast cancer is correlated to poor prognosis, due to cancer-related epithelial-to-mesenchymal transition (EMT) and poor chemotherapy response [106]. Conversely, another study displayed that the immunoreactivity for WT1, together with RSPO1 and P16, was significantly associated with a more favorable disease-free survival [107]. Furthermore, high levels of Wilms' Tumor 1 (WT1) protein and mRNA had been associated with aggressive phenotypes of breast tumors, because HER2/neuoncogene increases WT1 expression. Increased levels of WT1 are due to the engagement of Akt, resulting in HER2/neu overexpression [108].

2.8. WT1 Expression in Lung Carcinomas

WT1 expression was analyzed, by using immunohistochemical and quantitative real-time (qRT-PCR) analyses, in several types of lung carcinoma (41 adenocarcinomas, 13 squamous cell carcinomas, two large cell carcinomas and six small cell carcinomas). Data obtained from immunohistochemical analyses showed cytoplasmic WT1 immunoreactivity in 5/6 small cell carcinomas, 1/2 large cell carcinomas, 1/1 squamous cell carcinoma and in 4/5 adenocarcinomas. (In normal lung tissues, no immunoreactivity was observed). In the same study WT1 genomic DNA obtained from seven lung cancer tissues was PCR-amplified and examined for mutations by direct sequencing. The absence of mutations in all of the 10 exons of the WT1 gene was demonstrated, suggesting that the non-mutated, wild-type WT1 gene plays an important role in the tumorigenesis of de novo lung cancers, and may provide the rationale for new therapeutic strategies for lung cancer targeting the WT1 gene and its products [11].

2.9. WT1 Expression in Pancreatic Ductal Adenocarcinomas

WT1 expression was also reported in a series of pancreatic ductal adenocarcinomas. Oji et al. [13] showed that WT1 was expressed at the cytoplasmic level in 30/40 cases of pancreatic ductal carcinoma, while normal pancreatic cells adjacent to carcinoma cells were negative. No significant correlation was observed between WT1 expression and age, sex, T or N stage, tumor site and differentiation. These results suggest that the WT1 gene plays an important role in the tumorigenesis of pancreatic ductal adenocarcinoma [13]. Conversely, more recent studies have shown that the nuclear expression of WT1 in pancreatic ductal adenocarcinoma correlates with gender and tumor stage, while cytoplasmic staining correlates with gender, histological grade and perineural invasion. In addition, the same authors reported that a high nuclear expression of WT1 in pancreatic tumor tissues was significantly associated with poor overall survival, suggesting a possible role for it as a molecular biomarker of a poor prognosis among patients with pancreatic ductal adenocarcinoma [109].

2.10. WT1 Expression in Melanocytic Lesions

Several studies have reported the usefulness of WT1 in the differential diagnosis between nevi and melanomas. The first study on WT1 expression in melanocytic lesions dates back to 1997 [110], when it was observed that WT1 in melanoma, in the context of absent or mutated p53, acted as a transcriptional activator, whereas in the presence of wild-type p53, it acted as a repressor. Later, Wilsher and Cheerala [111] showed that WT1 (6F-H2) was a complementary marker of malignant melanoma. Indeed, by using immunohistochemistry, they demonstrated cytoplasmic WT1 expression in most invasive primary cutaneous melanomas, including spindle cell and desmoplastic melanomas, and in metastatic melanomas. However, its usefulness was limited by the fact that most Spitz nevi and a minority of dysplastic nevi expressed WT1. In another study, apart from demonstrating cytoplasmic, and more rarely, nuclear WT1 expression in melanoma, it was proven that the silencing of WT1 inhibited melanoma cell proliferation, supporting the role of WT1 cell proliferation in melanoma [21,112,113]. In contrast, Garrido-Ruiz et al. [114] reported a higher rate of WT1 staining in melanocytic nevi against melanomas, and an increased expression in advanced stages of melanoma progression. In addition, they supported an association of WT1 protein expression with a shorter overall survival. A significant expression of WT1 in desmoplastic (71%), compared with non-desmoplastic melanoma (47%), has also been recently observed. The same study reported that vertical growth phase melanomas exhibited an expression of WT1 more frequently than radial growth phase melanomas (46.5% vs. 16.0%) [115]. Finally, a study on 40 cases of desmoplastic melanomas showed a strong and diffuse cytoplasmic expression of WT1 (6F-H2 antibody) in all cases examined, suggesting the use of WT1 along with S-100p, SOX10, p75 and nestin as an optimal panel for the diagnosis of desmoplastic melanoma [116].

2.11. WT1 Expression in Colorectal Carcinoma

Colorectal cancer is one of the most commonly diagnosed cancers worldwide, accounting for an estimated 9.4% of all malignancies [117]. The treatment is surgery, but approximately 60% of patients experience local recurrence and/or distant metastases (Andre and Schmiegel, 2005). Despite advances in surgical techniques and in chemotherapy, around 20% of patients with colorectal carcinoma die from disease recurrence [117]. Thus, new diagnostic tools and therapeutic approaches are required. A previous study showed immunoreactivity in 89% of the cases examined [118]. In addition, in the same study, a quantitative real-time reverse transcription-polymerase chain reaction (RT-PCR) was performed that showed that WT1 mRNA was expressed in all (100%) of the 28 cases of colorectal adenocarcinoma. Moreover, WT1 mRNA expression levels were higher in 71% of the cases when compared to those of normal-appearing mucosal tissues. These results suggested an important role of WT1 in the tumorigenesis of primary colorectal adenocarcinoma, and that WT1 could be a new molecular target for the treatment of colorectal adenocarcinoma expressing WT1. However, no significant correlations were observed between WT1 mRNA expression levels and age, gender, site of tumors, T stage, N stage and M stage [118]. Miyata et al. recently evaluated the correlation between WT1 mRNA levels and other tumor-associated antigens with clinicopathological factors [119]. Notably, WT1 expression in colorectal carcinoma is significantly correlated with tumor progression, lymph node and distant metastasis, and clinical stage. These results suggest that WT1 could be an important novel independent marker for prognosis and tumor progression in colorectal adenocarcinoma [120].

2.12. WT1 Expression in Cerebral Tumors

Several authors have studied WT1 expression in cerebral neoplasms, including glial tumors and medulloblastomas [121]. The WT1 cytoplasmic expression using the anti-WT1 C-19 and anti-WT1 6F-H2 antibodies, in high-grade astrocytic tumors (glioblastoma and anaplastic astrocytoma), was significantly higher than that in low-grade ones (pilocytic astrocytoma and diffuse astrocytoma) (Figure 6) [122]. WT1 expression was also examined in anaplastic ependymomas, and anaplastic oligodendrogliomas, which showed diffuse cytoplasmic staining.

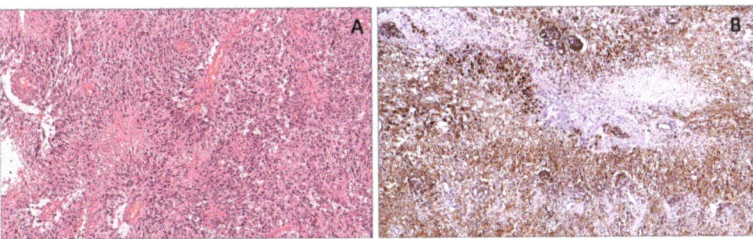

Figure 6. Glioblastoma multiforme showing pseudopalisading necrosis (**A**). Neoplastic cells showing strong and diffuse cytoplasmic expression of WT1 (*N-terminus*) (**B**).

Some authors correlated the expression of WT1 with the MIB-1 staining index because histological examination areas with features of anaplasia and high perivascular proliferation and cellularity show a strong WT1 protein expression [123]. A more recent article reported that in diffuse astrocytic tumors, high levels of WT1 expression are related to a higher World Health Organization (WHO) tumor grade, absence of IDH1 mutation, older age, but not related to O(6)- methyl guanine methyl transferase (MGMT) promoter methylation status. In addition, it would seem that WT1 expression is associated with a worse outcome in patients with diffuse astrocytoma, but not glioblastoma [124].

2.13. WT1 Gene Expression in Soft Tissue Sarcomas

Sotobori et al. [125] showed that WT1 mRNA expression levels in adult cases of soft tissue sarcomas were significantly higher than in normal soft tissues, and that the disease-specific survival rate for patients with elevated WT1 mRNA expression levels was found to be significantly worse in patients with low levels. Furthermore, their results demonstrated that the WT1 mRNA expression level is a significant prognostic indicator in patients with soft tissue sarcoma. On the contrary, other authors [126] evaluated WT1 protein and mRNA expression levels in various pediatric tumors, and showed that while WT1 protein was widely detected in these malignancies, WT1 mRNA expression varied widely in the different types of pediatric cancers. However, no significant relationship was evaluated between WT1 mRNA expression and clinical factors.

2.14. WT1 Expression in Malignant Peripheral Nerve Sheath Tumors

Malignant peripheral nerve sheath tumors (MPNSTs) are an aggressive and rare type of sarcoma, usually arising from peripheral nerves. They can occur sporadically or more frequently (up to 50% of cases) from pre-existing neurofibromas in the context of neurofibromatosis type 1 (NF1) [127]. Most MPNSTs are deeply localized, and often they are greater than 10 cm in maximum diameter by the time of presentation. Histologically, they show a spindle-cell fascicular appearance with abrupt alternations between cellular and more myxoid areas, suggesting neural differentiation. Some cases have a uniformly cellular and fascicular pattern reminiscent of a monophasic synovial sarcoma. In other cases, an abundant myxoid stroma can be observed, configuring the diagnosis of myxoid MPNST. Cells have a pale, poorly defined cytoplasm and narrow nuclei, often with a wavy or buckled configuration. In addition, the nuclei tend to be hyperchromatic, and at least focally pleomorphic with inconspicuous nucleoli. Mitoses are generally frequent. In about 10–15% of MPNSTs, especially in those arising in patients with NF1, heterologous differentiation can be present [128]. The most frequent divergent differentiation is the rhabdomyosarcomatous component, configuring the so-called malignant Triton tumor, which is associated with a poor prognosis. Less frequently, osteosarcomatous or chondrosarcomatous differentiation can be observed. Immunohistochemically, the S-100 protein is positive in about 50% of cases of MPNST [129,130].

Early studies on WT1 expression reported the positivity in Schwann cells of normal nerves. In peripheral nerve sheath tumors, including MPNSTs, neurofibromas and schwannomas, neoplastic cells expressed WT1 protein at the cytoplasmic level (Figure 7) [44]. A recent study by Kim et al. [131] evaluated WT1 expression in 87 cases of soft tissue sarcoma, including liposarcoma, MFH, rhabdomyosarcoma, leiomyosarcoma, MPNST, synovial sarcoma, fibrosarcoma and others. The authors observed cytoplasmic expression of WT1 (6F-H2) in 71% of the cases of malignant peripheral nerve sheath tumors, revealing no association between WT1 expression and overall survival or disease-free survival. Conversely, Ueda et al. [132] reported that the WT1 gene is frequently overexpressed in various types of soft tissue sarcoma [132], and that WT1 mRNA overexpression is significantly associated with a poor prognosis. This result was proved only in 4 out of 52 and 3 out of 36 samples, by immunoblotting [121] and immunohistochemistry. Therefore, further studies on the correlation between the protein and mRNA of the WT1 gene in larger cohorts are required, together with survival analysis, to validate the WT1 expression level as a prognostic factor. Parenti et al. [133] investigated WT1 expression in the MPNST sNF96.2 cell line, showing a strong WT1 staining in the nuclear and perinuclear areas of neoplastic cells. In addition, they studied the effects of silencing WT1 by RNA interference through Western Blot analysis and proliferation assays. The result was a reduction of cell growth in a time- and dose-dependent manner, suggesting that WT1 is involved in the development and progression of MPNSTs, and that it could be a potential therapeutic target for MPNSTs.

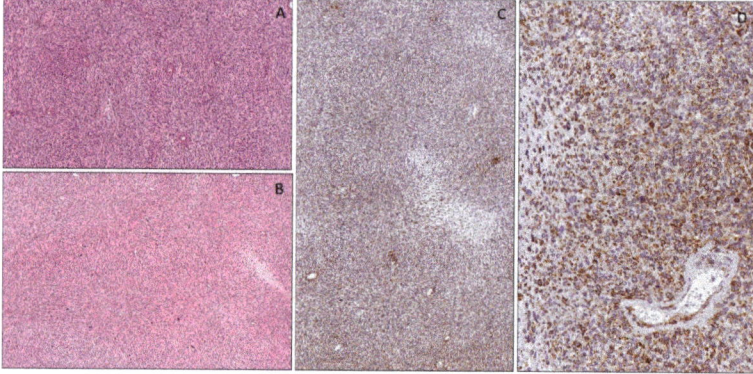

Figure 7. Peripheral nerve sheath tumor consisting of spindle cells arranged in a fascicular pattern (**A,B**). Immunohistochemical cytoplasmic expression of WT1 (*N-terminus*) in neoplastic cells at low (**C**) and high (**D**) magnification.

2.15. WT1 Expression in Desmoplastic Small Round Cell Tumors (DSRCTs)

DSRCTs are highly aggressive tumors, typically with intra-abdominal localization (pelvic peritoneum, mesentery, surface of the liver and omentum), but can arise in many other sites, including meninges, scalp, pleura, paranasal sinuses, parotid gland, pancreas, scrotum, ovary, kidney and bone [134]. These tumors are typical of pediatric and adolescent age, with a male predilection. Histologically, they are composed of round cells with scant cytoplasm, indistinct cell borders and hyperchromatic round to oval, or slightly angulated, nuclei that have finely granular chromatin and small nucleoli. The cells are arranged in variably-sized nests, trabeculae, or lobules, usually separated by a prominent fibro-sclerotic stroma. In some cases, necrosis in the central portion and calcification may be seen. Mitoses are usually observed. In rare cases neoplastic cells with glandular or pseudo-rosettes formation and rhabdoid or signet ring appearance have been reported [134]. Immunohistochemically, the neoplastic cells show a polyphenotypic profile, including desmin, vimentin and epithelial markers, such as epithelial membrane antigen and cytokeratin and WT1 (Figure 8) [134].

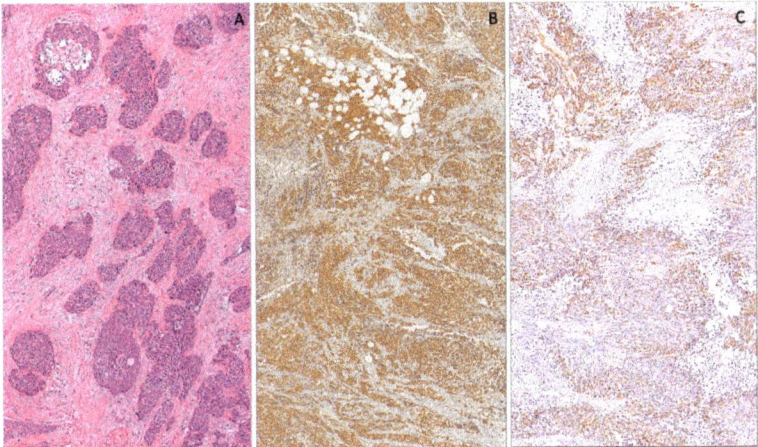

Figure 8. Desmoplastic small round cell tumor showing neoplastic cells arranged in variably-sized nests, separated by a prominent fibro-sclerotic stroma (**A**). Neoplastic cells showing diffuse nuclear expression with WT1 (*C-terminus*) (**B**) and cytoplasmic expression with WT1 (*N-terminus*) (**C**).

In most cases (>90%) of desmoplastic small round cell tumors, strong nuclear staining with antibodies directed against the *C-terminal* portion of WT1 protein (clone WT1 C19), due to a recurrent chromosomal translocation (11;22)(p13;q12) resulting in the EWSR1-WT1 fusion transcript, is observed [134–136]. In rare cases, unusual nuclear WT1 staining with *N-terminus* antibodies was described, and was due, probably, to novel fusion transcripts [35,43,137].

2.16. WT1 Expression in Malignant Rhabdoid Tumors

Malignant rhabdoid tumors are highly aggressive tumors that usually occur in the kidneys of children. Other sites are rarely affected, such as somatic soft tissues, liver, gastrointestinal tract, pelvis, retroperitoneum, abdomen, heart and central nervous system [138]. Interestingly, soft tissue localization prevails in fetuses, newborns and young children, while in adolescents, renal and nervous system sites, they are more frequent [138]. In some cases, tumors are metastatic at presentation and have a fatal course [138]. Histologically, they show solid or trabecular growth patterns composed of round/epithelioid to polygonal cells. Typically, neoplastic cells have abundant, deeply eosinophilic cytoplasm with a paranuclear eosinophilic, PAS-positive inclusion and large, round, vesicular nuclei with finely dispersed chromatin, containing a prominent eosinophilic nucleolus. Mitoses and necrosis are commonly seen. In some cases, minor tumor components consisting of smaller, round, undifferentiated cells with a scant cytoplasmic rim may be present or even prominent. Similarly to desmoplastic small round cell tumors, malignant rhabdoid tumors exhibit polyphenotipic profiles, with variable co-expression of different markers, including vimentin, cytokeratins, epithelial membrane antigen (EMA) and CD99 [138]. However, the complete absence of nuclear immunoreactivity for INI1 protein is the most useful diagnostic clue [139–142]. Tumors can express additional markers, such as muscle specific actin, alpha-smooth muscle actin, S100 protein, synapthophisin, and CD56. Occasionally, WT1 (clone WT-C19) can be expressed at nuclear or nucleo-cytoplasmic levels (Figure 9) [33,34,138]. We have experience of similar results also by using antibodies against the *N-terminal* portion (clone WT 6F-H2) [143].

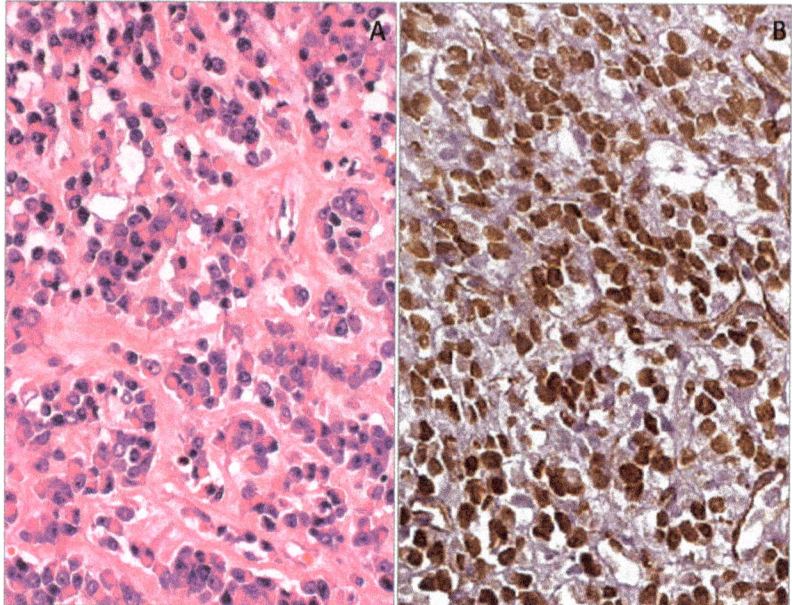

Figure 9. Malignant rhabdoid tumor of the kidney (**A**). Diffuse and strong nuclear WT1 (*N-terminus*) expression of neoplastic cell (**B**).

2.17. WT1 Expression in Rhabdomyosarcomas

Rhabdomyosarcomas (RMSs) are malignant tumors composed of cells that show evidence of skeletal muscle differentiation. Based on morphological, immunohistochemical and molecular features, at least four major subtypes can be recognized: (i) embryonal; (ii) alveolar; (iii) spindle cell/sclerosing; and (iv) pleomorphic. Embryonal, alveolar and spindle cell/sclerosing rhabdomyosarcomas are predominantly tumors of children and adolescents, while the pleomorphic subtype tends to occur in adults. Histologically, the typical pattern of embryonal rhabdomyosarcoma consists of small, round or spindle-shaped cells, admixed with variable numbers of round, strap-, or tadpole-shaped eosinophilic rhabdomyoblasts set in a myxoid stroma. In 20–30% of cases, cytoplasmic cross striations are present. Spindle cell/sclerosing rhabdomyosarcoma most commonly arises in the head and neck or paratesticular soft tissues, and shows a striking male predilection. Alveolar rhabdomyosarcoma is a distinct subtype of rhabdomyosarcoma usually associated with an aggressive behavior. It consists of larger, more rounded, undifferentiated cells with larger nuclei than those in the embryonal variant, admixed with variable numbers of eosinophilic rhabdomyoblasts and multinucleate giant cells with peripheral nuclei. These cells are most often arranged in an alveolar pattern. Spindle cell rhabdomyosarcomas are mainly composed of primitive-looking spindle, ovoid, or round cells, often associated with pseudovascular clefts, embedded in a prominent hyalinized collagenous stroma. Small foci of obvious rhabdomyoblastic differentiation may be evident. Immunohistochemically, regardless of histological type (embryonal, alveolar, spindle/sclerosing), albeit with a variable extension, desmin, myogenin and MyoD1 are considered the most sensitive and specific markers of skeletal muscle differentiation [144]. Several studies have reported a diffuse and strong cytoplasmic expression of WT1 *N-terminus* antibodies (cloneWT 6F-H2) in all variants of rhabdomyosarcomas, including embryonal, sclerosing/spindle cell and alveolar (Figure 10) [35,36,41,45,143,145]. These results are consistent with those reported in studies on WT1 expression in the cytoplasm of human developing myoblasts and myotubes during the early phases of skeletal myogenesis [37,41,42,46,52,146].

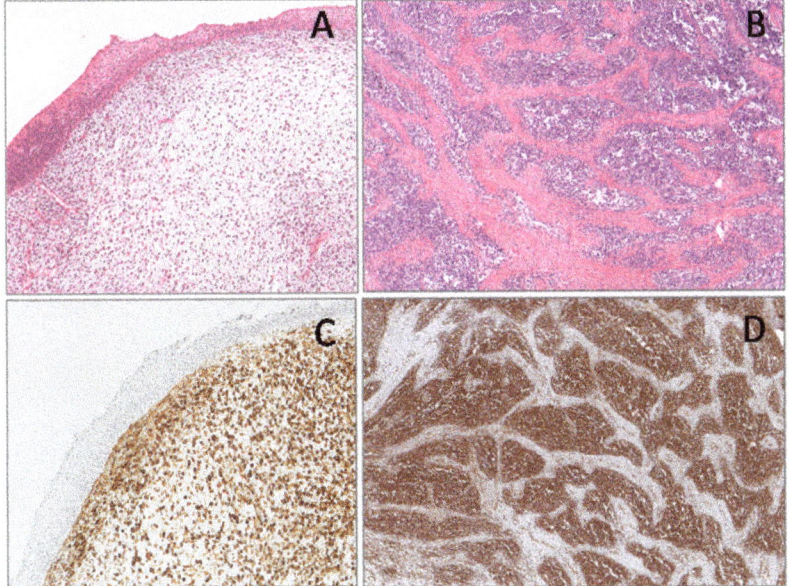

Figure 10. Embryonal rhabdomyosarcoma, botryoid type (**A**) and alveolar rhabdomyosarcoma (**B**). Neoplastic cells showing strong and diffuse cytoplasmic WT1 (*N-terminus*) staining (**C**,**D**).

2.18. WT1 Expression in Neuroblastic Tumors

Neuroblastic tumors arise in children and adolescents. They occur especially in the adrenal gland, retroperitoneum or, and more rarely, in the posterior mediastinum. On the basis of a different degree of differentiation of immature neuroblasts in mature ganglionic cells, three variants of neuroblastic tumors are identified: (i) neuroblastoma in which the schwannian stroma component is poor, including undifferentiated, poorly differentiated and differentiating neuroblastomas; (ii) ganglioneuroblastoma in which the schwannian stroma component is dominant, but foci of neuroblasts are still present, including intermixed and nodular ganglioneuroblastomas; (iii) ganglioneuroma in which the schwannian stroma is predominant and neuroblasts are absent, including maturing and mature ganglioneuromas [147]. Neuroblastoma consist of small, round cells, with scant cytoplasm and round, hyperchromatic nuclei, arranged around a fibrillar area (neuropil). The neuroblastoma is classified as poorly differentiated if ≤5% of the tumor cells show ganglionic differentiation, while, if the neuroblastic component shows ganglionic differentiation in more than 5% of the tumor cells, the neuroblastoma is classified as differentiating; the neuroblastoma is classified as undifferentiated when ganglionic differentiation is almost or completely absent [147]. Ganglioneuroblastoma is a neuroblastic tumor with intermediate features of differentiation between neuroblastoma and ganglioneuroma. Histologically, two variants are recognized, intermixed and nodular. In the former, the ganglioneuromatous component is associated with a collection of immature ganglion cells that are interspersed among the schwannian stroma, while in the latter, in addition to the ganglioneuromatous component, there is a well-circumscribed area of neuroblastoma [147]. When the tumor is composed of mature or maturing ganglion cells surrounded by fascicles of Schwann cells, it is called ganglioneuroma [147]. This tumor model perfectly summarizes what happens during developmental stages of a normal peripheral sympathetic nervous system [148–153]. In some studies, a focal and weak nuclear WT1 staining in neuroblastoma was reported [35,135,145]. Wang et al. showed WT1 expression preferentially in ganglioneuroblastoma and ganglioneuroma [154].

In our experience, by using antibodies against the *N-terminal* portion of the WT1 protein (clone WT6F-H2), a variable cytoplasmic WT1 staining was found only in the ganglion cell component of both ganglioneuroblastoma and ganglioneuroma, while the neuroblastic component was negative (Figure 11) [143].

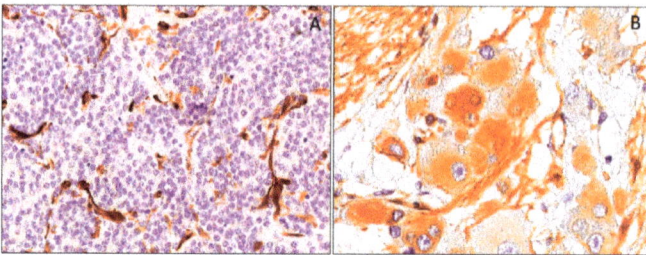

Figure 11. Neoplastic cells of poorly-differentiated neuroblastoma showing no immunohistochemical expression of WT1 (*N-terminus*) (**A**). Ganglion cell of a maturing ganglioneuroma showing heterogeneous cytoplasmic WT1 (*N-terminus*) expression (**B**).

2.19. Infantile-Type Fibromatoses

Young-type fibromatoses are a group of fibroblastic and myofibroblastic tumor and tumor-like lesions occurring in the soft tissues of children and adolescents. This group includes the fibrous hamartoma of infancy, myofibroma/myofibromatosis and lipofibromatosis. The biological behavior of these lesions is variable, with lesions showing a benign course such as fibrous hamartomatous of infancy, and lesions with a tendency to local recurrence such as myofibroma/myofibromatosis and lipofibromatosis. Although each of these entities exhibits characteristic morphological features, differential diagnostic problems may arise especially from small biopsy specimens. Interesting results have emerged from the study of WT1 in these lesions. All cases of young-type fibromatoses, including fibrous hamartoma of infancy, myofibroma/myofibromatosis and lipofibromatosis, exhibited a diffuse WT1 cytoplasmic staining. On the contrary, all cases of adult-type fibromatoses and nodular fasciitis, from which young-type fibromatoses are to be distinguished, are not immunoreactive for WT1 [39]. Amini Nik et al. [15], investigated the expression of WT1 mRNA and protein in desmoid-type fibromatoses. They found that the levels of WT1 mRNA, revealed by TaqMan quantitative PCR, in all examined miofibroblastic tumor cells, were from medium to high, while contiguous normal fibroblasts exhibited a lower expression. WT1 protein overexpression was confirmed by Western blot and immunohistochemistry analyses. These data suggest that WT1 may play a role in the tumorigenesis of desmoid-type fibromatoses.

2.20. Congenital/Infantile Fibrosarcoma

This is a malignant tumor currently classified in the category of intermediate neoplasms. It occurs in the first two years of life, with a significant number of cases diagnosed at birth or antenatally [155]. It occurs in the soft tissues of the trunk and distal extremities, with only rare cases reported in the retroperitoneum. Distant metastases rarely occur and when they do, prognosis is favorable [155]. Histologically, it shows a fascicular pattern, focally with a herring-bone configuration; it consists predominantly of spindle cells showing only a mild to focally moderate degree of nuclear atypia. Mitoses are usually numerous. The diagnosis of fibrosarcoma is frequently of exclusion, being mainly based on negative results for specific lineage markers such as desmin, myogenin, CD34, S-100, HMB-45, and cytokeratins. Fibrosarcoma may variably express, even if with focal extension, alpha-smooth muscle actin and/or desmin. We recently reported a series of congenital/infantile fibrosarcoma with a strong and diffuse cytoplasmic expression of WT1 by using antibodies against the *N-terminal* portion of the WT1 protein (cloneWT6F-H2) (Figure 12) [39,143]. Then the WT1 protein could be useful as an immunomarker to support a diagnosis of fibrosarcoma, mostly in daily practice, in distinguishing congenital/infantile fibrosarcoma from desmoid-type fibromatosis.

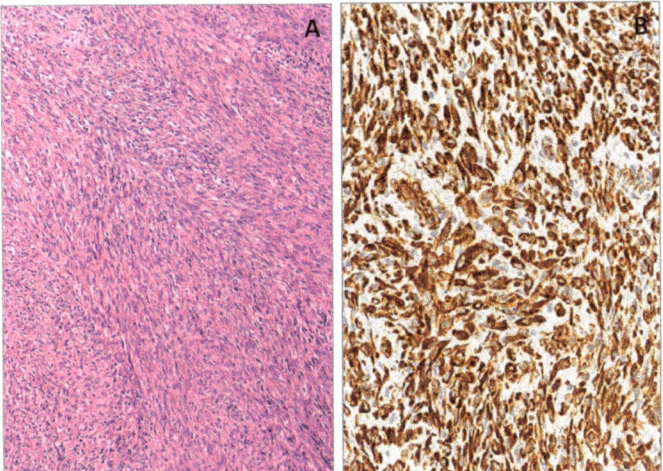

Figure 12. Congenital/infantile fibrosarcoma with herring-bone configuration (**A**). Neoplastic cells showing diffuse cytoplasmic WT1 (*N-terminus*) expression (**B**).

Although both tumors may show overlapping morphological and immunohistochemical features (expression of alpha-smooth muscle actin), desmoid-type fibromatosis is typically WT1-negative. However, the diagnosis of congenital/infantile fibrosarcoma is usually confirmed by the identification of the recurrent translocation t (12;15)(p13;q25) with an ETV6-NTRK3 gene fusion [156,157].

2.21. WT1 Expression in Vascular Tumors

Vascular lesions are a heterogeneous group of tumors, including benign and malignant tumors, as well as malformations. Vascular tumors and malformations can be diagnostically challenging. Although they may initially appear very similar, they have distinct clinical courses and management. To provide a correct diagnosis, several studies have been conducted to identify immunohistochemical markers. Among the antibodies studied, interesting results have emerged from the study of WT1 cytoplasmic expression. Based on the studies available in the literature that compare vascular lesions, both benign and malignant, with malformations, it emerged that almost all benign lesions, such as capillary hemangioma, pyogenic granulomas, cherry angiomas and tufted angiomas, are WT1-positive, while lymphangioma and cavernous hemangioma are negative. Malignant tumors, such as angiosarcomas, hemangioendotheliomas and Kaposi's sarcomas, are strongly WT1-positive (Figure 13). WT-1 expression in vascular malformations (angiokeratoma/verrucous hemangioma, combined vascular malformations, venous malformations, glomuvenous malformations, lymphatic malformations/lymphangioma, telangiectasia and targetoid hemosiderotic hemangioma) is generally completely negative or weak and focal positive. Interestingly, a strong and diffuse WT-1 staining was reported in a case of thrombosed vascular malformation with prominent endothelial hyperplasia [158–160]. WT1 expression in vascular tumors was also analyzed in fetal tissues, where a moderate to strong staining intensity in the cytoplasm of the endothelial cells of blood vessels was reported [37,52]. As WT1 staining has been obtained in the cytoplasm of embryonal/fetal endothelial cells, the reported cytoplasmic expression of this marker in many vascular tumors is not at all surprising.

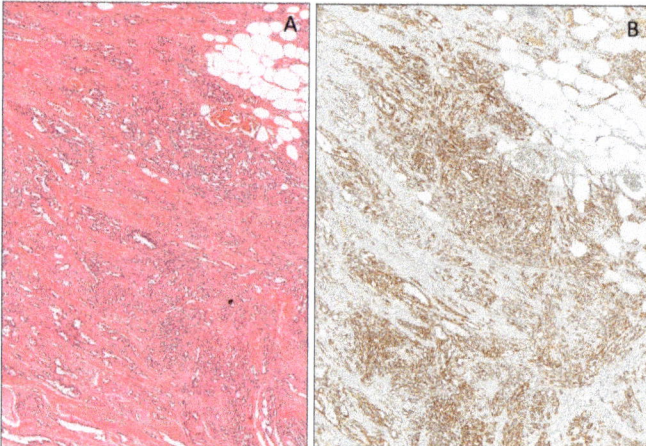

Figure 13. Angiosarcoma (**A**). Diffuse nuclear expression of WT1 (*N-terminus*) in neoplastic cells (**B**).

2.22. Mammary Myofibroblastoma, Epithelioid Cell Variant

Myofibroblastomais a rare, benign tumor composed of both fibroblastic and myofibroblastic cells [161–163], which localizes typically in the breast [163], vulvovaginal region [164,165] and soft tissues. It is composed of a proliferation of bland-looking spindle-shaped cells to epithelioid cells set in a predominant fibrous stroma. When the epithelioid cell component predominates, the myofibroblastoma is referred to as "epithelioid". It was observed that WT1 expression is limited to epithelioid-type myofibroblastoma, while all other variants (classic-type, collagenized/fibrotic-type, myxoid-type, lipomatous-type and palisaded/Schwannian-like) are completely negative [40]. Indeed, all cases reported of epithelioid-type myofibroblastomas exhibited a diffuse and strong WT1 cytoplasmic expression. In the evaluation of small breast biopsies, WT1 is an important marker, together with desmin, alpha-smooth muscle actin, Myogenin, MyoD1, h-caldesmon, S-100 protein, HMB45, EMA, Pancytokeratins and CD34, which are helpful in the differential diagnosis of lesions with epithelioid morphology.

Supplementary Materials: The supplementary materials are available online at http://www.mdpi.com/2076-3417/10/1/40/s1.

Author Contributions: Conceptualization, L.S. and G.M. (Gaetano Magro); Data curation, L.S., G.C., R.P., G.M.V., L.P., R.C., G.M. (Giuseppe Musumeci), G.M. (Gaetano Magro); Methodology, L.S., G.M.V. and G.M. (Gaetano Magro); Resources, G.M. (Gaetano Magro); Writing—original draft, L.S.; Writing—review & editing, L.S. and G.M. (Gaetano Magro). All authors have read and agreed to the published version of the manuscript.

Funding: This research received no external funding.

Conflicts of Interest: The authors declare no conflict of interest.

References

1. Call, K.M.; Glaser, T.; Ito, C.Y.; Buckler, A.J.; Pelletier, J.; Haber, D.A.; Rose, E.A.; Kral, A.; Yeger, H.; Lewis, W.H. Isolation and characterization of a zinc finger polypeptide gene at the human chromosome 11 Wilms' tumor locus. *Cell* **1990**, *60*, 509–520. [CrossRef]
2. Haber, D.A.; Buckler, A.J.; Glaser, T.; Call, K.M.; Pelletier, J.; Sohn, R.L.; Douglass, E.C.; Housman, D.E. An internal deletion within an 11p13 zinc finger gene contributes to the development of Wilms' tumor. *Cell* **1990**, *61*, 1257–1269. [CrossRef]
3. Gessler, M.; Poustka, A.; Cavenee, W.; Neve, R.L.; Orkin, S.H.; Bruns, G.A. Homozygous deletion in Wilms' tumours of a zinc-finger gene identified by chromosome jumping. *Nature* **1990**, *343*, 774–778. [CrossRef] [PubMed]

4. Mrowka, C.; Schedl, A. Wilms' tumor suppressor gene WT1: From structure to renal pathophysiologic features. *J. Am. Soc. Nephrol.* **2000**, *11* (Suppl. S16), S106–S115. [PubMed]
5. Bruening, W.; Pelletier, J. A non-AUG translational initiation event generates novel WT1 isoforms. *J. Biol. Chem.* **1996**, *271*, 8646–8654. [CrossRef] [PubMed]
6. Scharnhorst, V.; Dekker, P.; van der Eb, A.J.; Jochemsen, A.G. Internal translation initiation generates novel WT1 protein isoforms with distinct biological properties. *J. Biol. Chem.* **1999**, *274*, 23456–23462. [CrossRef]
7. Haber, D.A.; Sohn, R.L.; Buckler, A.J.; Pelletier, J.; Call, K.M.; Housman, D.E. Alternative splicing and genomic structure of the Wilms' tumor gene WT1. *Proc. Natl. Acad. Sci. USA* **1991**, *88*, 9618–9622. [CrossRef]
8. Sharma, P.M.; Bowman, M.; Madden, S.L.; Rauscher, F.J., 3rd; Sukumar, S. RNA editing in the Wilms' tumor susceptibility gene, WT1. *Genes. Dev.* **1994**, *8*, 720–731. [CrossRef]
9. Miwa, H.; Beran, M.; Saunders, G.F. Expression of the Wilms' tumor gene (WT1) in human leukemias. *Leukemia* **1992**, *6*, 405–409.
10. Oji, Y.; Ogawa, H.; Tamaki, H.; Oka, Y.; Tsuboi, A.; Kim, E.H.; Soma, T.; Tatekawa, T.; Kawakami, M.; Asada, M.; et al. Expression of the Wilms' tumor gene WT1 in solid tumors and its involvement in tumor cell growth. *Jpn. J. Cancer Res.* **1999**, *90*, 194–204. [CrossRef]
11. Oji, Y.; Miyoshi, S.; Maeda, H.; Hayashi, S.; Tamaki, H.; Nakatsuka, S.; Yao, M.; Takahashi, E.; Nakano, Y.; Hirabayashi, H.; et al. Overexpression of the Wilms' tumor gene WT1 in de novo lung cancers. *Int. J. Cancer* **2002**, *100*, 297–303. [CrossRef] [PubMed]
12. Koesters, R.; Linnebacher, M.; Coy, J.F.; Germann, A.; Schwitalle, Y.; Findeisen, P.; von Knebel Doeberitz, M. WT1 is a tumor-associated antigen in colon cancer that can be recognized by in vitro stimulated cytotoxic T cells. *Int. J. Cancer* **2004**, *109*, 385–392. [CrossRef] [PubMed]
13. Oji, Y.; Nakamori, S.; Fujikawa, M.; Nakatsuka, S.; Yokota, A.; Tatsumi, N.; Abeno, S.; Ikeba, A.; Takashima, S.; Tsujie, M.; et al. Overexpression of the Wilms' tumor gene WT1 in pancreatic ductal adenocarcinoma. *Cancer Sci.* **2004**, *95*, 583–587. [CrossRef] [PubMed]
14. Loeb, D.M.; Evron, E.; Patel, C.B.; Sharma, P.M.; Niranjan, B.; Buluwela, L.; Weitzman, S.A.; Korz, D.; Sukumar, S. Wilms' tumor suppressor gene (WT1) is expressed in primary breast tumors despite tumor-specific promoter methylation. *Cancer Res.* **2001**, *61*, 921–925.
15. Amini Nik, S.; Hohenstein, P.; Jadidizadeh, A.; Van Dam, K.; Bastidas, A.; Berry, R.L.; Patek, C.E.; Van der Schueren, B.; Cassiman, J.J.; Tejpar, S. Upregulation of Wilms' tumor gene 1 (WT1) in desmoid tumors. *Int. J. Cancer* **2005**, *114*, 202–208. [CrossRef]
16. Shimizu, M.; Toki, T.; Takagi, Y.; Konishi, I.; Fujii, S. Immunohistochemical detection of the Wilms' tumor gene (WT1) in epithelial ovarian tumors. *Int. J. Gynecol. Pathol.* **2000**, *19*, 158–163. [CrossRef]
17. Andersson, C.; Oji, Y.; Ohlson, N.; Wang, S.; Li, X.; Ottander, U.; Lundin, E.; Sugiyama, H.; Li, A. Prognostic significance of specific anti-WT1 IgG antibody level in plasma in patients with ovarian carcinoma. *Cancer Med.* **2014**, *3*, 909–918. [CrossRef]
18. Oji, Y.; Suzuki, T.; Nakano, Y.; Maruno, M.; Nakatsuka, S.; Jomgeow, T.; Abeno, S.; Tatsumi, N.; Yokota, A.; Aoyagi, S.; et al. Overexpression of the Wilms' tumor gene WT1 in primary astrocytic tumors. *Cancer Sci.* **2004**, *95*, 822–827. [CrossRef]
19. Menssen, H.D.; Bertelmann, E.; Bartelt, S.; Schmidt, R.A.; Pecher, G.; Schramm, K.; Thiel, E. Wilms' tumor gene (WT1) expression in lung cancer, colon cancer and glioblastoma cell lines compared to freshly isolated tumor specimens. *J. Cancer Res. Clin. Oncol.* **2000**, *126*, 226–232. [CrossRef]
20. Athale, U.H.; Shurtleff, S.A.; Jenkins, J.J.; Poquette, C.A.; Tan, M.; Downing, J.R.; Pappo, A.S. Use of reverse transcriptase polymerase chain reaction for diagnosis and staging of alveolar rhabdomyosarcoma, Ewing sarcoma family of tumors, and desmoplastic small round cell tumor. *J. Pediatr. Hematol. Oncol.* **2001**, *23*, 99–104. [CrossRef]
21. Wagner, N.; Michiels, J.F.; Schedl, A.; Wagner, K.D. The Wilms' tumour suppressor WT1 is involved in endothelial cell proliferation and migration: Expression in tumour vessels in vivo. *Oncogene* **2008**, *27*, 3662–3672. [CrossRef] [PubMed]
22. Wagner, K.D.; Cherfils-Vicini, J.; Hosen, N.; Hohenstein, P.; Gilson, E.; Hastie, N.D.; Michiels, J.F.; Wagner, N. The Wilms' tumour suppressor Wt1 is a major regulator of tumour angiogenesis and progression. *Nat. Commun.* **2014**, *5*, 5852. [CrossRef] [PubMed]
23. Lee, S.B.; Haber, D.A. Wilms tumor and the WT1 gene. *Exp. Cell. Res.* **2001**, *264*, 74–99. [CrossRef] [PubMed]

24. Little, M.; Holmes, G.; Walsh, P. WT1: What has the last decade told us? *Bioessays* **1999**, *21*, 191–202. [CrossRef]
25. Davies, R.; Moore, A.; Schedl, A.; Bratt, E.; Miyahawa, K.; Ladomery, M.; Miles, C.; Menke, A.; van Heyningen, V.; Hastie, N. Multiple roles for the Wilms' tumor suppressor, WT1. *Cancer Res.* **1999**, *59*, 1747s–1750s.
26. Hastie, N.D. Life, sex, and WT1 isoforms–three amino acids can make all the difference. *Cell* **2001**, *106*, 391–394. [CrossRef]
27. Niksic, M.; Slight, J.; Sanford, J.R.; Caceres, J.F.; Hastie, N.D. The Wilms' tumour protein (WT1) shuttles between nucleus and cytoplasm and is present in functional polysomes. *Hum. Mol. Genet.* **2004**, *13*, 463–471. [CrossRef]
28. Scholz, H.; Kirschner, K.M. A role for the Wilms' tumor protein WT1 in organ development. *Physiology* **2005**, *20*, 54–59. [CrossRef]
29. Roberts, S.G. Transcriptional regulation by WT1 in development. *Curr. Opin. Genet. Dev.* **2005**, *15*, 542–547. [CrossRef]
30. Hohenstein, P.; Hastie, N.D. The many facets of the Wilms' tumour gene, WT1. *Hum. Mol. Genet.* **2006**, *15*, 196–201. [CrossRef]
31. Wagner, K.D.; El Maï, M.; Ladomery, M.; Belali, T.; Leccia, N.; Michiels, J.F.; Wagner, N. Altered VEGF splicing isoform balance in tumor endothelium involves activation of splicing factors Srpk1 and Srsf1 by the Wilms' tumor suppressor Wt1. *Cells* **2019**, *8*, 41. [CrossRef] [PubMed]
32. Amin, E.M.; Oltean, S.; Hua, J.; Gammons, M.V.; Hamdollah-Zadeh, M.; Welsh, G.I.; Cheung, M.K.; Ni, L.; Kase, S.; Rennel, E.S.; et al. WT1 mutants reveal SRPK1 to be a downstream angiogenesis target by altering VEGF splicing. *Cancer Cell* **2011**, *20*, 768–780. [CrossRef] [PubMed]
33. Ramani, P.; Cowell, J.K. The expression pattern of Wilms' tumour gene (WT1) product in normal tissues and paediatric renal tumours. *J. Pathol.* **1996**, *179*, 162–168. [CrossRef]
34. Charles, A.K.; Mall, S.; Watson, J.; Berry, P.J. Expression of the Wilms' tumour gene WT1 in the developing human and in paediatric renal tumours: An immunohistochemical study. *Mol. Pathol.* **1997**, *50*, 138–144. [CrossRef] [PubMed]
35. Carpentieri, D.F.; Nichols, K.; Chou, P.M.; Matthews, M.; Pawel, B.; Huff, D. The expression of WT1 in the differentiation of rhabdomyosarcoma from other pediatric small round blue cell tumors. *Mod. Pathol.* **2002**, *15*, 1080–1086. [CrossRef] [PubMed]
36. Bisceglia, M.; Vairo, M.; Galliani, C.; Lastilla, G.; Parafioriti, A.; De Maglio, G. Immunohistochemical investigation of WT1 expression in 117 embryonal tumors. *Pathologica* **2011**, *103*, 182–183.
37. Parenti, R.; Perris, R.; Vecchio, G.M.; Salvatorelli, L.; Torrisi, A.; Gravina, L.; Magro, G. Immunohistochemical expression of Wilms' tumor protein (WT1) in developing human epithelial and mesenchymal tissues. *Acta Histochem.* **2013**, *115*, 70–75. [CrossRef]
38. Parenti, R.; Puzzo, L.; Vecchio, G.M.; Gravina, L.; Salvatorelli, L.; Musumeci, G.; Vasquez, E.; Magro, G. Immunolocalization of Wilms' Tumor protein (WT1) in developing human peripheral sympathetic and gastroenteric nervous system. *Acta Histochem.* **2014**, *116*, 48–54. [CrossRef]
39. Magro, G.; Salvatorelli, L.; Vecchio, G.M.; Musumeci, G.; Rita, A.; Parenti, R. Cytoplasmic expression of Wilms' tumor transcription factor-1 (WT1): A useful immunomarker for young-type fibromatoses and infantile fibrosarcoma. *Acta Histochem.* **2014**, *116*, 1134–1140. [CrossRef]
40. Magro, G.; Longo, F.; Salvatorelli, L.; Vecchio, G.M.; Parenti, R. Wilms' tumor protein (WT1) in mammary myofibroblastoma: An immunohistochemical study. *Acta Histochem.* **2014**, *116*, 905–910. [CrossRef]
41. Magro, G.; Salvatorelli, L.; Puzzo, L.; Musumeci, G.; Bisceglia, M.; Parenti, R. Oncofetal expression of Wilms' tumor 1 (WT1) protein in human fetal, adult and neoplastic skeletal muscle tissues. *Acta Histochem.* **2015**, *117*, 492–504. [CrossRef] [PubMed]
42. Magro, G.; Longo, F.R.; Angelico, G.; Spadola, S.; Amore, F.F.; Salvatorelli, L. Immunohistochemistry as potential diagnostic pitfall in the most common solid tumors of children and adolescents. *Acta Histochem.* **2015**, *117*, 397–414. [CrossRef] [PubMed]
43. Nakatsuka, S.; Oji, Y.; Horiuchi, T.; Kanda, T.; Kitagawa, M.; Takeuchi, T.; Kawano, K.; Kuwae, Y.; Yamauchi, A.; Okumura, M.; et al. Immunohistochemical detection of WT1 protein in a variety of cancer cells. *Mod. Pathol.* **2006**, *19*, 804–814. [CrossRef] [PubMed]

44. Schittenhelm, J.; Thiericke, J.; Nagel, C.; Meyermann, R.; Beschorner, R. WT1 expression in normal and neoplastic cranial and peripheral nerves is independent of grade of malignancy. *Cancer Biomark.* **2010**, *7*, 73–77. [CrossRef] [PubMed]
45. Bisceglia, M.; Magro, G.; Carosi, I.; Cannazza, V.; Ben Dor, D. Primary embryonal rhabdomyosarcoma of the prostate in adults: Report of a case and review of the literature. *Int. J. Surg. Pathol.* **2011**, *19*, 831–837. [CrossRef]
46. Salvatorelli, L.; Bisceglia, M.; Vecchio, G.; Parenti, R.; Galliani, C.; Alaggio, R. A comparative immunohistochemical study of oncofetalcy-toplasmic WT1 expression in human fetal, adult and neoplasticskeletal muscle. *Pathologica* **2011**, *103*, 186.
47. Singh, A.; Mishra, A.K.; Ylaya, K.; Hewitt, S.M.; Sharma, K.C.; Saxena, S. Wilms' tumor-1, claudin-1 and ezrin are useful immunohistochemical markers that help to distinguish schwannoma from fibroblastic meningioma. *Pathol. Oncol. Res.* **2012**, *18*, 383–389. [CrossRef]
48. Pritchard-Jones, K.; Fleming, S.; Davidson, D.; Bickmore, W.; Porteous, D.; Gosden, C.; Bard, J.; Buckler, A.; Pelletier, J.; Housman, D. The candidate Wilms' tumour gene is involved in genitourinary development. *Nature* **1990**, *346*, 194–197. [CrossRef]
49. Sharma, P.M.; Yang, X.; Bowman, M.; Roberts, V.; Sukumar, S. Molecular-cloning of rat Wilms' tumor complementary DNA and a study of messenger RNA expression in the urogenital system and the brain. *Cancer Res.* **1992**, *52*, 6407–6412.
50. Armstrong, J.F.; Pritchard-Jones, K.; Bickmore, W.A.; Hastie, N.D.; Bard, J.B. The expression of the Wilms' tumour gene, WT1, in the developing mammalian embryo. *Mech. Dev.* **1993**, *4*, 85–97. [CrossRef]
51. Mundlos, S.; Pelletier, J.; Darveau, A.; Bachmann, M.; Winterpacht, A.; Zabel, B. Nuclear localization of the protein encoded by the Wilms' tumor gene WT1 in embryonic and adult tissues. *Development* **1993**, *119*, 1329–1341. [PubMed]
52. Parenti, R.; Salvatorelli, L.; Musumeci, G.; Parenti, C.; Giorlandino, A.; Motta, F.; Magro, G. Wilms' tumor 1 (WT1) protein expression in human developing tissues. *Acta Histochem.* **2015**, *117*, 386–396. [CrossRef] [PubMed]
53. Davies, J.A.; Ladomery, M.; Hohenstein, P.; Michael, L.; Shafe, A.; Spraggon, L.; Hastie, N. Development of an siRNA-based method for repressing specific genes in renal organ culture and its use to show that the Wt1 tumour suppressor is required for nephron differentiation. *Hum. Mol. Genet.* **2004**, *13*, 235–246. [CrossRef] [PubMed]
54. Miller-Hodges, E.; Hohenstein, P. WT1 in disease: Shifting the epithelial-mesenchymal balance. *J. Pathol.* **2012**, *226*, 229–240. [CrossRef]
55. Kreidberg, J.A.; Sariola, H.; Loring, J.M.; Maeda, M.; Pelletier, J.; Housman, D.; Jaenisch, R. WT-1 is required for early kidney development. *Cell* **1993**, *74*, 679–691. [CrossRef]
56. Wagner, N.; Wagner, K.D.; Scholz, H.; Kirschner, K.M.; Schedl, A. Intermediate filament protein nestin is expressed in developing kidney and heart and might be regulated by the Wilms' tumor suppressor Wt1. *Am. J. Physiol. Regul. Integr. Comp. Physiol.* **2006**, *291*, R779–R787. [CrossRef]
57. Wagner, K.D.; Wagner, N.; Vidal, V.P.; Schley, G.; Wilhelm, D.; Schedl, A.; Englert, C.; Scholz, H. The Wilms' tumor gene Wt1 is required for normal development of the retina. *EMBO J.* **2002**, *21*, 1398–1405. [CrossRef]
58. Clark, A.J.; Ware, J.L.; Chen, M.Y.; Graf, M.R.; Van Meter, T.E.; Dos Santos, W.G.; Fillmore, H.L.; Broaddus, W.C. Effect of WT1 gene silencing on the tumorigenicity of human glioblastoma multiforme cells. *J. Neurosurg.* **2010**, *112*, 18–25. [CrossRef]
59. Johannessen, C.M.; Reczek, E.E.; James, M.F.; Brems, H.; Legius, E.; Cichowski, K. The NF1 tumor suppressor critically regulates TSC2 and mTOR. *Proc. Natl. Acad. Sci. USA* **2005**, *102*, 8573–8578. [CrossRef]
60. Moore, A.W.; McInnes, L.; Kreidberg, J.; Hastie, N.D.; Schedl, A. YAC complementation shows a requirement for Wt1 in the development of epicardium, adrenal gland and throughout nephrogenesis. *Development* **1999**, *126*, 1845–1857.
61. Martínez-Estrada, O.M.; Lettice, L.A.; Essafi, A.; Guadix, J.A.; Slight, J.; Velecela, V.; Hall, E.; Reichmann, J.; Devenney, P.S.; Hohenstein, P.; et al. Wt1 is required for cardiovascular progenitor cell formation through transcriptional control of Snail and E-cadherin. *Nat. Genet.* **2010**, *42*, 89–93. [CrossRef] [PubMed]
62. Wagner, N.; Wagner, K.D.; Theres, H.; Englert, C.; Schedl, A.; Scholz, H. Coronary vessel development requires activation of the TrkB neurotrophin receptor by the Wilms' tumor transcription factor Wt1. *Genes Dev.* **2005**, *19*, 2631–2642. [CrossRef] [PubMed]

63. Chau, Y.Y.; Hastie, N.D. The role of Wt1 in regulating mesenchyme in cancer, development, and tissue homeostasis. *Trends Genet.* **2012**, *28*, 515–524. [CrossRef] [PubMed]
64. Al-Hussain, T.; Ali, A.; Akhtar, M. Wilms tumor: An update. *Adv. Anat. Pathol.* **2014**, *21*, 166–173. [CrossRef] [PubMed]
65. Beckwith, J.B. Wilms' tumor and other renal tumors of childhood: A selective review from the National Wilms' Tumor Study Pathology Center. *Hum. Pathol.* **1983**, *14*, 481–492. [CrossRef]
66. Charles, A.K.; Brown, K.W.; Berry, P.J. Microdissecting the genetic events in nephrogenic rests and Wilms' tumor development. *Am. J. Pathol.* **1998**, *153*, 991–1000. [CrossRef]
67. Marsden, H.B.; Lawler, W. Primary renal tumours in the first year of life. A population based review. *Virchows. Arch. A Pathol. Anat. Histopathol.* **1983**, *399*, 1–9.
68. Garvin, A.J.; Surrette, F.; Hintz, D.S.; Rudisill, M.T.; Sens, M.A.; Sens, D.A. The in vitro growth and characterization of the skeletal muscle component of Wilms' tumor. *Am. J. Pathol.* **1985**, *121*, 298–310.
69. Wigger, H.J. Fetal rhabdomyomatous nephroblastoma-a variant of Wilms' tumor. *Hum. Pathol.* **1976**, *7*, 613–623. [CrossRef]
70. Attanoos, R.L.; Gibbs, A.R. Pathology of malignant mesothelioma. *Histopathology* **1997**, *30*, 403–418. [CrossRef]
71. McCaughey, W.T.; Al-Jabi, M. Differentiation of serosal hyperplasia and neoplasia in biopsies. *Pathol. Annu.* **1986**, *21*, 271–293. [PubMed]
72. Klebe, S.; Brownlee, S.A.; Mahar, A.; Burchette, J.L.; Sporn, T.A.; Vollmer, R.T.; Roggli, V.L. Sarcomatoid mesothelioma: A clinical-pathologic correlation of 326 cases. *Mod. Pathol.* **2010**, *23*, 470–479. [CrossRef] [PubMed]
73. Oates, J.; Edwards, C. HBME-1, MOC-31, WT1 and calretinin: An assessment of recently described markers for mesothelioma and adenocarcinoma. *Histopathology* **2000**, *36*, 341–347. [CrossRef] [PubMed]
74. Ordóñez, N.G. Value of thyroid transcription factor-1, E-cadherin, BG8, WT1, and CD44S immunostaining in distinguishing epithelial pleural mesothelioma from pulmonary and non pulmonary adenocarcinoma. *Am. J. Surg. Pathol.* **2000**, *24*, 598–606. [CrossRef]
75. Ordóñez, N.G. The immunohistochemical diagnosis of mesothelioma: A comparative study of epithelioid mesothelioma and lung adenocarcinoma. *Am. J. Surg. Pathol.* **2003**, *27*, 1031–1051. [CrossRef]
76. Ordóñez, N.G. The diagnostic utility of immunohistochemistry in distinguishing between mesothelioma and renal cell carcinoma: A comparative study. *Hum. Pathol.* **2004**, *35*, 697–710. [CrossRef]
77. Kushitani, K.; Takeshima, Y.; Amatya, V.J.; Furonaka, O.; Sakatani, A.; Inai, K. Differential diagnosis of sarcomatoid mesothelioma from true sarcoma and sarcomatoid carcinoma using immunohistochemistry. *Pathol. Int.* **2008**, *58*, 75–83. [CrossRef]
78. Tsuta, K.; Kato, Y.; Tochigi, N.; Hoshino, T.; Takeda, Y.; Hosako, M.; Maeshima, A.M.; Asamura, H.; Kondo, T.; Matsuno, Y. Comparison of different clones (WT49 versus 6F-H2) of WT-1 antibodies for immunohistochemical diagnosis of malignant pleural mesothelioma. *Appl. Immunohistochem. Mol. Morphol.* **2009**, *17*, 126–130. [CrossRef]
79. Harwood, T.R.; Gracey, D.R.; Yokoo, H. Pseudomesotheliomatous carcinoma of the lung. A variant of peripheral lung. *Cancer Am. J. Clin. Pathol.* **1976**, *65*, 159–167. [CrossRef]
80. Goldstein, N.S.; Bassi, D.; Uzieblo, A. WT1 is an integral component of an antibody panel to distinguish pancreaticobiliary and some ovarian epithelial neoplasms. *Am. J. Clin. Pathol.* **2001**, *116*, 246–252. [CrossRef]
81. Lee, B.H.; Hecht, J.L.; Pinkus, J.L.; Pinkus, G.S. WT1, estrogen receptor, and progesterone receptor as markers for breast or ovarian primary sites in metastatic adenocarcinoma to body fluids. *Am. J. Clin. Pathol.* **2002**, *117*, 745–750. [CrossRef]
82. Hashi, A.; Yuminamochi, T.; Murata, S.; Iwamoto, H.; Honda, T.; Hoshi, K. Wilms' tumor gene immunoreactivity in primary serous carcinomas of the fallopian tube, ovary, endometrium, and peritoneum. *Int. J. Gynecol. Pathol.* **2003**, *22*, 374–377. [CrossRef]
83. Logani, S.; Oliva, E.; Amin, M.B.; Folpe, A.L.; Cohen, C.; Young, R.H. Immunoprofile of ovarian tumors with putative transitional cell (urothelial) differentiation using novel urothelial markers: Histogenetic and diagnostic implications. *Am. J. Surg. Pathol.* **2003**, *27*, 1434–1441. [CrossRef]
84. Hecht, J.L.; Lee, B.H.; Pinkus, J.L.; Pinkus, G.S. The value of Wilms' tumor susceptibility gene 1 in cytologic preparations as a marker for malignant mesothelioma. *Cancer* **2002**, *96*, 105–109. [CrossRef]
85. Goldstein, N.S.; Uzieblo, A. WT1 immunoreactivity in uterine papillary serous carcinomas is different from ovarian serous carcinomas. *Am. J. Clin. Pathol.* **2002**, *117*, 541–545. [CrossRef]

86. Al-Hussaini, M.; Stockman, A.; Foster, H.; McCluggage, W.G. WT-1 assists in distinguishing ovarian from uterine serous carcinoma and in distinguishing between serous and endometrioid ovarian carcinoma. *Histopathology* **2004**, *44*, 109–115. [CrossRef]
87. Acs, G.; Pasha, T.; Zhang, P.J. WT1 is differentially expressed in serous, endometrioid, clear cell, and mucinous carcinomas of the peritoneum, fallopian tube, ovary, and endometrium. *Int. J. Gynecol. Pathol.* **2004**, *23*, 110–118. [CrossRef]
88. Gilks, C.B. Subclassification of ovarian surface epithelial tumors based on correlation of histologic and molecular pathologic data. *Int. J. Gynecol. Pathol.* **2004**, *23*, 200–205. [CrossRef]
89. Waldstrøm, M.; Grove, A. Immunohistochemical expression of Wilms' tumor gene protein in different histologic subtypes of ovarian carcinomas. *Arch. Pathol. Lab. Med.* **2005**, *129*, 85–88.
90. Taube, E.T.; Denkert, C.; Sehouli, J.; Kunze, C.A.; Dietel, M.; Braicu, I.; Letsch, A.; Darb-Esfahani, S. Wilms' tumor protein 1 (WT1)—Not only a diagnostic but also a prognostic marker in high-grade serous ovarian carcinoma. *Gynecol. Oncol.* **2016**, *140*, 494–502. [CrossRef]
91. Norris, H.J.; Taylor, H.B. Prognosis of granulosa-theca tumors of the ovary. *Cancer* **1968**, *21*, 255–263. [CrossRef]
92. Young, R.H.; Scully, R.E. Ovarian sex cord-stromal tumors with bizarre nuclei: A clinicopathologic analysis of 17 cases. *Int. J. Gynecol. Pathol.* **1983**, *1*, 325–335. [CrossRef]
93. Gaffey, M.J.; Frierson, H.F., Jr.; Iezzoni, J.C.; Mills, S.E.; Clement, P.B.; Gersell, D.J.; Shashi, V.; von Kap-Herr, C.; Young, R.H. Ovarian granulosa cell tumors with bizarre nuclei: An immunohistochemical analysis with fluorescence in situ hybridization documenting trisomy 12 in the bizarre component [corrected]. *Mod. Pathol.* **1996**, *9*, 308–315.
94. Young, R.H. Sex cord-stromal tumors of the ovary and testis: Their similarities and differences with consideration of selected problems. *Mod. Pathol.* **2005**, *18*, S81–S98. [CrossRef]
95. Arora, D.S.; Cooke, I.E.; Ganesan, T.S.; Ramsdale, J.; Manek, S.; Charnock, F.M.; Groome, N.P.; Wells, M. Immunohistochemical expression of inhibin/activin subunits in epithelial and granulosa cell tumours of the ovary. *J. Pathol.* **1997**, *181*, 413–418. [CrossRef]
96. Cathro, H.P.; Stoler, M.H. The utility of calretinin, inhibin, and WT1 immunohistochemical staining in the differential diagnosis of ovarian tumors. *Hum. Pathol.* **2005**, *36*, 195–201. [CrossRef]
97. Deavers, M.T.; Malpica, A.; Liu, J.; Broaddus, R.; Silva, E.G. Ovarian sex cord-stromal tumors: An immunohistochemical study including a comparison of calretinin and inhibin. *Mod. Pathol.* **2003**, *16*, 584–590. [CrossRef]
98. He, H.; Luthringer, D.J.; Hui, P.; Lau, S.K.; Weiss, L.M.; Chu, P.G. Expression of CD56 and WT1 in ovarian stroma and ovarian stromal tumors. *Am. J. Surg. Pathol.* **2008**, *32*, 884–890. [CrossRef]
99. Zhao, C.; Bratthauer, G.L.; Barner, R.; Vang, R. Diagnostic utility of WT1 immunostaining in ovarian Sertoli cell tumor. *Am. J. Surg. Pathol.* **2007**, *31*, 1378–1386. [CrossRef]
100. Zhao, C.; Vinh, T.N.; McManus, K.; Dabbs, D.; Barner, R.; Vang, R. Identification of the most sensitive and robust immunohistochemical markers in different categories of ovarian sex cord-stromal tumors. *Am. J. Surg. Pathol.* **2009**, *33*, 354–366. [CrossRef]
101. Nasomyon, T.; Samphao, S.; Sangkhathat, S.; Mahattanobon, S.; Graidist, P. Correlation of Wilms' tumor 1 isoforms with HER2 and ER-α and its oncogenic role in breast Cancer. *AntiCancer Res.* **2014**, *34*, 1333–1342.
102. Domfeh, A.B.; Carley, A.L.; Striebel, J.M.; Karabakhtsian, R.G.; Florea, A.V.; McManus, K.; Beriwal, S.; Bhargava, R. WT1 immunoreactivity in breast carcinoma: Selective expression in pure and mixed mucinous subtypes. *Mod. Pathol.* **2008**, *21*, 1217–1223. [CrossRef]
103. Hwang, H.; Quenneville, L.; Yaziji, H.; Gown, A.M. Wilms tumor gene product: Sensitive and contextually specific marker of serous carcinomas of ovarian surface epithelial origin. *Appl. Immunohistochem. Mol. Morphol.* **2004**, *12*, 122–126. [CrossRef]
104. Lee, A.H.; Paish, E.C.; Marchio, C.; Sapino, A.; Schmitt, F.C.; Ellis, I.O.; Reis-Filho, J.S. The expression of Wilms' tumour-1 and Ca125 in invasive micropapillary carcinoma of the breast. *Histopathology* **2007**, *51*, 824–828. [CrossRef]
105. Oh, E.J.; Koo, J.S.; Kim, J.Y.; Jung, W.H. Correlation between solid papillary carcinoma and associated invasive carcinoma according to expression of WT1 and several MUCs. *Pathol. Res. Pract.* **2014**, *210*, 953–958. [CrossRef]

106. Artibani, M.; Sims, A.H.; Slight, J.; Aitken, S.; Thornburn, A.; Muir, M.; Brunton, V.G.; Del-Pozo, J.; Morrison, L.R.; Katz, E.; et al. WT1 expression in breast cancer disrupts the epithelial/mesenchymal balance of tumour cells and correlates with the metabolic response to docetaxel. *Sci. Rep.* **2017**, *7*, 45255. [CrossRef]
107. Choi, E.J.; Yun, J.A.; Jeon, E.K.; Won, H.S.; Ko, Y.H.; Kim, S.Y. Prognostic significance of RSPO1, WNT1, P16, WT1, and SDC1 expressions in invasive ductal carcinoma of the breast. *World J. Surg. Oncol.* **2013**, *11*, 314. [CrossRef]
108. Tuna, M.; Chavez-Reyes, A.; Tari, A.M. HER2/neu increases the expression of Wilms' Tumor 1 (WT1) protein to stimulate S-phase proliferation and inhibit apoptosis in breast cancer cells. *Oncogene* **2005**, *24*, 1648–1652. [CrossRef]
109. Li, B.Q.; Huang, S.; Shao, Q.Q.; Sun, J.; Zhou, L.; You, L.; Zhang, T.P.; Liao, Q.; Guo, J.C.; Zhao, Y.P. WT1-associated protein is a novel prognostic factor in pancreatic ductal adenocarcinoma. *Oncol. Lett.* **2017**, *13*, 2531–2538. [CrossRef]
110. Rodeck, U.; Bossler, A.; Kari, C.; Humphreys, C.W.; Györfi, T.; Maurer, J.; Thiel, E.; Menssen, H.D. Expression of the WT1 Wilms' tumor gene by normal and malignant human melanocytes. *Int. J. Cancer* **1994**, *59*, 78–82. [CrossRef]
111. Wilsher, M.; Cheerala, B. WT1 as a complementary marker of malignant melanoma: An immunohistochemical study of whole sections. *Histopathology* **2007**, *51*, 605–610. [CrossRef]
112. Wagner, N.; Panelos, J.; Massi, D.; Wagner, K.D. The Wilms' tumor suppressor WT1 is associated with melanoma proliferation. *Pflug. Arch.* **2000**, *455*, 839–847. [CrossRef]
113. Michiels, J.F.; Perrin, C.; Leccia, N.; Massi, D.; Grimaldi, P.; Wagner, N. PPARbeta activation inhibits melanoma cell proliferation involving repression of the Wilms' tumour suppressor WT1. *Pflug. Arch.* **2010**, *459*, 689–703. [CrossRef]
114. Garrido-Ruiz, M.C.; Rodriguez-Pinilla, S.M.; Pérez-Gómez, B.; Rodriguez-Peralto, J.L. WT1 expression in nevi and melanomas: A marker of melanocytic invasion into the dermis. *J. Cutan. Pathol.* **2010**, *37*, 542–548. [CrossRef]
115. Garrido Ruiz, M.C.; Requena, L.; Kutzner, H.; Ortiz, P.; Pérez-Gómez, B.; Rodriguez-Peralto, J.L. Desmoplastic melanoma: Expression of epithelial-mesenchymal transition-related proteins. *Am. J. Dermatopathol.* **2014**, *36*, 238–242. [CrossRef]
116. Plaza, J.A.; Bonneau, P.; Prieto, V.; Sangueza, M.; Mackinnon, A.; Suster, D.; Bacchi, C.; Estrozi, B.; Kazakov, D.; Kacerovska, D.; et al. Desmoplastic melanoma: An updated immunohistochemical analysis of 40 cases with a proposal for an additional panel of stains for diagnosis. *J. Cutan. Pathol.* **2016**, *43*, 313–323. [CrossRef]
117. Siegel, R.; Ma, J.; Zou, Z.; Jemal, A. Cancer statistics. *CA Cancer J. Clin.* **2014**, *64*, 9–29. [CrossRef]
118. Oji, Y.; Yamamoto, H.; Nomura, M.; Nakano, Y.; Ikeba, A.; Nakatsuka, S.; Abeno, S.; Kiyotoh, E.; Jomgeow, T.; Sekimoto, M.; et al. Overexpression of the Wilms' tumor gene WT1 in colorectal adenocarcinoma. *Cancer Sci.* **2003**, *94*, 712–717. [CrossRef]
119. Miyata, Y.; Kumagai, K.; Nagaoka, T.; Kitaura, K.; Kaneda, G.; Kanazawa, H.; Suzuki, S.; Hamada, Y.; Suzuki, R. Clinicopathological significance and prognostic value of Wilms' tumor gene expression in colorectal Cancer. *Cancer Biomark.* **2015**, *15*, 789–797. [CrossRef]
120. Aslan, A.; Erdem, H.; Celik, M.A.; Sahin, A.; Cankaya, S. Investigation of Insulin-Like Growth Factor-1 (IGF-1), P53, and Wilms' Tumor 1 (WT1) Expression Levels in the Colon Polyp Subtypes in Colon Cancer. *Med. Sci. Monit.* **2019**, *25*, 5510–5517. [CrossRef]
121. Nakahara, Y.; Okamoto, H.; Mineta, T.; Tabuchi, K. Expression of the Wilms' tumor gene product WT1 in glioblastomas and medulloblastomas. *Brain Tumor. Pathol.* **2004**, *21*, 113–116. [CrossRef] [PubMed]
122. Schittenhelm, J.; Mittelbronn, M.; Nguyen, T.D.; Meyermann, R.; Beschorner, R. WT1 expression distinguishes astrocytic tumor cells from normal and reactive astrocytes. *Brain. Pathol.* **2008**, *18*, 344–353. [CrossRef] [PubMed]
123. Hashiba, T.; Izumoto, S.; Kagawa, N.; Suzuki, T.; Hashimoto, N.; Maruno, M.; Yoshimine, T. Expression of WT1 protein and correlation with cellular proliferation in glial tumors. *Neurol. Med. Chir.* **2007**, *47*, 165–170. [CrossRef] [PubMed]
124. Rauscher, J.; Beschorner, R.; Gierke, M.; Bisdas, S.; Braun, C.; Ebner, F.H.; Schittenhelm, J. WT1 expression increases with malignancy and indicates unfavourable outcome in astrocytoma. *J. Clin. Pathol.* **2014**, *67*, 556–561. [CrossRef]

125. Sotobori, T.; Ueda, T.; Oji, Y.; Naka, N.; Araki, N.; Myoui, A.; Sugiyama, H.; Yoshikawa, H. Prognostic significance of Wilms' tumor gene (WT1) mRNA expression in soft tissue sarcoma. *Cancer* **2006**, *106*, 2233–2240. [CrossRef]
126. Oue, T.; Ueharaa, S.; Yamanakaa, H.; Takamaa, Y.; Ojib, Y.; Fukuzawa, M. Expression of Wilms' tumor 1 gene in a variety of pediatric tumors. *J. Ped. Surg.* **2011**, *46*, 2233–2238. [CrossRef]
127. Weiss, S.W.; Goldblum, J.R. *Enzinger and Weiss's Soft Tissue Tumors*, 5th ed.; Mosby, J.S., Ed.; Elsevier: Amsterdam, The Netherlands, 2008; pp. 903–925.
128. Ducatman, B.S.; Scheithauer, B.W. Malignant peripheral nerve sheath tumors showing. *Cancer* **1984**, *54*, 1049–1057. [CrossRef]
129. Wick, M.R.; Swanson, P.E.; Scheithauer, B.W.; Manivel, J.C. Malignant peripheral nerve sheath tumor. An immunohistochemical study of 62 cases. *Am. J. Clin. Pathol.* **1987**, *87*, 425–433. [CrossRef]
130. Johnson, T.L.; Lee, M.W.; Meis, J.M.; Zarbo, R.J.; Crissman, J. Immunohistochemical characterization of malignant peripheral nerve sheath tumors. *Surg. Pathol.* **1991**, *4*, 121–135.
131. Kim, A.; Park, E.Y.; Kim, K.; Lee, J.H.; Shin, D.H.; Kim, J.Y.; Park, D.Y.; Lee, C.H.; Sol, M.Y.; Choi, K.U.; et al. Prognostic significance of WT1 expression in soft tissue sarcoma. *World J. Surg. Oncol.* **2014**, *12*, 214. [CrossRef]
132. Ueda, T.; Oji, Y.; Naka, N.; Nakano, Y.; Takahashi, E.; Koga, S.; Asada, M.; Ikeba, A.; Nakatsuka, S.; Abeno, S.; et al. Overexpression of the Wilms' tumor gene WT1 in human bone and soft-tissue sarcomas. *Cancer Sci.* **2003**, *94*, 271–276. [CrossRef]
133. Parenti, R.; Cardile, V.; Graziano, A.C.; Parenti, C.; Venuti, A.; Bertuccio, M.P.; Furno, D.L.; Magro, G. Wilms' tumor gene 1 (WT1) silencing inhibits proliferation of malignant peripheral nerve sheath tumor sNF96.2 cell line. *PLoS ONE* **2014**, *9*, e114333. [CrossRef]
134. Antonescu, C.R.; Ladanyi, M. Desmoplastic small round cell tumour. In *WHO Classification of Tumours of Soft Tissue and Bone*; Fletcher, C.D.M., Bridge, J.A., Hogendoorn, P.C.W., Mertens, F., Eds.; IARC: Lyon, France, 2013; pp. 225–227.
135. Barnoud, R.; Sabourin, J.C.; Pasquier, D.; Ranchère, D.; Bailly, C.; Terrier-Lacombe, M.J.; Pasquier, B. Immunohistochemical expression of WT1 by desmoplastic small round cell tumor: A comparative study with other small round cell tumors. *Am. J. Surg. Pathol.* **2000**, *24*, 830. [CrossRef] [PubMed]
136. Hill, D.A.; Pfeifer, J.D.; Marley, E.F.; Dehner, L.P.; Humphrey, P.A.; Zhu, X.; Swanson, P.E. WT1 staining reliably differentiates desmoplastic small round cell tumor from Ewing sarcoma/primitive neuroectodermal tumor. An immunohistochemical and molecular diagnostic study. *Am. J. Clin. Pathol.* **2000**, *114*, 345–353. [CrossRef]
137. Murphy, A.J.; Bishop, K.; Pereira, C.; Chilton-MacNeill, S.; Ho, M.; Zielenska, M.; Thorner, P.S. A new molecular variant of desmoplastic small round cell tumor: Significance of WT1 immunostaining in this entity. *Hum. Pathol.* **2008**, *39*, 1763–1770. [CrossRef]
138. Alaggio, R.; Coffin, C.M.; Vargas, S.O. Soft tissue tumors of uncertain origin. *Pediatr. Dev. Pathol.* **2012**, *15* (Suppl. S1), 267–305. [CrossRef]
139. Hoot, A.C.; Russo, P.; Judkins, A.R.; Perlman, E.J.; Biegel, J.A. Immunohistochemical analysis of hSNF5/INI1 distinguishes renal and extra-renal malignant rhabdoid tumors from other pediatric soft tissue tumors. *Am. J. Surg. Pathol.* **2004**, *28*, 1485–1491. [CrossRef]
140. Sigauke, E.; Rakheja, D.; Maddox, D.L.; Hladik, C.L.; White, C.L.; Timmons, C.F.; Raisanen, J. Absence of expression of SMARCB1/INI1 in malignant rhabdoid tumors of the central nervous system, kidneys and soft tissue: An immunohistochemical study with implications for diagnosis. *Mod. Pathol.* **2006**, *19*, 717–725. [CrossRef]
141. Judkins, A.R. Immunohistochemistry of INI1 expression: A new tool for old challenges in CNS and soft tissue pathology. *Adv. Anat. Pathol.* **2007**, *14*, 335–339. [CrossRef]
142. Machado, I.; Noguera, R.; Santonja, N.; Donat, J.; Fernandez-Delgado, R.; Acevedo, A.; Baragaño, M.; Navarro, S. Immunohistochemical study as a tool in differential diagnosis of pediatric malignant rhabdoid tumor. *Appl. Immunohistochem. Mol. Morphol.* **2010**, *18*, 150–158. [CrossRef]
143. Salvatorelli, L.; Parenti, R.; Leone, G.; Musumeci, G.; Vasquez, E.; Magro, G. Wilms tumor 1 (WT1) protein: Diagnostic utility in pediatric tumors. *Acta Histochem.* **2015**, *117*, 367–378. [CrossRef] [PubMed]
144. Parham, D.M.; Alaggio, R.; Coffin, C.M. Myogenic tumors in children and adolescents. *Pediatr. Dev. Pathol.* **2012**, *15* (Suppl. S1), 211–238. [CrossRef] [PubMed]

145. Sebire, N.J.; Gibson, S.; Rampling, D.; Williams, S.; Malone, M.; Ramsay, A.D. Immunohistochemical findings in embryonal small round cell tumors with molecular diagnostic confirmation. *Appl. Immunohistochem. Mol. Morphol.* **2005**, *13*, 1–5. [CrossRef] [PubMed]
146. Musumeci, G.; Castrogiovanni, P.; Coleman, R.; Szychlinska, M.A.; Salvatorelli, L.; Parenti, R.; Magro, G.; Imbesi, R. Somitogenesis: From somite to skeletal muscle. *Acta Histochem.* **2015**, *117*, 313–328. [CrossRef] [PubMed]
147. Rosai, J. *Rosai and Ackerman's Surgical Pathology*, 10th ed.; Elsevier: New York, NY, USA, 2011.
148. Magro, G.; Grasso, S.; Emmanuele, C. Immunohistochemical distribution of S-100 protein and type IV collagen in human embryonic and fetal sympathetic neuroblasts. *Histochem. J.* **1995**, *27*, 694–701. [CrossRef] [PubMed]
149. Magro, G.; Ruggieri, M.; Fraggetta, F.; Grasso, S.; Viale, G. Cathepsin D is a marker of ganglion cell differentiation in the developing and neoplastic human peripheral sympathetic nervous tissues. *Virchows Arch.* **2000**, *437*, 406–412. [CrossRef]
150. Magro, G.; Grasso, S. Immunohistochemical identification and comparison of glial cell lineage in fetal, neonatal, adult and neoplastichumanadrenal medulla. *Histochem. J.* **1997**, *29*, 293–299. [CrossRef]
151. Magro, G.; Grasso, S. The glial cell in the ontogenesis of the human peripheral sympathetic nervous system and in neuroblastoma. *Pathologica* **2001**, *93*, 505–516.
152. De Preter, K.; Vandesompele, J.; Heimann, P.; Yigit, N.; Beckman, S.; Schramm, A.; Eggert, A.; Stallings, R.L.; Benoit, Y.; Renard, M.; et al. Human fetal neuroblast and neuroblastoma transcriptome analysis confirms neuroblast origin and highlights neuroblastoma candidate genes. *Genome Biol.* **2007**, *8*, 401. [CrossRef]
153. Hoehner, J.C.; Hedborg, F.; Eriksson, L.; Sandstedt, B.; Grimelius, L.; Olsen, L.; Påhlman, S. Developmental gene expression of sympathetic nervous system tumors reflects their histogenesis. *Lab. Investig.* **1998**, *78*, 29–45.
154. Wang, L.L.; Perlman, E.J.; Vujanic, G.M.; Zuppan, C.; Brundler, M.A.; Cheung, C.R.; Calicchio, M.L.; Dubois, S.; Cendron, M.; Murata-Collins, J.L.; et al. Desmoplastic small round cell tumor of the kidney in childhood. *Am. J. Surg. Pathol.* **2007**, *31*, 576–584. [CrossRef] [PubMed]
155. Coffin, C.M.; Alaggio, R. Fibroblastic and myofibroblastic tumors in children and adolescents. *Pediatr. Dev. Pathol.* **2012**, *15*, 127–180. [CrossRef]
156. Bourgeois, J.M.; Knezevich, S.R.; Mathers, J.A.; Sorensen, P.M. Molecular detection of the ETV6-NTRK3 gene fusion differentiates congenital fibrosarcoma from other childhood spindle cell tumors. *Am. J. Surg. Pathol.* **2000**, *24*, 937–946. [CrossRef] [PubMed]
157. Sheng, W.Q.; Hisaoka, M.; Okamoto, S.; Tanaka, A.; Meis-Kindblom, J.M.; Kindblom, L.G.; Ishida, T.; Nojima, T.; Hashimoto, H. Congenital–infantile fibrosarcoma: A clinico-pathologic study of 10 cases and molecular detection of the ETV6-NTRK3 fusion transcripts using paraffin embedded tissues. *Am. J. Clin. Pathol.* **2001**, *115*, 348–355. [CrossRef] [PubMed]
158. Galfione, S.K.; Ro, J.Y.; Ayala, A.G.; Ge, Y. Diagnostic utility of WT-1 cytoplasmic stain in variety of vascular lesions. *Int. J. Clin. Exp. Pathol.* **2014**, *7*, 2536–2543. [PubMed]
159. Timár, J.; Mészáros, L.; Orosz, Z.; Albini, A.; Rásó, E. WT1 expression in angiogenic tumours of the skin. *Histopathology* **2005**, *47*, 67–73. [CrossRef]
160. Al Dhaybi, R.; Powell, J.; McCuaig, C.; Kokta, V. Differentiation of vasculartumors from vascular malformations by expression of Wilms'tumor 1 gene: Evaluation of 126 cases. *J. Am. Acad. Dermatol.* **2010**, *63*, 1052–1057. [CrossRef]
161. Magro, G.; Bisceglia, M.; Michal, M.; Eusebi, V. Spindle cell lipoma-like tumor, solitary fibrous tumor and myofibroblastoma ofthe breast: A clinic pathological analysis of 13 cases in favor of a unifying histologic concept. *Virchows Arch.* **2002**, *440*, 249–260. [CrossRef]
162. Magro, G.; Gurrera, A.; Bisceglia, M. H-caldesmon expression in myofibroblastoma of the breast: Evidence supporting the distinctionfrom leiomyoma. *Histopathology* **2003**, *42*, 233–238. [CrossRef]
163. Magro, G.; Greco, P.; Alaggio, R.; Gangemi, P.; Ninfo, V. Polypoid angiomyofibroblastoma-like tumor of the oral cavity: A hitherto unreported soft tissue tumor mimicking embryonal rhabdomyosarcoma. *Pathol. Res. Pract.* **2008**, *204*, 837–843. [CrossRef]

164. Magro, G. Stromal tumors of the lower female genital tract: Histo-genetic, morphological and immunohistochemical similaritieswith the "benign spindle cell tumors of the mammary stroma". *Pathol. Res. Pract.* **2007**, *203*, 827–829. [CrossRef] [PubMed]
165. Magro, G.; Caltabiano, R.; Kacerovská, D.; Vecchio, G.M.; Kazakov, D.; Michal, M. Vulvovaginal myofibroblastoma: Expanding themorphological and immunohistochemical spectrum. A clinico-pathologic study of 10 cases. *Hum. Pathol.* **2012**, *43*, 243–253. [CrossRef] [PubMed]

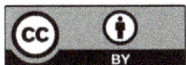
© 2019 by the authors. Licensee MDPI, Basel, Switzerland. This article is an open access article distributed under the terms and conditions of the Creative Commons Attribution (CC BY) license (http://creativecommons.org/licenses/by/4.0/).

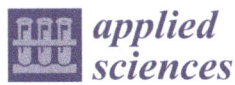

Review

Matrix Metalloproteinases and Temporomandibular Joint Disorder: A Review of the Literature

Logan Herm, Ardit Haxhia, Flavio de Alcantara Camejo, Lobat Tayebi and Luis Eduardo Almeida *

Surgical Sciences Department, Oral Surgery, School of Dentistry, Marquette University, Milwaukee, WI 53233, USA; logan.herm@marquette.edu (L.H.); ardit.haxhia@marquette.edu (A.H.); flavio.dealcantaracamejo@marquette.edu (F.d.A.C.); lobat.tayebi@marquette.edu (L.T.)
* Correspondence: luis.almeida@marquette.edu

Received: 30 September 2019; Accepted: 21 October 2019; Published: 24 October 2019

Abstract: Temporomandibular disorders (TMD) are progressive degenerative disorders that affect the components of the temporomandibular joint (TMJ), characterized by pain and limitations in function. Matrix metalloproteinases (MMP) are enzymes involved in physiological breakdown of tissue that can have a pathological effect from an increase in activity during inflammation. A PubMed search of the current literature (within the past 10 years) was conducted to identify human studies involving matrix metalloproteinases activity in TMJ components of patients with TMD. Two separate searches results in 34 studies, six of which met inclusion criteria. Immunohistochemistry and gene analysis were used to evaluate MMP expression in the study groups. This review showed the strongest evidence for involvement of MMP-1, MMP-2, and MMP-9 in TMD; however, limitations included low sample sizes and a lack of recent clinical studies. Future research with more definitive conclusions could allow for additional pharmaceutical targets in MMP when treating patients with temporomandibular disorders.

Keywords: matrix metalloproteinases; temporomandibular joint disorder; temporomandibular joint

1. Introduction

The temporomandibular joint (TMJ) is classified as a ginglymoarthrodial joint, allowing for rotational and translational movements in normal function. Its primary components include the glenoid fossa of the temporal bone, the articular disc, the head of the mandibular condyle, and masticatory muscles. This joint is capable of remodeling even after growth has stopped, allowing it to make structural changes and adapt to different physiological demands [1].

Temporomandibular disorders (TMD) are a group of degenerative disorders involving the components of the TMJ, which can lead to displacement of the disc, joint remodeling, and eventually osteoarthritis [2]. Disc displacement can occur anteriorly, posteriorly, medially, or laterally; however, it is most commonly displaced anteriorly [3]. TMD affects around 25% of the population, and it is characterized by orofacial pain, restricted range of motion, joint dysfunction, and ultimately, a decreased quality of life [2,4]. The etiology of TMD is still a topic of discussion; however, some known risk factors include trauma and microtrauma, malocclusion, and psychological factors, such as stress and anxiety [5].

The progression of TMD is classified primarily based on the location of the disc and its mobility during mandibular movement. In a normal functioning joint, the disc remains between the head of the mandibular condyle and the glenoid fossa through the full range of movement. In early stage TMD, the disc is displaced anteriorly when the mandible is closed and reduces to a normal location upon opening, classified as anterior disc displacement with reduction (ADDwR). In late stages of TMD, the disc is anteriorly displaced in both closed and open positions, classified as anterior disc displacement without reduction (ADDwoR). These later stages tend to be associated with more pain and limitation in mandibular mobility [2].

A more advanced staging guide to the internal derangements of TMD was created by Wilkes in 1989, placing patients into five categories based on clinical, radiographic (tomographic, arthrographic, and magnetic resonance imaging) and findings during surgery, including gross surface and anatomic changes to the disc and other components of the TMJ [6]. In the first stage, the early stage, patients present with clicking of the joint, but no pain, limited range of motion, or other symptoms. Radiographically and surgically, the disc is displaced slightly anteriorly, but all other aspects of the joint are normal. In Wilke's early/intermediate stage, the patient presents with additional symptoms, including episodes of pain, tenderness, and mechanical problems associated with the joint. Radiographically and surgically, the disc is displaced anteriorly, with slight deformation of its posterior aspect. In the intermediate stage there are more occurrences of pain, mechanical problems, including locking and decreased range of motion. In Wilke's intermediate/late stage of TMD, the patient has a chronic pain and decreased range of motion. Radiographically and surgically, an increased severity in comparison to the intermediate stage is noted, along with remodeling of the hard tissue surfaces of the joint. The disc, however, has yet to be perforated up to this stage. In the final stage, the late stage, patients present with crepitus and grinding in the joint with mandibular movement, chronic pain, restricted range of motion, and an overall decrease in function. Radiographically and surgically, the disc and hard tissues of the joint have undergone significant deformation, remodeling, and arthritic changes have occurred, including perforations of the attachments and erosion of articulating surfaces [6].

Matrix metalloproteinases (MMPs) are the major enzymes involved in extracellular matrix (ECM) and basement membrane remodeling and degradation, along with other enzymes, such as a disintegrin and metalloproteinases (with or without thrombospondin), and plasminogen activators, among others [7–9]. These enzymes are seen in both physiological and pathological processes, including embryogenesis, apoptosis, bone remodeling, inflammation, arthritis, and cancer [7,8]. However, the role of MMPs is not limited to the ECM, as they have also been shown to play a role in regulating inflammatory response, namely by processing chemokines, growth factors, receptors, proteases, and other molecules and proteins [9]. They are a family of 26 endopeptidases that degrade collagen, gelatin, proteoglycans, and other ECM components, and they are regulated at the level of their gene expression (cytokines, growth factors, hormones, and others), posttranslational activation, and endogenous inhibition (tissue inhibitors of metalloproteinases [TIMP]) [8,10]. As inflammation occurs, however, processes involving these enzymes shift from physiological to pathological, and MMP activity results in excess tissue breakdown and damage [11].

Some MMPs have been suggested as being involved in angiogenesis, apoptosis, and osteoarthritis, processes which are seen in temporomandibular joint disorders [7]. Angiogenesis, found mostly in the synovial membrane in TMD, allows for new vessel formation to combat the hypoxia associated with an increase in the intra-articular pressure seen in TMD [12]. Chondrocytes undergo apoptosis in the early stages of TMD as the disc begins to remodel, and eventual cartilage degradation occurs, leading to osteoarthritic changes [4]. With evidence of the involvement of MMPs in these processes, and with the processes playing a crucial role in the progression of TMD, it would seem that MMP activity would be increased in joints of patients with the disorder. This paper aims to review the current scientific literature in order to investigate potential links between various MMPs and TMD.

2. Methodology

2.1. Search Protocol

Two independent electronic searches were conducted by two reviewers using PubMed to find relevant literature using Medical Subjective Headings (MeSH) Terms. The MeSH terms included in each search were:

1. "Temporomandibular Joint Disorders/enzymology" (Mesh) **OR** "Temporomandibular Joint Disorders/metabolism" (Mesh) **OR** "Temporomandibular Joint Disorders/pathology" (Mesh)) **AND** "Humans" (Mesh)) **AND** "Immunohistochemistry" (Mesh)) **AND** "Matrix Metalloproteinases" (Mesh)
2. "Temporomandibular Joint Disorders" (MeSH Major Topic) **AND** "Matrix Metalloproteinases" [MeSH Major Topic]) **AND** "Humans" (MeSH Terms)

2.2. Selection Protocol

Inclusion and exclusion criteria were determined before the search results were evaluated. Inclusion criteria used in selection included the following:

1. English language;
2. Living human subjects;
3. Publication within the past 10 years (since 2009);
4. Studies that evaluated samples of TMD and the level of MMP in the disease.

Exclusion criteria used in selection included the following:

1. Case studies;
2. Pilot studies;
3. Literature reviews.

2.3. Data Analysis

The data collected from each selected study, summarized in Table 1, included MMP type assessed in the study, sample size and groups, mean age involved in study, TMJ assessment, and the results of the study. Since the studies differed significantly in their methodology, a direct data analysis was unable to be conducted, and further evaluation of the quality of the included studies, such as statistical power, was not done beyond looking at the sample size.

Table 1. Studies that fit the inclusion criteria and published within the past 10 years [11,13–17]. Anterior disc displacement with reduction (ADDwR); anterior disc displacement without reduction (ADDwoR); matrix metalloproteinases (MMP); temporomandibular joint (TMJ).

Included Researcher's Characteristics and Main Results					
Authors	Experimental Sample	Age of Experimental Sample (Mean)	MMP Assessed and Method	TMJ Assessment	Result
Perotto et al., 2018	Group 1: Healthy 8 Samples Group 2: ADDwR 21 Samples Group 3: ADDwoR 10 Samples	33.59	MMP-13 Immuno-Histochemical Staining (IHC)	Clinical Examination, Symptoms, Panorex	No significant different in MMP-13 expression
Almeida et al., 2014	45 Samples from 33 Subjects	32.26	MMP-2, MMP-9 IHC	Clinical Examination, Symptoms, Panorex	Upregulation of MMP-2. No significant difference in MMP-9 expression.
Loreto et al., 2013	25 Samples from 25 Subjects	34.2	MMP-7, MMP-9 IHC	Clinical Examination, Symptoms, MRI	Upregulation of both MMP-7 and MMP-9.
Planello et al., 2011	115 Samples from 115 Subjects	42.82	MMP-1, MMP-3, MMP-9 DNA Purification, PCR, Genotype Analysis	CT Imaging, MRI, History of Symptoms	Upregulation of MMP-1. No association with MMP-3 and MMP-9.
Milosevic et al., 2015	100 Samples from 100 Subjects	37.12	MMP-9 DNA Extraction, Genotype Analysis, PCR	Clinical Evaluation, History of Symptoms	Upregulation of MMP-9.

Table 1. Cont.

Authors	Experimental Sample	Age of Experimental Sample (Mean)	MMP Assessed and Method	TMJ Assessment	Result
Luo et al., 2015	Group A: 185 Healthy Group B: 141 ADDwR Group C1: 115 ADDwoR w/o OA Group C2: 206 ADDwoR w/ OA	Group A: 33.49 Group B: 36.64 Group C: 37.22	MMP-1 DNA Sampling, Genotype Analysis	Clinical and Radiographic Examinations, Symptoms	Upregulation of MMP-1 in ADDwoR with or without TMJ osteoarthritis.

3. Results

3.1. General Outcomes

Initial searches using the MeSH terms indicated above resulted in 34 studies, nine of which were duplicates and three of which were unable to be accessed. After removing duplicates and inaccessible studies, 22 studies remained. One study was not included due to samples being cadaveric, one focused on interleukins (IL) and used unspecified MMPs as markers for IL, two were animal studies, and two others were literature reviews. All other studies satisfied both the English language and the living human subject inclusion criteria, leaving 16 total studies. After including only studies published within the past 10 years, 6 studies remained, all of which were accepted based on all other indicated inclusion and exclusion criteria. Studies with researcher's characteristics and main results excluded from this review due to date of publication are included in Table 2 for additional comparison.

Table 2. Studies that fit all inclusion criteria, but were published more than 10 years ago [18–27].

Authors	Experimental Samples	Age of Experimental Samples (Mean)	MMP Assessed and Method	TMJ Assessment	Result
Tiilikainen et al., 2005	54 Samples from 54 Subjects	36.3	MMP-3, MMP-8 IHC	Clinical Examination, CT, MRI, Symptoms	No significant difference between severity of TMD in expression of MMP-3 or MMP-8.
Ishimaru et al., 2000	94 Samples	31.33	MMP-1, MMP-3 IHC	Clinical Examination, Panorex, Arthrograms, Visual Analog Score Calculations	Upregulation of both MMP-1 and MMP-3.
Kanyama et al., 2000	10 Samples from 10 Subjects	29.7	MMP-1, MMP-2, MMP-3, MMP-9 IHC	Clinical Examination, MRI, Symptoms	Upregulation of MMP-1, MMP-2, MMP-3 and MMP-9.
Marchetti et al., 1999	11 Subjects	No Mean Range: 26–43	MMP-2 IHC	MRI and Macroscopic Examination	Upregulation of MMP-2.
Yoshida et al., 1999	16 Subjects	41.12	MMP-3 IHC	-	Upregulation of MMP-3.
Fujita et al., 2008	54 Samples from 50 Patients	36.2	MMP-3 Enzymography, Western Blot Analysis, Immuno-precipitation	Clinical and Radiographic Examinations,	Upregulation of MMP-3.
Srinivas et al., 2000	44 Subjects	36	MMP-2, MMP-8, MMP-9 Enzyme Activity, Western Immunoblotting	Symptoms, Clinical and Radiographic Examination, Surgical Observation	Upregulation of MMP-2, MMP-8, and MMP-9
Yoshida et al., 2006	44 Samples from 35 Subjects	36.6	MMP-2, MMP-9 Sample Collection, MRI, Western Immunoblotting	Clinical Examination, MRI, Symptoms	Upregulation of MMP-2 and MMP-9.

Table 2. *Cont.*

			Excluded Researcher's Characteristics and Main Results		
Authors	Experimental Samples	Age of Experimental Samples (Mean)	MMP Assessed and Method	TMJ Assessment	Result
Mizui et al., 2001	86 Subjects	Range: 19–84	MMP-2 Proteolytic Activity, Enzymogram	Radiographic Analysis	Upregulation of MMP-2.
Tanaka et al., 2001	41 Samples from 38 Subjects	34.8	MMP-2, MMP-9 Enzyme Activity, Immuno-blotting, Gelatinolytic Activity	Symptoms, Clinical and Radiographic Exam	MMP-2 and MMP-9 were upregulated more in ADDwoR than in ADDwR.

3.2. Description of Included Studies

In 2018, Perotto et al. used 39 disc samples from 27 patients to look at MMP-13 expression in TMD. Exclusion criteria for subjects Perotto's study included use of orthodontic appliances, chronic anti-inflammatory use, history of diseases causing impaired immune function, such as HIV, diabetes, or any use of immunosuppressive therapy. The patients, with a mean age of 33.59, then filled out a pain questionnaire, had a clinical examination, and radiographs or CT imaging was performed for diagnostic purposes, placing patients into groupings of either ADDwR or ADDwoR. Surgery was performed on patients and samples were obtained and underwent immunohistological staining to analyze for MMP-13 activity. The researchers did not find a significant difference in expression of MMP-13 in samples from patients with TMD, in either the ADDwR or the ADDwoR groupings, when compared to the control group.

Almeida et al. (2014) analyzed activity of two matrix metalloproteinases and their protein levels in TMD, both MMP-2 and MMP-9. In this study, 45 disc samples from 33 patients (mean age of 32.36 years) were analyzed using immunohistological staining. Diagnosis was made using a pain questionnaire and clinical examination, grouping patients into ADDwR and ADDwoR, and selected patients were treated surgically following unsuccessful non-surgical treatment. Following immunohistochemical staining of samples obtained during surgery, MMP-2 was found to be significantly increased in samples from subjects with TMD when compared to the control. It was also found that there was an increase in MMP-2 in samples from patients with ADDwoR when compared to ADDwR, suggesting a correlation between progression of TMD and MMP-2 levels. Levels of MMP-9 showed no significant difference between the TMD disc samples when compared with control disc samples.

Loreto et al. (2013) used immunohistochemical staining to look at MMP-7 and MMP-9 in disc samples from subjects with TMD. They used 25 disc samples from 25 patients (mean age of 34), which were obtained surgically following unsuccessful non-surgical intervention after diagnosis using a history of present illness, clinical examination, and MRI. They assessed the severity of the disease by looking at unassisted maximum mouth opening and using a visual analog scale to assess pain. Following staining, both MMP-7 and MMP-9 were found to be expressed at levels significantly higher in samples from patients with TMD when compared to control samples.

Planello et al. (2011) analyzed the frequency of polymorphisms in genes coding for MMP-1, MMP-3, and MMP-9 proteinases in patients with TMJ degeneration. The study was conducted on 232 individuals, 115 of which had TMJ degeneration and a mean age of 42.82. To diagnose the study group, the researchers used MRI and/or CT scans to image one or both mandibular condyles. Genomic DNA was gathered from epithelial buccal cells and a PCR reaction was performed for MMP-1, MMP-3, and MMP-9 coding genes. A genotype analysis using restriction fragment length polymorphisms was performed, and the frequency of each allele was determined in both groups. Compared to the control group, there was a statistically significant association between the MMP-1 genotype and the TMJ degeneration group. No association was found between the MMP-3 and MMP-9 genotypes and TMJ degeneration.

Milosevic et al. (2015) studied polymorphisms of multiple genes in order to investigate their role in TMD. The study included 182 healthy individuals and 100 patients with TMD, with a mean age of 37.12. The TMD in the study group was assessed using clinical signs and symptoms. Genomic DNA was gathered from buccal swabs and genotyping was conducted in order to evaluate MMP-9 polymorphisms, as well as other enzyme polymorphisms outside the scope of this review. The researchers found a significant difference in genotype and allele frequency in the MMP-9 gene of TMD patients when compared to the control group.

Luo et al. (2015) studied polymorphisms of MMP-1 genes in healthy individuals and patients with articular disc derangement and TMJ osteoarthritis. The researchers split patients into three groups, as follows: Group A included 185 healthy individuals; Group B included 141 patients with unilateral ADDwR; and Group C included 321 patients with ADDwoR, 115 of which did not present TMJ osteoarthritis (C1) and 206 of which presented TMJ osteoarthritis (C2). These patients were diagnosed through clinical and radiographic examinations. Genomic DNA was extracted from buccal swabs and a PCR analysis was conducted in order to assess variations in the MMP-1 gene. Comparisons between the groups showed a variety of allele distributions. Groups A and B did not show a significant statistical difference. Groups A and C showed a noticeable statistical difference with an odds ratio of 2.455 after adjusting for age. When observing the subgroups in Group C, Group C1 had no difference with group B, while Group C2 had a significant statistical difference and an odds ratio of 1.912. Groups C1 and C2 showed no significant statistical difference. Overall, their findings suggest the MMP-1 gene is upregulated in patients with ADDwoR, and the presence of TMJ osteoarthritis had no influence.

4. Discussion

Differences in study design, groupings of samples, and MMPs analyzed prevented direct analysis of data in the present studies. Three studies, those of Perotto, Almeida, and Luo, not only grouped samples on the presence and absence of TMD, but also in the degree to which the disease had progressed, either ADDwR or ADDwoR. Many of the studies analyzed different MMPs, and there were different techniques used to test for expression of the MMP, including immunohistochemical staining and PCR. Four of the included studies, those of Almeida, Loreto, Planello, and Milosevic, analyzed the same MMP, MMP-9, and while Almeida and Planello found that there was no significant different in samples from subjects with TMD, Loreto and Milosevic found an increase in expression. The Kanyama study in 2000, the Srinivas study in 2000, the Yoshida study in 2006, and the Tanaka study in 2001, which were excluded due to date of publication, found that MMP-9 was upregulated in disc samples from subjects with TMD. The inconclusiveness as to whether or not there is a correlation between the levels of MMP-9 expression and TMD of some of the studies can likely be contributed to the small sample size in each.

Aside from MMP-9, the only other overlap of MMP in the included studies was MMP-1, which was found to be upregulated in TMD samples in both the study conducted by Planello, as well as the study conducted by Luo. Aside from these two MMPs, there is no additional overlap between MMPs analyzed in the included studies; however, there is some ability to compare with the studies excluded due to date of publication. MMP-2, which was found by Almeida to be upregulated in disc samples from subjects with TMD, was also found to have higher expression in TMD samples by Kanyama, Marchetti, Srinivas, Mizui, and Tanaka.

Based on the information present in the included studies, it is difficult to draw a definitive conclusion with respect to the involvement of most MMPs in TMD, even when the studies that were excluded due to date of publication are considered. The strongest evidence for MMP involvement in TMD lies with MMP-1, MMP-2, and MMP-9; however, there were limitations in all of the studies, the biggest being sample size, which ranged from only 25 to 141 samples in the included studies.

5. Conclusions

Despite the high prevalence of TMD in the population, current treatment modalities tend to have a poor long-term success and few patients seek treatment [2]. The available modalities are diverse, ranging from non-invasive techniques, such as physical therapy, ultrasound, low-level laser therapy, and splints, to minimally invasive techniques, such as corticosteroid injections, arthrocentesis of the joint, with or without platelet-rich plasma or hyaluronic acid injections, and arthroscopic surgery, to invasive procedures for the more advanced stage of TMD, which include discectomy, disc replacement, and the most invasive, total joint replacement [2,28,29]. It is recommended that attempts at treatment begin with non-invasive techniques and progress to invasive techniques, as risks with the invasive techniques involving open joint surgery can include facial nerve and optic lesions, transarticular and intracranial perforations, and pre-auricular hematoma, among others [3]. Further limitations and complications of arthroscopy, arthrocentesis, and orthognathic surgery used for treatment of TMD include arteriovenous fistula, pseudoaneurysm, infection, broken instruments in the joint, and condylar resorption [30,31]. Additionally, bruxism and dysfunctional oral habits have been shown to be risk factors for recurrent TMD symptoms after orthognathic surgery [32]. Due to limitations and complications of surgery, it is necessary to develop more efficacious techniques in non-invasive and pharmaceutical therapies for treating TMD.

Some of the pharmaceutical therapies for TMD include botox and cyclobenzaprine, which induce muscle relaxation, NSAIDs, and corticosteroids, which reduce pain and inflammation, and tricyclic antidepressants, which work to reduce pain [33]. However, these agents work to target the effects that TMD has on the patient rather than an underlying cause. To the researchers' knowledge, there are currently no pharmaceutical agents that are used to target an element of the underlying pathogenesis of TMD, such as MMPs, to stop the progression of this debilitating disorder.

There is ongoing pharmaceutical research to uncover potential MMP inhibitors for therapeutic use in different disease processes, such as cancer [34]. Thus far, however, limitations have prevented identification of a suitable therapeutic agent. The poorly understood specificity of their biological substrates makes it difficult to target specific MMPs, which causes detrimental problems, as MMPs are vital to survival [34]. There have been additional problems in its use, some of which include problems with oral bioavailability, toxicity, and metabolic stability [34,35]. Despite the unsuccessful attempts, knowledge of MMPs continues to evolve and the use of new and future technological advances, including use of CRISPR-Cas9 and MMP-activatable optical probes, make the use of MMP as a pharmaceutical target more hopeful [34,35]. If and when a successful pharmaceutical agent is discovered targeting MMPs, having a good understanding of the specific MMPs involved in TMD progression could provide an expedited route to applying the therapy to TMD treatment.

More studies with larger sample sizes are needed to analyze the involvement of specific MMPs in TMD. With more concrete evidence of its role, and because of the nature of the enzymes, MMPs could prove to provide a better understanding of the progression of TMD and be a valuable pharmaceutical target for therapy.

Author Contributions: Conceptualization, F.d.A.C. and L.E.A.; Methodology, L.H., A.H.; Software, Not applicable; Validation, L.E.A., L.H., and A.H.; Formal Analysis, Not applicable; Investigation, L.H., A.H. and F.d.A.C.; Resources, L.H., A.H.; Data Curation, L.H., A.H.; Writing—Original Draft Preparation, L.H., A.H.; Writing—Review & Editing, L.E.A., L.H., A.H., F.d.A.C. and L.T.; Visualization, L.E.A.; Supervision, F.d.A.C., L.T. and L.E.A.; Project Administration, L.E.A.; Funding Acquisition, Not applicable.

Funding: This research received no external funding.

Acknowledgments: There are no acknowledgements and no funding was used for this review.

Conflicts of Interest: No conflicts of interest.

References

1. Mathew, A.L.; Sholapurkar, A.A.; Pai, K.M. Condylar Changes and Its Association with Age, TMD, and Dentition Status: A Cross-Sectional Study. *Int. J. Dent.* **2011**, *2011*, 1–7. [CrossRef] [PubMed]
2. Murphy, M.K.; MacBarb, R.F.; Wong, M.E.; Athanasiou, K.A. Temporomandibular Joint Disorders: A Review of Etiology, Clinical Management, and Tissue Engineering Strategies. *Int. J. Oral Maxillofac. Implant.* **2013**, *28*, e393–e414. [CrossRef] [PubMed]

3. Poluha, R.L.; Canales, G.D.L.T.; Costa, Y.M.; Grossmann, E.; Bonjardim, L.R.; Conti, P.C.R. Temporomandibular joint disc displacement with reduction: A review of mechanisms and clinical presentation. *J. Appl. Oral Sci.* **2019**, *27*, 1–9. [CrossRef] [PubMed]
4. Wang, X.; Zhang, J.; Gan, Y.; Zhou, Y. Current Understanding of Pathogenesis and Treatment of TMJ Osteoarthritis. *J. Dent. Res.* **2015**, *94*, 666–673. [CrossRef]
5. Sójka, A.; Stelcer, B.; Roy, M.; Mojs, E.; Pryliński, M. Is there a relationship between psychological factors and TMD? *Brain Behav.* **2019**, *9*, 1–11. [CrossRef]
6. Wilkes, C.H. Internal Derangements of the Temporomandibular Joint: Pathological Variations. *Arch. Otolaryngol. Head Neck Surg.* **1989**, *115*, 469–477. [CrossRef]
7. Amălinei, C.; Căruntu, I.D.; Giuşcă, S.E.; Bălan, R.A. Matrix metalloproteinases involvement in pathologic conditions. *Rom. J. Morphol. Embryol. Rev. Roum. Morphol. Embryol.* **2010**, *51*, 215–228.
8. Peng, W.-J.; Yan, J.-W.; Wan, Y.-N.; Wang, B.-X.; Tao, J.-H.; Yang, G.-J.; Pan, H.-F.; Wang, J. Matrix Metalloproteinases: A Review of Their Structure and Role in Systemic Sclerosis. *J. Clin. Immunol.* **2012**, *32*, 1409–1414. [CrossRef]
9. Butler, G.; Overall, C. Matrix metalloproteinase processing of signaling molecules to regulate inflammation. *Periodontology* **2000**, *63*, 123–148. [CrossRef]
10. Verma, R.P.; Hansch, C. Matrix metalloproteinases (MMPs): Chemical–biological functions and (Q)SARs. *Bioorg. Med. Chem.* **2007**, *15*, 2223–2268. [CrossRef]
11. Almeida, L.E.; Caporal, K.; Ambros, V.; Azevedo, M.; Noronha, L.; Leonardi, R.; Trevilatto, P.C. Immunohistochemical expression of matrix metalloprotease-2 and matrix metalloprotease-9 in the disks of patients with temporomandibular joint dysfunction. *J. Oral Pathol. Med.* **2014**, *44*, 75–79. [CrossRef] [PubMed]
12. Ke, J.; Liu, Y.; Long, X.; Li, J.; Fang, W.; Meng, Q.; Zhang, Y. Up-regulation of vascular endothelial growth factor in synovial fibroblasts from human temporomandibular joint by hypoxia. *J. Oral Pathol. Med.* **2007**, *36*, 290–296. [CrossRef] [PubMed]
13. Perotto, J.H.; Camejo, F.D.A.; Doetzer, A.D.; Almeida, L.E.; Azevedo, M.; Olandoski, M.; Noronha, L.; Trevilatto, P.C. Expression of MMP-13 in human temporomandibular joint disc derangement and osteoarthritis. *Cranio* **2017**, *36*, 161–166. [CrossRef] [PubMed]
14. Loreto, C.; Leonardi, R.; Musumeci, G.; Pannone, G.; Castorina, S. An Ex Vivo Study on Immunohistochemical Localization of MMP-7 and MMP-9 in Temporomandibular Joint Discs with Internal Derangement. *Eur. J. Histochem.* **2013**, *57*, e12. [CrossRef] [PubMed]
15. Planello, A.C.; Campos, M.I.G.; Meloto, C.B.; Secolin, R.; Rizatti-Barbosa, C.M.; Line, S.R.P.; De Souza, A.P.; Rizatti-Barbosa, C.M. Association of matrix metalloproteinase gene polymorphism with temporomandibular joint degeneration. *Eur. J. Oral Sci.* **2011**, *119*, 1–6. [CrossRef]
16. Milosevic, N.; Nikolic, N.; Djordjevic, I.; Todorović, A.; Lazić, V.; Milašin, J. Association of Functional Polymorphisms in Matrix Metalloproteinase-9 and Glutathione S-Transferase T1 Genes with Temporomandibular Disorders. *J. Oral Facial Pain Headache* **2015**, *29*, 279–285. [CrossRef]
17. Luo, S.; Deng, M.; Long, X.; Li, J.; Xu, L.; Fang, W. Association between polymorphism of MMP-1 promoter and the susceptibility to anterior disc displacement and temporomandibular joint osteoarthritis. *Arch. Oral Boil.* **2015**, *60*, 1675–1680. [CrossRef]
18. Tiilikainen, P.; Pirttiniemi, P.; Kainulainen, T.; Pernu, H.; Raustia, A. MMP-3 and -8 expression is found in the condylar surface of temporomandibular joints with internal derangement. *J. Oral Pathol. Med.* **2005**, *34*, 39–45. [CrossRef]
19. Ishimaru, J.-I.; Oguma, Y.; Goss, A. Matrix metalloproteinase and tissue inhibitor of metalloproteinase in serum and lavage synovial fluid of patients with temporomandibular joint disorders. *Br. J. Oral Maxillofac. Surg.* **2000**, *38*, 354–359. [CrossRef]
20. Kanyama, M.; Kuboki, T.; Kojima, S.; Fujisawa, T.; Hattori, T.; Takigawa, M.; Yamashita, A. Matrix metalloproteinases and tissue inhibitors of metalloproteinases in synovial fluids of patients with temporomandibular joint osteoarthritis. *J. Orofac. Pain* **2000**, *14*, 20–30.
21. Marchetti, C.; Cornaglia, I.; Casasco, A.; Bernasconi, G.; Baciliero, U.; Stetler-Stevenson, W. Immunolocalization of gelatinase-A (matrix metalloproteinase-2) in damaged human temporomandibular joint discs. *Arch. Oral Boil.* **1999**, *44*, 297–304. [CrossRef]

22. Yoshida, H.; Yoshida, T.; Iizuka, T.; Sakakura, T.; Fujita, S. The localization of matrix metalloproteinase-3 and tenascin in synovial membrane of the temporomandibular joint with internal derangement. *Oral Dis.* **1999**, *5*, 50–54. [CrossRef] [PubMed]
23. Fujita, H.; Morisugi, T.; Tanaka, Y.; Kawakami, T.; Kirita, T.; Yoshimura, Y. MMP-3 activation is a hallmark indicating an early change in TMJ disorders, and is related to nitration. *Int. J. Oral Maxillofac. Surg.* **2009**, *38*, 70–78. [CrossRef] [PubMed]
24. Srinivas, R.; Sorsa, T.; Tjäderhane, L.; Niemi, E.; Raustia, A.; Pernu, H.; Teronen, O.; Salo, T. Matrix metalloproteinases in mild and severe temporomandibular joint internal derangement synovial fluid. *Oral Surg. Oral Med. Oral Pathol. Oral Radiol. Endodontol.* **2001**, *91*, 517–525. [CrossRef] [PubMed]
25. Yoshida, K.; Takatsuka, S.; Hatada, E.; Nakamura, H.; Tanaka, A.; Ueki, K.; Nakagawa, K.; Okada, Y.; Yamamoto, E.; Fukuda, R. Expression of matrix metalloproteinases and aggrecanase in the synovial fluids of patients with symptomatic temporomandibular disorders. *Oral Surg. Oral Med. Oral Pathol. Oral Radiol. Endodontol.* **2006**, *102*, 22–27. [CrossRef]
26. Mizui, T.; Ishimaru, J.-I.; Miyamoto, K.; Kurita, K. Matrix metalloproteinase-2 in synovial lavage fluid of patients with disorders of the temporomandibular joint. *Br. J. Oral Maxillofac. Surg.* **2001**, *39*, 310–314. [CrossRef]
27. Tanaka, A.; Kumagai, S.; Kawashiri, S.; Takatsuka, S.; Nakagawa, K.; Yamamoto, E.; Matsumoto, N. Expression of matrix metalloproteinase-2 and -9 in synovial fluid of the temporomandibular joint accompanied by anterior disc displacement. *J. Oral Pathol. Med.* **2001**, *30*, 59–64. [CrossRef]
28. Fernandes, G.; Gonçalves, D.; Conti, P. Musculoskeletal Disorders. *Dent. Clin. N. Am.* **2018**, *62*, 553–564. [CrossRef]
29. Zotti, F.; Albanese, M.; Rodella, L.F.; Nocini, P.F. Platelet-Rich Plasma in treatment of Temporomandibular Joint: Narrative Review. *Int. J. Mol. Sci.* **2019**, *20*, 277. [CrossRef]
30. Catherine, Z.; Breton, P.; Bouletreau, P. Condylar resorption after orthognathic surgery: A systematic review. *Rev. Stomatol. Chir. Maxillo Faciale Chir. Orale* **2016**, *117*, 3–10. [CrossRef]
31. Laskin, D.M. Arthroscopy versus Arthrocentesis for Treating Internal Derangements of the Temporomandibular Joint. *Oral Maxillofac. Surg. Clin. N. Am.* **2018**, *30*, 325–328. [CrossRef] [PubMed]
32. Bruguiere, F.; Sciote, J.J.; Roland-Billecart, T.; Raoul, G.; Machuron, F.; Ferri, J.; Nicot, R. Pre-operative parafunctional or dysfunctional oral habits are associated with the temporomandibular disorders after orthognathic surgery: An observational cohort study. *J. Oral Rehabil.* **2018**, *46*, 321–329. [CrossRef] [PubMed]
33. Ouanounou, A.; Goldberg, M.; Haas, D.A. Pharmacotherapy in Temporomandibular Disorders: A Review. *J. Can. Dent. Assoc.* **2017**, *83*, 1–8.
34. Vandenbroucke, R.E.; Libert, C. Is there new hope for therapeutic matrix metalloproteinase inhibition? *Nat. Rev. Drug Discov.* **2014**, *13*, 904–927. [CrossRef]
35. Winer, A.; Adams, S.; Mignatti, P. Matrix Metalloproteinase Inhibitors in Cancer Therapy: Turning Past Failures into Future Successes. *Mol. Cancer Ther.* **2018**, *17*, 1147–1155. [CrossRef]

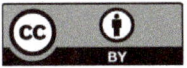

© 2019 by the authors. Licensee MDPI, Basel, Switzerland. This article is an open access article distributed under the terms and conditions of the Creative Commons Attribution (CC BY) license (http://creativecommons.org/licenses/by/4.0/).

Review

The Telocytes in the Subepicardial Niche

Cristian Bogdan Iancu [1], Mugurel Constantin Rusu [1,*], Laurențiu Mogoantă [2], Sorin Hostiuc [3] and Oana Daniela Toader [4]

1. Division of Anatomy, Faculty of Dental Medicine, "Carol Davila" University of Medicine and Pharmacy, RO-050474 Bucharest, Romania; crisbo6@gmail.com
2. Department of Histology, University of Medicine and Pharmacy Craiova, RO-200349 Craiova, Romania; laurentiu_mogoanta@yahoo.com
3. Department of Legal Medicine and Bioethics, Faculty of Dental Medicine, "Carol Davila" University of Medicine and Pharmacy, RO-050474 Bucharest, Romania; soraer@gmail.com
4. Department XIII of Obstetrics, Gynecology and Neonatology, "Polizu" Clinical Hospital, "Carol Davila" University of Medicine and Pharmacy, RO-050474 Bucharest, Romania; oana.toader@yahoo.com
* Correspondence: anatomon@gmail.com; Tel.: +40-722-363-705

Received: 3 March 2019; Accepted: 15 April 2019; Published: 18 April 2019

Abstract: A great interest has developed over the last several years in research on interstitial Cajal-like cells (ICLCs), later renamed to telocytes (TCs). Such studies are restricted by diverse limitations. We aimed to critically review (sub)epicardial ICLCs/TCs and to bring forward supplemental immunohistochemical evidence on (sub)epicardial stromal niche inhabitants. We tested the epicardial expressions of CD117/c-kit, CD34, Cytokeratin 7 (CK7), Ki67, Platelet-Derived Growth Factor Receptor (PDGFR)-α and D2-40 in adult human cardiac samples. The mesothelial epicardial cells expressed D2-40, CK7, CD117/c-kit and PDGFR-α. Subepicardial D2-40-positive lymphatic vessels and isolated D2-40-positive and CK7-positive subepicardial cells were also found. Immediate submesothelial spindle-shaped cells expressed Ki-67. Submesothelial stromal cells and endothelial tubes were PDGFR-α-positive and CD34-positive. The expression of CD34 was pan-stromal, so a particular stromal cell type could not be distinguished. The stromal expression of CD117/c-kit was also noted. It seems that epicardial TCs could not be regarded as belonging to a unique cell type until (pre)lymphatic endothelial cells are inadequately excluded. Markers such as CD117/c-kit or CD34 seem to be improper for identifying TCs as a distinctive cell type. Care should be taken when using the immunohistochemical method and histological interpretations, as they may not produce accurate results.

Keywords: heart; pericardium; cytokeratin; c-kit; PDGFR; initial lymphatics

---

1. Introduction

Telocytes (TCs) were proposed in 2010 as being stromal cells morphologically different from other interstitial resident cells [1]. They were previously considered interstitial Cajal-like cells (ICLCs) [2–10]. Telocytes are small-sized cells residing in stem niches; they project long, slender, and moniliform prolongations, which are known as telopodes [11–14]. In recent years, TCs have been noted in almost all organs and tissues in the human body [15,16]. To date, no selective marker has been found for TCs [17]. The immunophenotype of TCs 'is similar to that of interstitial, endothelial, smooth muscle, mast and haematopoietic stem cells and neurons' [18]. Increasing evidence strongly suggests that, rather than being a distinctive cell type, TCs are just a cell morphology [11] of other TC-like cell types (fibroblasts, immune cells, endothelial cells, stem cells, etc.) [19–21], or a morphology resulted if thin, flat, pancake-like cells are cut and documented on two-dimensional slices [22]. Nevertheless, TCs, as a group, could simply be the result of a lack of uniformity and consensus in the terminology relating to CD34-positive stromal cells used by different research teams [23]. Telocytes do not appear in the *Terminologia Histologica* [24,25].

The cardiac lymph is drained through the initial lymphatics from the subendocardial plexus to Sappey's subepicardial plexus by intramyocardial channels; precollecting vessels drain the subepicardial plexus into collecting vessels running alongside the major coronary branches [26]. When cardiac ICLCs/TCs were documented previously, they were not distinguished from lymphatic endothelial cells [26].

Following our research on the general background of TCs, we decided to critically review and provide new immunohistochemical evidence on (sub)epicardial stromal niche inhabitants. Very few studies have attempted to characterize epicardial ICLCs/TCs in different species and by different methods [10,27–29] or to test whether or not such stromal inhabitants of a niche supplied by the overlying mesothelium belong to Sappey's subepicardial plexus. We found no previously existing evidence indicating a potential mesothelial origin of (sub)epicardial ICLCs/TCs. We therefore applied an epithelial and a lymphatic marker within a panel of antibodies that also included c-kit and CD34, commonly used markers for ICLCs/TCs [10,30–33], but also hematopoietic markers, to document potentially overlooked cells discrimination when TCs were found in the subepicardial niche.

2. Materials and Methods

We performed a retrospective immunohistochemical study on archived paraffin-embedded samples of adult human cardiac tissue (seven cases) resulting from donor cadavers who died of non-cardiac diseases, with age ranges from 54 to 65 years. The study was tacitly approved by the responsible authorities where the work was carried out, and it was conducted in accordance with the general principles of medical research, as stated in the Declaration of Helsinki.

The paraffin-embedded samples were processed with an automatic histoprocessor (Diapath, Martinengo, BG, Italy) with paraffin embedding. Sections were cut manually at 3 μm and mounted on SuperFrost® electrostatic slides for immunohistochemistry (Thermo Scientific, Menzel-Gläser, Braunschweig, Germany). Histological evaluations used 3-μm-thick sections stained with hematoxylin and eosin. Internal negative controls resulted when the primary antibodies were not applied on slides.

The following antibodies have been used in immunohistochemical reactions: CD117/c-kit (Y145 clone), rabbit monoclonal antibody, Biocare Medical, Concord, CA, USA; CD34 (QBEnd/10 clone), mouse monoclonal antibody, Biocare Medical, Concord, CA, USA; Cytokeratin 7/CK7 (OV-TL 12/30 clone), mouse monoclonal antibody, Biocare Medical, Concord, CA, USA; Ki67 (MIB clone), mouse monoclonal antibody, Biocare Medical, Concord, CA, USA; Platelet-Derived Growth Factor Receptor (PDGFR)-α (C-9 clone), mouse monoclonal antibody, Santa Cruz Biotechnology Inc. CA, USA; D2-40 Lymphatic Marker (D2-40 clone) and mouse monoclonal antibody, Biocare Medical, Concord, CA, USA.

In all cases, the tissues were deparaffinized and rehydrated prior to labelling and then treated according to the protocol to block endogenous enzymes or to unmask the antigens. For CD34, Ki67, CK7, D2-40 Lymphatic Marker and CD117/c-kit, the endogenous peroxidase was blocked using a stabilized hydrogen peroxide compound (Peroxidazed 1-Biocare Medical, Concord, CA, USA). The samples labelled with PDGFR-α antibody were heated at 95 °C for 5 min in sodium citrate buffer, pH 6.0, to unmask the antigen. The next steps were performed according to manufacturer's instructions. Briefly, the separate protocols are indicated below.

CD34: The samples were pretreated enzymatically using a trypsin kit (Carezyme I-Biocare Medical Concord, CA, USA). To reduce nonspecific background staining, a Background Punisher Kit (Biocare Medical, Concord, CA, USA) was used for 10 min at room temperature (RT). Next, the primary antibody was added at a dilution of 1:50 for one hour at RT. A two-step detection system was used: Universal Horseradish Peroxidase (HRP) Detection Kit (Biocare Medical Concord, CA, USA), employing a DAB (3,3'-diaminobenzidine) substrate for HRP-based detection.

Ki67, CK7, D2-40 Lymphatic Marker, and CD117/c-kit: Pretreatment for epitope retrieval was performed at a high temperature in a controlled environment using a Decloaking Chamber (Biocare

Medical, Concord, CA, USA) and a retrieval solution at pH 6 (Revealer Decloaker-Biocare Medical, Concord, CA, USA); these solutions are specially formulated for superior pH stability at high temperatures. Blocking endogenous biotin and reducing nonspecific background was done similarly to CD34 staining. Subsequently, primary antibodies were added at a specified dilution (1:100 for Ki67, CK7, and D2-40 Lymphatic Marker and 1:200 in the case of CD117/c-kit) for half an hour to one hour at RT. Next, a secondary probe and an enzyme-labelled tertiary polymer were added consecutively at RT for 10 min each. These two steps belong to the MACH 4™ Universal Alkaline Phosphatase Polymer Detection Kit (Biocare Medical, Concord, CA, USA).

CD117/c-kit was treated with an enzyme-labelled secondary polymer, at RT, according to the MACH 2 Universal Alkaline Phosphatase Polymer Detection Kit (Biocare Medical, Concord, CA, USA). Finally, a HRP-based detection system employing a DAB substrate (Biocare's DAB) was used.

PDGFR-α: The specimens were incubated for 1 h in UltraCruz® Blocking Reagent (Santa Cruz Biotechnology Inc. CA, USA), followed by adding up the primary antibody at a dilution of 1:50 for 30 min at room temperature. After three washes with PBS, the slides were incubated for 45 min with biotin-conjugated secondary antibody diluted in UltraCruz® Blocking Reagent and next with avidin-biotin complex, using the A and B reagents from the ImmunoCruz® ABC Kit (Santa Cruz Biotechnology Inc. CA, USA) for another 30 min. A peroxidase substrate and a chromogen mixture system employing hydrogen peroxide and DAB chromophore were used for detection.

The negative controls included omission of either the first- or the second-step reagent and substitution of the first-step reagent with an irrelevant isotype-matched antibody.

In all cases, the sections were counterstained with haematoxylin and rinsed with purified, deionised water.

The slides were analysed and sorted using a calibrated station for scaling numerous microphotographs. We used a Zeiss working station composed of an AxioImager M1 microscope and an AxioCam HRc camera, both integrated by AxioVision imaging software capable of image acquisition, processing, analysis, and interpretation (Carl Zeiss AG, Oberkochen, Germany).

3. Results

We accurately identified the epicardial histology of hematoxylin and eosin-stained slides. The single-cell mesothelial layer of epicardium covers the subepicardial stroma consisting of subepicardial fat embedding microvessels, nerves (occasionally with intrinsic solitary neurons) and microganglia, and isolated cells, both spindle-shaped and rounded.

On several samples, the epicardium appeared to be denuded of mesothelial cells. When hypertrophied mesothelial epicardial cells were present, they expressed D2-40 (Figure 1), CK7 (Figure 2), CD117/c-kit (Figure 3) and PDGFR-α (Figure 4). We did not observe the mesothelial expression of CD34.

Immediately beneath the mesothelial layer, lumina-presenting, thin, lymphatic vessels with circumferential dispositions were labelled with the D2-40 marker (Figure 1). Moreover, large lymphatic vessels with nuclei bulging into lumina (Figure 1) and isolated D2-40-expressing rounded cells with eccentric nuclei and small protrusions (Figure 1) were found embedded within the submesothelial fat of the samples. We noted that the endothelial cells of longitudinally cut lymphatic vessels could have a TC-like appearance, but the identification of lumina made the distinction between these cell types (Figure 1).

Rounded CK7-positive isolated subepicardial cells were identified on the slides (Figure 2). Moreover, immediate submesothelial spindle-shaped cells expressed the proliferation marker Ki-67 (Figure 2). Stromal cells and endothelial tubes in the submesothelial stroma were found expressing PDGFR-α (Figure 4) as well as CD34 (Figure 5). The expression of CD34 seemed pan-stromal, so no particular stromal cell type could be identified. The stromal expression of CD117/c-kit was also observed in the slides (Figure 3).

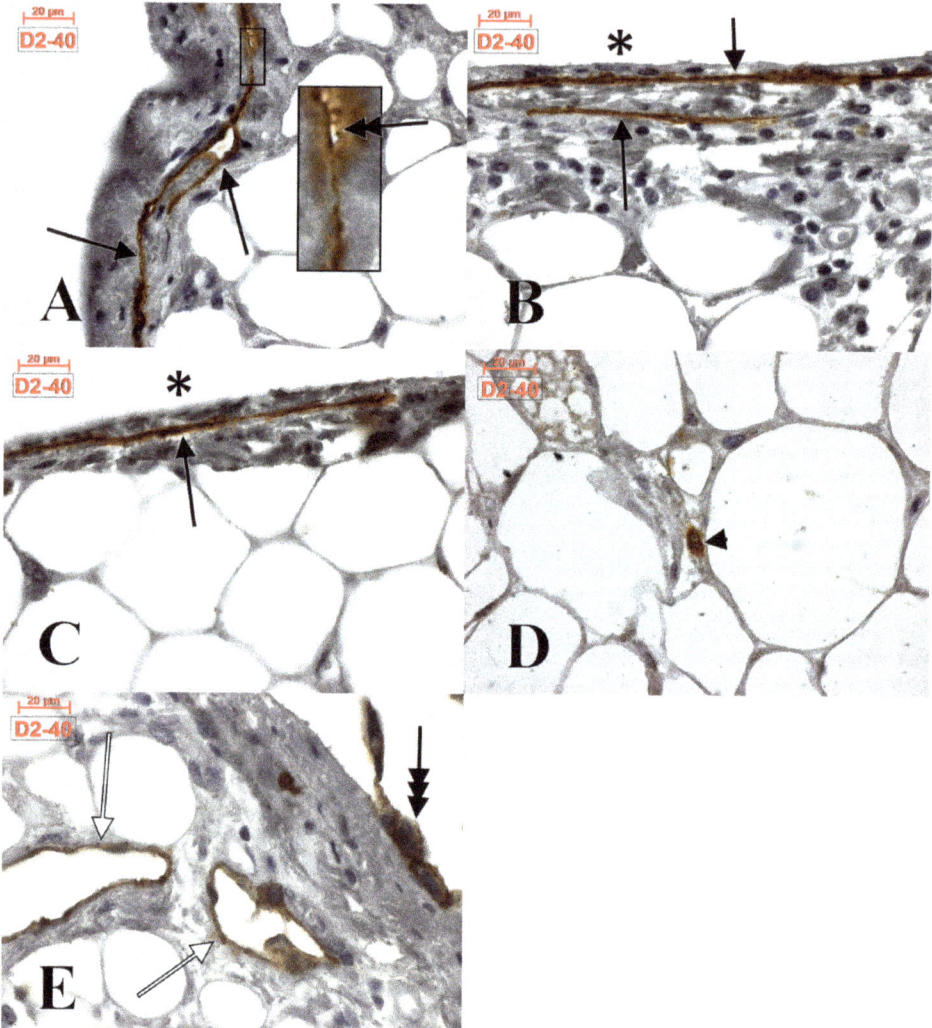

Figure 1. Human adult cardiac wall (**A–D**: left atrial wall, **E**: left atrial appendage). Epicardial and subepicardial expression of podoplanin (D2-40). Thin subepicardial lymphatics express D2-40 (**A–C**, arrows). When they are tangentially cut, they could be confused with telopodes (**A**, inset, digitally magnified) if the narrow lumen (double-headed arrow) is overlooked. The arrowhead in (**D**) indicates a D2-40-expressing isolated cell embedded within the subepicardial fat. Although epicardium was largely denuded of epithelium (*) in the studied samples, there were found areas covered by D2-40 + hypertrophied mesothelial cells (E, triple-headed arrow). Large lymph collectors with intraluminally bulged endothelial cells were found embedded within the subepicardial fat (E, white arrows).

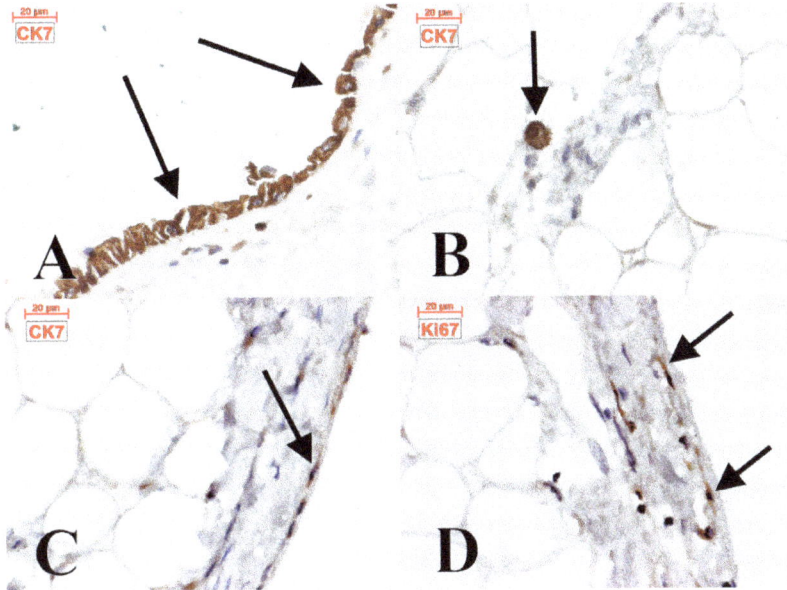

Figure 2. Human adult cardiac wall. Cytokeratin 7 is expressed in epicardial (mesothelial) cells (**A**, arrows), as well as in isolated subepicardial round cells (**B**, arrow) and in immediate subepicardial spindle-shaped slender cells (**C**, arrow). These last also express Ki67 (**D**, arrows), the proliferative marker.

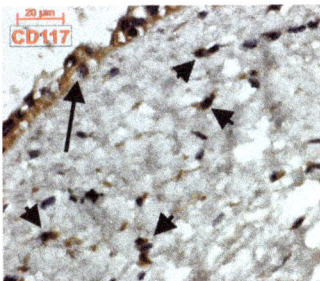

Figure 3. Human adult cardiac wall. CD117/c-kit has epicardial (mesothelial) (arrow) and subepicardial (arrowheads) expression.

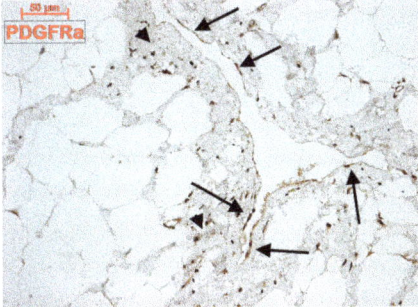

Figure 4. Human adult cardiac wall. Epicardial (mesothelial) (arrows) and subepicardial (arrowheads) expression of Platelet-Derived Growth Factor Receptor (PDGFRα).

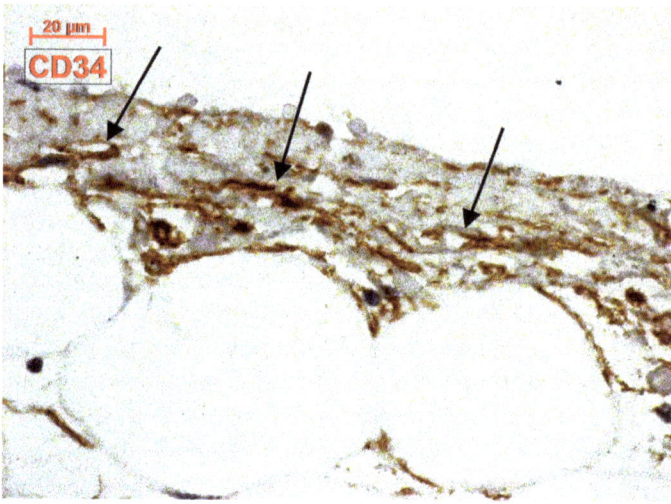

Figure 5. Human adult cardiac wall. Immediate submesothelial expression of CD34 includes nascent endothelial tubes (arrows).

4. Discussion

4.1. The Epicardial Lymphatics

The cardiac lymph is drained through the initial lymphatics from the subendocardial lymphatic plexus to Sappey's subepicardial lymphatic plexus via intramyocardial lymphatic channels; precollecting vessels from the subepicardial plexus further drain into collecting vessels neighboring the major coronary branches [26]. Here, we detected the immediate submesothelial location of Sappey's subepicardial lymphatic plexus, which consists of lymphatic vessels with circumferential dispositions. As lymphatics were overlooked in tissue samples in which cardiac ICLCs/TCs were discriminated [26], the molecular anatomy of the epicardial niche must be revisited.

4.2. C-Kit-Positive Cardiac Cells

The c-kit protein (CD117) is a type III tyrosine-protein kinase that recognises the stem cell factor (SCF) ligand [34]. During development, the c-kit receptor is expressed both in cardiac progenitors capable of cardiomyogenesis and in others with divergent evolution patterns [35]. This receptor–ligand interaction activates signaling pathways that are responsible for cellular proliferation, development and differentiation. We found c-kit expressed equally in epicardial mesothelial and subepicardial stromal cells, which could indicate the presence of a stem/progenitor niche and transdifferentiation processes.

The cardiac stem cells expressing c-kit have been studied extensively (see [35]). Approximately 1.1–1.8% of the myocardial cell population in humans are c-kit-positive [36,37]. Approximately half of these cells are multipotent cells, and the other half are early committed cells [38]. Interestingly, most of the detected c-kit-positive cells were found to also express two other proteins: CD45 and CD34, the pan-leukocyte and endothelial/hematopoietic progenitor markers, respectively [39,40]. With rare exceptions, freshly isolated c-kit-positive cells do not express myocytes (α-sarcomeric actin, cardiac myosin, desmin, α-cardiac actinin and connexin 43), endothelial cells (von Willebrand factor, CD31 and vimentin), smooth muscle cells (α-smooth muscle actin and desmin) or fibroblast cytoplasmic proteins (fibronectin, procollagen I and vimentin) [41]. In vitro, isolated, c-kit-positive cardiac stem cells are spindle-shaped, like cardiac fibroblasts, and co-express GATA4 and NKX2.5 [36,42].

The pattern of markers displayed by c-kit-positive cells raised doubts with regards to their origin. Beltrami et al. found that endothelial progenitor cells (EPCs) express both c-kit and CD34, while c-kit-positive stromal cells are negative for the endothelial/hematopoietic progenitor marker CD34 [41]. They are also different from bone-marrow-derived cells, which express CD45 [41]. Interestingly, several studies demonstrated that most c-kit-positive stromal cardiac cells are mast cells that co-express CD45 [43,44], while c-kit-positive/CD45 stromal cells express mRNA of the endothelial lineage [45]. Accordingly, either c-kit-expressing TCs will not express CD34 or CD34-positive TCs are not c-kit-expressing cells. The expressions of c-kit and CD34 in cardiac interstitia are mutually exclusive and not concomitant. If they are found to be concomitant, the immunohistochemical method and its results should be checked or repeated to avoid producing inaccurate data (Figure 6).

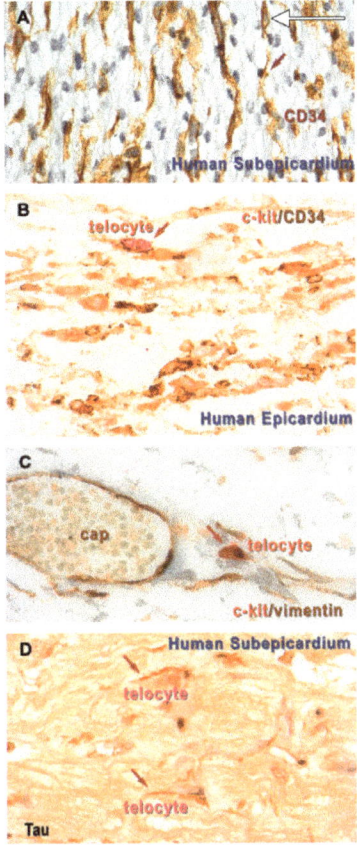

Figure 6. Reprinted with permission from John Wiley and Sons (License Number: 4562340930830) from [27]. The original legend in the *.pdf version of the article indicates "*Figure 3(A) Immunostaining for CD34 (brown). CD34 positivity might be expressed by telocytes and endothelial cells. (B) Localization of double positive cells for c-Kit (red) and CD34 (brown). (C) Human epicardium, deep layer. Vimentin positivity is stronger than c-Kit positivity by sandwich method. (D) Cells expressing τ protein (arrows). (A–D) Original magnification, 40X*". One could observe from the figure and the legend that the thin arrow added by the authors in (**A**) was not assigned to endothelial tubes, nor was it regarded as a telocyte, but it rather belongs to an endothelial tube (we added an additional white arrow). The cells indicated as "telocytes" in (**B,C**) do not display the peculiar telopodes. The expression of Tau-protein demonstrated in (**D**) is rather pan-tissular due to a consistent background staining. The double-labelling result in (**B**) indicating a c-kit+/CD34+ phenotype of telocytes (TCs) is highly speculative due to an invalid immunohistochemical method that determined the pan-labelling of the slide.

4.3. What Are (Sub)epicardial TCs?

Stem cells can originate from the epithelial–mesenchymal transformation (EMT) of epicardial mesothelial cells (EMCs) in the adult human heart [46,47]. Epicardium-derived cells (EPDCs) are known to express CD117/c-kit [46], which matches with our results. Immunofluorescence of the ICLCs found subepicardial TCs immediately beneath the CD34-positive epicardial mesothelium, which were either CD34-positive/c-kit-positive or purely c-kit-positive [10]. It appears that subepicardial ICLCs/TCs are EPDCs. This is reinforced by our discovery of proliferative immediate submesothelial Ki-67-positive spindle-shaped cells. Such submesothelial ICLCs were further documented through transmission electron microscopy (TEM) by the same research group; beneath them, 'isolated smooth muscle cells' were found [29]. In that study [29], subepicardial ICLCs were speculated through TEM without the aid of any antibodies. Further studies of the subepicardial niche were performed by Popescu et al., who reported an enlarged panel of markers useful for the identification of subepicardial TCs, such as vimentin, S100 protein, tau protein, CD57 and nestin [27]. This last antibody was listed in the report's Materials and Methods section but was not documented in the Results section of that article [27]. A polyclonal antibody was then used against CD117/c-kit [27], but that immunohistochemical method included an antigen retrieval stage (though this procedure may produce nonspecific staining results) [48]. Completely and nonspecifically stained slides were then used to sample the findings on the subepicardial TCs (Figure 6), so the respective evidence could not convince. This is demonstrative of the highly subjective manner in which TCs were assigned molecular phenotypes in the past. As we discussed previously, a lack of evidence for telepodes does not exclude the possibility of a TC morphology being present [20]. Notably, the possible expression of tau protein in TCs was speculated (Figure 6) but not discussed further in that study [27], although the presence of this protein would have indicated the presence of microtubular content in TCs. This, in turn, may have been perplexing; when this research team identified the ultrastructural anatomy of TCs [1], microtubules were not listed.

In another study, epicardial ICLCs were found to be positive for c-kit and/or CD34, or they co-expressed c-kit and vimentin [10]. In a subsequent study, epicardial TCs were found to co-express either c-kit and CD34 or c-kit and vimentin [27]. In both these studies, Popescu et al. did not examine the epicardial expressions of lymphatic markers, mast cell markers or CD45. The expression of c-kit combined with the expressions of well-known endothelial markers, such as CD34 and vimentin, could not exclude TCs from the possibility of being of the endothelial lineage. It was suggested to use CD31 to discriminate the endothelial cells from TCs [49]. We also noted the striking histological resemblance of c-kit-positive epicardial 'telocytes' (Figure 2B in [27]) to c-kit-positive mast cells (Figure 1D in [50]). Both appear as large and degranulating cells. All these observations support recent and consistent evidence for TCs' failure to be categorized as a distinctive cell type [11,24,26].

4.4. The Epicardial and Subepicardial Expression of Podoplanin

Although in the central nervous system (CNS) and thymus, endothelial cells and pericytes result from ectoderm-derived neural crest cells, they are mesoderm- and mesothelium-derived in coelomic organs [51]. This supports the (re)activated mechanism of mesothelial-to-endothelial/pericitary transformation in epicardial cells, which is actually an epithelial–mesenchymal transformation (EMT), ensuring that either subepicardial vasculogenesis or subepicardial lymphvasculogenesis occurs. This reasonably correlates with our evidence of podoplanin-expressing mesothelial cells and submesothelial lymphatics and isolated cells. We also found PDGFR-α-expressing epicardial mesothelial cells; this is normal, as signaling through both PDGFRs, α and β, is needed for epicardial EMT and the formation of EPDCs [52]. In these regards, testing the PDGFR expression in mesothelial cells would support a potential of EMT in the samples studied. PDGFR-α is crucial in the differentiation of cardiac fibroblasts from EPDCs [53], so a PDGFR-α-positive subepicardial stroma would clearly indicate a subepicardium with reparatory potential, regardless of whether the respective stromal cells do or do not have telopodes. A strong expression of PDGFR-α in human adult cardiac tissue was demonstrated in the interstitial cells of the subepicardium, myocardium, endocardium, coronary smooth muscle and endothelial cells, as we also found, and cardiomyocytes express this marker [13,54]. PDGFR-α was not tested in previous studies on epicardial and subepicardial TCs, although Crețoiu and Popescu indicated that 'CD34/PDGFR[-]α double immunohistochemistry can orientate the diagnosis' [55]. This double expression was used for TC identification in other normal and pathological non-cardiac tissues [56–60]. Cardiac TCs were indicated to have a CD34-positive/PDGFR-α-positive phenotype [61], but this resulted in cell cultures that did not use any sorting molecules; cells were sorted solely based on morphological criteria. Moreover, the rodent hearts analysed 'were minced into 1 mm^3 pieces and incubated on an orbital shaker' [61], which could not permit the discrimination of epicardium-specific cells from other cell populations in those cardiac samples.

Podoplanin (or GP36, E11 antigen, oncofetal antigens M2A and T1A-2, aggrus) is a mucin-type transmembrane glycoprotein first identified as podoplanin in podocytes [62–64] but as the E11 antigen in osteoblasts and osteocytes [65,66]. Podoplanin is homologous to the oncofetal antigen M2A, which is recognized by the D2-40 antibody [67]. Lymphatic endothelial cells express high levels of podoplanin [68]. Podoplanin has homologues in humans, mice, rats, dogs and hamsters and is relatively well-conserved between species [68]. Podoplanin is a cell morphological regulator [67] and is required for normal heart development, specifically for EMT in epicardium-derived cells [68], and our evidence reasonably suggests that this role of podoplanin also exists in adult tissues. During development, podoplanin is expressed in the epithelial lining of the coelomic wall of the pericardio–peritoneal canal and in the cells lining the pleural and pericardial cavities [66]. Podoplanin is expressed in epithelial and mesothelial cells, such as those in the intestinal epithelium, alveolar type I cells, podocytes, the mesothelium of the visceral peritoneum [66] and, as we demonstrated, in epicardial mesothelial cells.

Several markers could be used to identify lymphatic endothelial cells on slides, such as CD31 (the pan-endothelial marker), podoplanin (D2-40), Vascular Endothelial Growth Factor Receptor-3 (VEGFR-3), Lymphatic Vascular Endothelial Hyaluronan Receptor-1 (LYVE-1) and Prospero related homeobox1 (PROX1) [69]. Therefore, further co-staining experiments could be helpful in better assessing the lymphatic anatomy of subepicardium. CD31 was noted as useful in discriminating between TCs and endothelial cells, as both are known to express CD34 [70]. It was recently demonstrated that pre-lymphatic interstitial spaces are lined by TC-like endothelial cells that express vimentin, CD34 and D2-40 but do not express other lymphatic markers, such as CD31, ERG (avian v-ets erythroblastosis virus E26 oncogene homolog) or LYVE-1 [71]. Therefore, neither CD31 nor lymphatic markers other than podoplanin/D2-40 could disprove the relationship between TCs and the lymph drainage pathway.

The processes of EMT allow epithelial cells to become mobile mesenchymal cells after the epithelial adherens junctions loosen through E-cadherin loss [66]. Podoplanin can be presented as an inhibitor of E-cadherin, thus stimulating the EMT process, which involves the epicardium in myocardial differentiation [66]. Therefore, expression of D2-40 in mesothelial cells, such as we found, could be indicative of the EMT potential of D2-40-positive mesothelial cells. Such transdifferentiations could support the potential for cardiac lymphatic vasculature to increase in major cardiac pathological changes, such as acute and chronic ischaemia, progressive atherosclerosis, myocarditis and hypertrophy [72].

4.5. Processes of Epicardial Transdifferentiation

The transition of a cell from an epithelial to a mesenchymal phenotype, or EMT, has been shown to play critical roles in several physiological and pathological contexts, from embryogenesis to fibrosis and cancer progression [73]. The postnatal mammalian epicardium is a dormant single-cell layer [74]. After an injury, the adult epicardium is activated, which involves the induction of a developmental gene program, EMT and migration [75]. Several genes are involved in epicardial activation, including WT1 (Wilms' tumour 1), TBX18 and RALDH2 [74]. Human EPDCs closely resemble submesothelial fibroblasts and express cardiac marker genes, such as GATA4 and cardiac troponin T [76]. EPDCs display intense β-catenin staining, which supports their epithelial nature [76]. The reactivation of the epicardium occurs in ischaemia, with the re-expression of developmental genes and renewed EMT [77].

We have brought forward evidence of CK7 expression in EMCs as well as in isolated subepicardial stromal cells that could be viewed as EPDCs. To our knowledge, the CK7 marker has not been tested previously on human cardiac samples. CK7 should therefore be included in the list of known markers of EPDCs, such as β-catenin, CD44, CD46, CD90, CD105, HLA-ABC [76] and WT1 [78]. The expression of CD117/c-kit was also associated with EPDCs [46]. We also found c-kit expressed in mesothelial cells, which could indicate that the stem/progenitor phenotype of future EPDCs could be acquired prior to the stromal migration of the epithelial cells. During human cardiogenesis, ventricular and atrial epicardia exhibit different pan-cytokeratin expression patterns and cell arrangements; atrial epicardial cells are distributed in a stochastic fashion on the surface with a diffuse cytokeratin expression throughout the cytoplasm, whereas ventricular epicardial cells exhibit a spindle-cell morphology and preferential alignment, being orientated side-by-side with strong cytokeratin staining outlining the cell membrane and cytoskeletal filaments [79]. Polyclonal anti-keratin antibodies were used to stain the mesothelial and mesenchymal cells of the proepicardium, as well as epicardium, in quail embryos [80,81], and not in human samples.

Adult EPDCs can form tube-like structures [75]. Tangentially cut tube-like structures, if tangentially cut, could appear on slides or grids as TC-like cells [82]. We found such D2-40-expressing tubes immediately beneath the podoplanin-expressing epicardial mesothelium, which strongly suggests that subepicardial lymphatics could acquire an epicardial-based support for their maintenance.

In a static two-dimensional TEM study of epicardial ICLCs, Gherghiceanu and Popescu observed that mesenchymal cells, 'guided by ICLCs, were found migrating from [the] sub-epicardial area in the mesothelial layer'; that is, they were 'migrating under the basal lamina of the epicardial mesothelial cell' [29]. The authors also speculated that 'epithelial–mesenchymal transition is not a common process involved in cardiac regeneration in vivo' [29]. That concept inspired us to document the processes of mesenchymal–epithelial transition (MET) mentioned by this TEM study.

TGFβ-induced EMT could be reversed through inhibition of the Smad2 signaling pathway [83]. Serum-free culture media, as well as TGFβ receptor inhibitors, notch receptor inhibitors or Rho-associated coiled-coil protein kinase (ROCK) inhibitors could inhibit EMT in differentiated epithelial cells or could induce MET in dedifferentiated epithelial cells [84].

The metanephric mesenchyme suffers an epithelial transformation regulated by WNT4 [85]. During this transformation, the WNT4 signal can be replaced by other members of the WNT gene family, including WNT1, WNT3A, WNT7A and WNT7B [86]. WNT proteins are also involved in cardiac development and differentiation [87]. The classic canonical WNT signaling pathway involves β-catenin [87]. The epicardial retinoic X receptor α is required for the EMT of epicardial cells, as the loss of that receptor results in damaged myocardial growth and coronary artery formation. WNT9B is downstream of the epicardial retinoic X receptor α, which in turn regulates FGFβ expression in the myocardium [87,88]. The in vitro EMT of human adult epicardial cells is regulated by TGFβ-signaling and WT-1 [78]. Gherghiceanu and Popescu's TEM discovery of isolated smooth muscle cells in the subepicardial space was appreciated as 'quite unique' and able to explain why EPDCs generate smooth muscle cells in cultures [29]. This is not a novelty, as both human and rat epicardial cells could be transdifferentiated to smooth muscle cells [76], and TGFβ stimulates the process of transdifferentiation [89].

Interestingly, during cardiac development, the atrial and ventricular epicardia behave differently under ex vivo conditions: only the ventricular EPDCs spontaneously undergo EMT (that is, growing with a spindle-like morphology and diminishing the expressions of WT-1, GATA5, TBX18 and TCF21) [79].

5. Conclusions

As the epicardium may undergo several different transdifferentiation processes, it is hazardous to designate intermediate cell stages as specific cell types. Epicardial ICLCs/TCs cannot be regarded as a particular cell type as (pre)lymphatic endothelial cells are inadequately excluded. Markers such as CD117/c-kit and CD34 seem to be unsuitable for identifying TCs as a distinctive cell type. The identification of TCs on two-dimensional slides should be regarded with caution, and researchers using the immunohistochemical method and related protocols should be careful to avoid gathering and promoting nonspecific or inaccurate results.

Author Contributions: Conceptualization, C.B.I. and M.C.R.; methodology, L.M.; software, S.H. and M.C.R.; validation, M.C.R., S.H. and L.M.; investigation, C.B.I., O.D.T.; writing—original draft preparation, C.B.I.; writing—review and editing, M.C.R. and S.H.

Funding: This research received no external funding.

Conflicts of Interest: The authors declare no conflict of interest.

References

1. Popescu, L.M.; Faussone-Pellegrini, M.S. TELOCYTES—A case of serendipity: The winding way from Interstitial Cells of Cajal (ICC), via Interstitial Cajal-Like Cells (ICLC) to TELOCYTES. *J. Cell. Mol. Med.* **2010**, *14*, 729–740. [CrossRef] [PubMed]
2. Ciontea, S.M.; Radu, E.; Regalia, T.; Ceafalan, L.; Cretoiu, D.; Gherghiceanu, M.; Braga, R.I.; Malincenco, M.; Zagrean, L.; Hinescu, M.E.; et al. C-kit immunopositive interstitial cells (Cajal-type) in human myometrium. *J. Cell. Mol. Med.* **2005**, *9*, 407–420. [CrossRef] [PubMed]
3. Cretoiu, D.; Ciontea, S.M.; Popescu, L.M.; Ceafalan, L.; Ardeleanu, C. Interstitial Cajal-like cells (ICLC) as steroid hormone sensors in human myometrium: Immunocytochemical approach. *J. Cell. Mol. Med.* **2006**, *10*, 789–795. [CrossRef]
4. Gherghiceanu, M.; Hinescu, M.E.; Andrei, F.; Mandache, E.; Macarie, C.E.; Faussone-Pellegrini, M.S.; Popescu, L.M. Interstitial Cajal-like cells (ICLC) in myocardial sleeves of human pulmonary veins. *J. Cell. Mol. Med.* **2008**, *12*, 1777–1781. [CrossRef] [PubMed]
5. Gherghiceanu, M.; Hinescu, M.E.; Popescu, L.M. Myocardial interstitial Cajal-like cells (ICLC) in caveolin-1 KO mice. *J. Cell. Mol. Med.* **2009**, *13*, 202–206. [CrossRef]
6. Hinescu, M.E.; Gherghiceanu, M.; Mandache, E.; Ciontea, S.M.; Popescu, L.M. Interstitial Cajal-like cells (ICLC) in atrial myocardium: Ultrastructural and immunohistochemical characterization. *J. Cell. Mol. Med.* **2006**, *10*, 243–257. [CrossRef]
7. Hinescu, M.E.; Popescu, L.M. Interstitial Cajal-like cells (ICLC) in human atrial myocardium. *J. Cell. Mol. Med.* **2005**, *9*, 972–975. [CrossRef]
8. Kostin, S.; Popescu, L.M. A distinct type of cell in myocardium: Interstitial Cajal-like cells (ICLCs). *J. Cell. Mol. Med.* **2009**, *13*, 295–308. [CrossRef]
9. Pieri, L.; Vannucchi, M.G.; Faussone-Pellegrini, M.S. Histochemical and ultrastructural characteristics of an interstitial cell type different from ICC and resident in the muscle coat of human gut. *J. Cell. Mol. Med.* **2008**, *12*, 1944–1955. [CrossRef]
10. Suciu, L.; Popescu, L.M.; Regalia, T.; Ardelean, A.; Manole, C.G. Epicardium: Interstitial Cajal-like cells (ICLC) highlighted by immunofluorescence. *J. Cell. Mol. Med.* **2009**, *13*, 771–777. [CrossRef]
11. Iancu, C.B.; Rusu, M.C.; Mogoanta, L.; Hostiuc, S.; Grigoriu, M. Myocardial Telocyte-Like Cells: A Review Including New Evidence. *Cells Tissues Organs* **2019**. [CrossRef]
12. Rusu, M.C.; Folescu, R.; Manoiu, V.S.; Didilescu, A.C. Suburothelial interstitial cells. *Cells Tissues Organs* **2014**, *199*, 59–72. [CrossRef]
13. Rusu, M.C.; Hostiuc, S.; Vrapciu, A.D.; Mogoanta, L.; Manoiu, V.S.; Grigoriu, F. Subsets of telocytes: Myocardial telocytes. *Ann. Anat.* **2017**, *209*, 37–44. [CrossRef]
14. Grigoriu, F.; Hostiuc, S.; Vrapciu, A.D.; Rusu, M.C. Subsets of telocytes: The progenitor cells in the human endocardial niche. *Rom. J. Morphol. Embryol.* **2016**, *57*, 767–774.
15. Varga, I.; Polak, S.; Kyselovic, J.; Kachlik, D.; Danisovic, L.; Klein, M. Recently Discovered Interstitial Cell Population of Telocytes: Distinguishing Facts from Fiction Regarding Their Role in the Pathogenesis of Diverse Diseases Called "Telocytopathies". *Medicina* **2019**, *55*, 56. [CrossRef]
16. Dobra, M.A.; Vrapciu, A.D.; Pop, F.; Petre, N.; Rusu, M.C. The molecular phenotypes of ureteral telocytes are layer-specific. *Acta Histochem.* **2017**. [CrossRef]

17. Vannucchi, M.G.; Traini, C. The telocytes/myofibroblasts 3-D network forms a stretch receptor in the human bladder mucosa. Is this structure involved in the detrusor overactive diseases? *Ann. Anat.* **2018**, *218*, 118–123. [CrossRef] [PubMed]
18. Mitrofanova, L.B.; Gorshkov, A.N.; Konovalov, P.V.; Krylova, J.S. Telocytes in the human sinoatrial node. *J. Cell. Mol. Med.* **2017**. [CrossRef] [PubMed]
19. Rusu, M.C.; Hostiuc, S. Telocytes and telocytes-like cells. Past, present, and above all future. *Ann. Anat.* **2019**. [CrossRef]
20. Petrea, C.E.; Craitoiu, S.; Vrapciu, A.D.; Manoiu, V.S.; Rusu, M.C. The telopode- and filopode-projecting heterogeneous stromal cells of the human sclera niche. *Ann. Anat.* **2018**, *218*, 129–140. [CrossRef] [PubMed]
21. Petrea, C.E.; Rusu, M.C.; Manoiu, V.S.; Vrapciu, A.D. Telocyte-Like Cells Containing Weibel-Palade Bodies in Rat Lamina Fusca. *Ann. Anat.* **2018**, *218*, 88–94. [CrossRef] [PubMed]
22. Neuhaus, J.; Schroppel, B.; Dass, M.; Zimmermann, H.; Wolburg, H.; Fallier-Becker, P.; Gevaert, T.; Burkhardt, C.J.; Do, H.M.; Stolzenburg, J.U. 3D-electron microscopic characterization of interstitial cells in the human bladder upper lamina propria. *Neurourol. Urodyn.* **2018**, *37*, 89–98. [CrossRef]
23. Diaz-Flores, L.; Gutierrez, R.; Garcia, M.P.; Saez, F.J.; Diaz-Flores, L., Jr.; Valladares, F.; Madrid, J.F. CD34+ stromal cells/fibroblasts/fibrocytes/telocytes as a tissue reserve and a principal source of mesenchymal cells. Location, morphology, function and role in pathology. *Histol. Histopathol.* **2014**, *29*, 831–870. [CrossRef]
24. Varga, I.; Kyselovič, J.; Danišovič, Ľ.; Gálfiová, P.; Kachlík, D.; Polák, Š.; Klein, M. Recently discovered interstitial cells termed telocytes: Distinguishing cell-biological and histological facts from fictions. *Biologia* **2018**. [CrossRef]
25. Varga, I.; Danisovic, L.; Kyselovic, J.; Gazova, A.; Musil, P.; Miko, M.; Polak, S. The functional morphology and role of cardiac telocytes in myocardium regeneration. *Can. J. Physiol. Pharmacol.* **2016**. [CrossRef]
26. Rusu, M.C.; Hostiuc, S. Critical review: Cardiac telocytes vs cardiac lymphatic endothelial cells. *Ann. Anat.* **2019**, *222*, 40–54. [CrossRef] [PubMed]
27. Popescu, L.M.; Manole, C.G.; Gherghiceanu, M.; Ardelean, A.; Nicolescu, M.I.; Hinescu, M.E.; Kostin, S. Telocytes in human epicardium. *J. Cell. Mol. Med.* **2010**, *14*, 2085–2093. [CrossRef] [PubMed]
28. Popescu, L.M.; Gherghiceanu, M.; Manole, C.G.; Faussone-Pellegrini, M.S. Cardiac renewing: Interstitial Cajal-like cells nurse cardiomyocyte progenitors in epicardial stem cell niches. *J. Cell. Mol. Med.* **2009**, *13*, 866–886. [CrossRef]
29. Gherghiceanu, M.; Popescu, L.M. Human epicardium: Ultrastructural ancestry of mesothelium and mesenchymal cells. *J. Cell. Mol. Med.* **2009**, *13*, 2949–2951. [CrossRef]
30. Rusu, M.C.; Pop, F.; Hostiuc, S.; Dermengiu, D.; Lala, A.I.; Ion, D.A.; Manoiu, V.S.; Mirancea, N. The human trigeminal ganglion: C-kit positive neurons and interstitial cells. *Ann. Anat.* **2011**, *193*, 403–411. [CrossRef]
31. Suciu, L.; Popescu, L.M.; Gherghiceanu, M.; Regalia, T.; Nicolescu, M.I.; Hinescu, M.E.; Faussone-Pellegrini, M.S. Telocytes in human term placenta: Morphology and phenotype. *Cells Tissues Organs* **2010**, *192*, 325–339. [CrossRef]
32. Chang, Y.; Li, C.; Lu, Z.; Li, H.; Guo, Z. Multiple immunophenotypes of cardiac telocytes. *Exp. Cell Res.* **2015**, *338*, 239–244. [CrossRef]
33. Petre, N.; Rusu, M.C.; Pop, F.; Jianu, A.M. Telocytes of the mammary gland stroma. *Folia Morphol.* **2016**, *75*, 224–231. [CrossRef]
34. Iancu, C.B.; Iancu, D.; Rentea, I.; Hostiuc, S.; Dermengiu, D.; Rusu, M.C. Molecular signatures of cardiac stem cells. *Rom. J. Morphol. Embryol.* **2015**, *56*, 1255–1262.
35. Keith, M.C.; Bolli, R. "String Theory" of c-kitpos Cardiac Cells: A New Paradigm Regarding the Nature of These Cells That May Reconcile Apparently Discrepant Results. *Circ. Res.* **2015**, *116*, 1216–1230. [CrossRef]
36. Bearzi, C.; Rota, M.; Hosoda, T.; Tillmanns, J.; Nascimbene, A.; De Angelis, A.; Yasuzawa-Amano, S.; Trofimova, I.; Siggins, R.W.; Lecapitaine, N.; et al. Human cardiac stem cells. *Proc. Natl. Acad. Sci. USA* **2007**, *104*, 14068–14073. [CrossRef]
37. Choi, S.H.; Jung, S.Y.; Asahara, T.; Suh, W.; Kwon, S.-M.; Baek, S.H. Direct comparison of distinct cardiomyogenic induction methodologies in human cardiac-derived c-kit positive progenitor cells. *Tissue Eng. Regen. Med.* **2012**, *9*, 311–319. [CrossRef]
38. Bearzi, C.; Cascapera, S.; Nascimbene, A.; Casarsa, C.; Rastaldo, R.; Hosoda, T.; De Angelis, A.; Rota, M.; Quaini, F.; Urbanek, K.; et al. Late-Breaking Basic Science Abstracts. Late Breaking Developments in Stem Cell Biology and Cardiac Growth Regulation. *Circulation* **2005**, *111*, 1720–1724.

39. Ye, J.; Boyle, A.; Shih, H.; Sievers, R.E.; Zhang, Y.; Prasad, M.; Su, H.; Zhou, Y.; Grossman, W.; Bernstein, H.S.; et al. Sca-1+ cardiosphere-derived cells are enriched for Isl1-expressing cardiac precursors and improve cardiac function after myocardial injury. *PLoS ONE* **2012**, *7*, e30329. [CrossRef]
40. Barile, L.; Messina, E.; Giacomello, A.; Marban, E. Endogenous cardiac stem cells. *Prog. Cardiovasc. Dis.* **2007**, *50*, 31–48. [CrossRef]
41. Beltrami, A.P.; Barlucchi, L.; Torella, D.; Baker, M.; Limana, F.; Chimenti, S.; Kasahara, H.; Rota, M.; Musso, E.; Urbanek, K.; et al. Adult cardiac stem cells are multipotent and support myocardial regeneration. *Cell* **2003**, *114*, 763–776. [CrossRef]
42. Choi, S.H.; Jung, S.Y.; Suh, W.; Baek, S.H.; Kwon, S.M. Establishment of Isolation and Expansion Protocols for Human Cardiac C-kit-Positive Progenitor Cells for Stem Cell Therapy. *Transplant. Proc.* **2013**, *45*, 420–426. [CrossRef]
43. Zhou, Y.; Pan, P.; Yao, L.; Su, M.; He, P.; Niu, N.; McNutt, M.A.; Gu, J. CD117-positive cells of the heart: Progenitor cells or mast cells? *J. Histochem. Cytochem.* **2010**, *58*, 309–316. [CrossRef]
44. Veinot, J.P.; Prichett-Pejic, W.; Song, J.; Waghray, G.; Parks, W.; Mesana, T.G.; Ruel, M. CD117-positive cells and mast cells in adult human cardiac valves-observations and implications for the creation of bioengineered grafts. *Cardiovasc. Pathol.* **2006**, *15*, 36–40. [CrossRef]
45. Sandstedt, J.; Jonsson, M.; Lindahl, A.; Jeppsson, A.; Asp, J. C-kit+ CD45- cells found in the adult human heart represent a population of endothelial progenitor cells. *Basic Res. Cardiol.* **2010**, *105*, 545–556. [CrossRef]
46. Di Meglio, F.; Castaldo, C.; Nurzynska, D.; Romano, V.; Miraglia, R.; Bancone, C.; Langella, G.; Vosa, C.; Montagnani, S. Epithelial-mesenchymal transition of epicardial mesothelium is a source of cardiac CD117-positive stem cells in adult human heart. *J. Mol. Cell. Cardiol.* **2010**, *49*, 719–727. [CrossRef]
47. Bronnum, H.; Andersen, D.C.; Schneider, M.; Nossent, A.Y.; Nielsen, S.B.; Sheikh, S.P. Islet-1 is a dual regulator of fibrogenic epithelial-to-mesenchymal transition in epicardial mesothelial cells. *Exp. Cell Res.* **2013**, *319*, 424–435. [CrossRef]
48. Min, K.W. Interstitial cells of Cajal (pICC) in the pancreas. *J. Cell. Mol. Med.* **2005**, *9*, 737–739. [CrossRef]
49. Manetti, M.; Guiducci, S.; Ruffo, M.; Rosa, I.; Faussone-Pellegrini, M.S.; Matucci-Cerinic, M.; Ibba-Manneschi, L. Evidence for progressive reduction and loss of telocytes in the dermal cellular network of systemic sclerosis. *J. Cell. Mol. Med.* **2013**, *17*, 482–496. [CrossRef]
50. Metzger, R.; Rolle, U.; Fiegel, H.C.; Franke, F.E.; Muenstedt, K.; Till, H. C-kit receptor in the human vas deferens: Distinction of mast cells, interstitial cells and interepithelial cells. *Reproduction* **2008**, *135*, 377–384. [CrossRef]
51. Armulik, A.; Genove, G.; Betsholtz, C. Pericytes: Developmental, physiological, and pathological perspectives, problems, and promises. *Dev. Cell* **2011**, *21*, 193–215. [CrossRef]
52. Smith, C.L.; Baek, S.T.; Sung, C.Y.; Tallquist, M.D. Epicardial-derived cell epithelial-to-mesenchymal transition and fate specification require PDGF receptor signaling. *Circ. Res.* **2011**, *108*, e15–e26. [CrossRef]
53. Rudat, C.; Norden, J.; Taketo, M.M.; Kispert, A. Epicardial function of canonical Wnt-, Hedgehog-, Fgfr1/2-, and Pdgfra-signalling. *Cardiovasc. Res.* **2013**, *100*, 411–421. [CrossRef]
54. Chong, J.J.; Reinecke, H.; Iwata, M.; Torok-Storb, B.; Stempien-Otero, A.; Murry, C.E. Progenitor cells identified by PDGFR-alpha expression in the developing and diseased human heart. *Stem Cells Dev.* **2013**, *22*, 1932–1943. [CrossRef]
55. Cretoiu, S.M.; Popescu, L.M. Telocytes revisited. *Biomol. Concepts* **2014**, *5*, 353–369. [CrossRef]
56. Manole, C.G.; Gherghiceanu, M.; Simionescu, O. Telocyte dynamics in psoriasis. *J. Cell. Mol. Med.* **2015**, *19*, 1504–1519. [CrossRef]
57. Wang, F.; Bei, Y.; Zhao, Y.; Song, Y.; Xiao, J.; Yang, C. Telocytes in pregnancy-induced physiological liver growth. *Cell. Physiol. Biochem.* **2015**, *36*, 250–258. [CrossRef]
58. Marini, M.; Mencucci, R.; Rosa, I.; Favuzza, E.; Guasti, D.; Ibba-Manneschi, L.; Manetti, M. Telocytes in normal and keratoconic human cornea: An immunohistochemical and transmission electron microscopy study. *J. Cell. Mol. Med.* **2017**, *21*, 3602–3611. [CrossRef]
59. Milia, A.F.; Ruffo, M.; Manetti, M.; Rosa, I.; Conte, D.; Fazi, M.; Messerini, L.; Ibba-Manneschi, L. Telocytes in Crohn's disease. *J. Cell. Mol. Med.* **2013**, *17*, 1525–1536. [CrossRef]
60. Vannucchi, M.G.; Traini, C.; Manetti, M.; Ibba-Manneschi, L.; Faussone-Pellegrini, M.S. Telocytes express PDGFRalpha in the human gastrointestinal tract. *J. Cell. Mol. Med.* **2013**, *17*, 1099–1108. [CrossRef]

61. Zhou, Q.; Wei, L.; Zhong, C.; Fu, S.; Bei, Y.; Huica, R.I.; Wang, F.; Xiao, J. Cardiac telocytes are double positive for CD34/PDGFR-alpha. *J. Cell. Mol. Med.* **2015**, *19*, 2036–2042. [CrossRef]
62. Breiteneder-Geleff, S.; Matsui, K.; Soleiman, A.; Meraner, P.; Poczewski, H.; Kalt, R.; Schaffner, G.; Kerjaschki, D. Podoplanin, novel 43-kd membrane protein of glomerular epithelial cells, is down-regulated in puromycin nephrosis. *Am. J. Pathol.* **1997**, *151*, 1141–1152.
63. Al-Rawi, M.A.; Mansel, R.E.; Jiang, W.G. Molecular and cellular mechanisms of lymphangiogenesis. *Eur. J. Surg. Oncol.* **2005**, *31*, 117–121. [CrossRef]
64. Adamczyk, L.A.; Gordon, K.; Kholova, I.; Meijer-Jorna, L.B.; Telinius, N.; Gallagher, P.J.; van der Wal, A.C.; Baandrup, U. Lymph vessels: The forgotten second circulation in health and disease. *Virchows Arch.* **2016**, *469*, 3–17. [CrossRef]
65. Wetterwald, A.; Hoffstetter, W.; Cecchini, M.G.; Lanske, B.; Wagner, C.; Fleisch, H.; Atkinson, M. Characterization and cloning of the E11 antigen, a marker expressed by rat osteoblasts and osteocytes. *Bone* **1996**, *18*, 125–132. [CrossRef]
66. Mahtab, E.A.; Wijffels, M.C.; Van Den Akker, N.M.; Hahurij, N.D.; Lie-Venema, H.; Wisse, L.J.; Deruiter, M.C.; Uhrin, P.; Zaujec, J.; Binder, B.R.; et al. Cardiac malformations and myocardial abnormalities in podoplanin knockout mouse embryos: Correlation with abnormal epicardial development. *Dev. Dyn.* **2008**, *237*, 847–857. [CrossRef]
67. Sawa, Y. New trends in the study of podoplanin as a cell morphological regulator. *Jpn. Dent. Sci. Rev.* **2010**, *46*, 165–172. [CrossRef]
68. Astarita, J.L.; Acton, S.E.; Turley, S.J. Podoplanin: Emerging functions in development, the immune system, and cancer. *Front. Immunol.* **2012**, *3*, 283. [CrossRef]
69. Karunamuni, G.; Yang, K.; Doughman, Y.Q.; Wikenheiser, J.; Bader, D.; Barnett, J.; Austin, A.; Parsons-Wingerter, P.; Watanabe, M. Expression of lymphatic markers during avian and mouse cardiogenesis. *Anat. Rec.* **2010**, *293*, 259–270. [CrossRef]
70. Manetti, M.; Rosa, I.; Messerini, L.; Guiducci, S.; Matucci-Cerinic, M.; Ibba-Manneschi, L. A loss of telocytes accompanies fibrosis of multiple organs in systemic sclerosis. *J. Cell. Mol. Med.* **2014**, *18*, 253–262. [CrossRef]
71. Benias, P.C.; Wells, R.G.; Sackey-Aboagye, B.; Klavan, H.; Reidy, J.; Buonocore, D.; Miranda, M.; Kornacki, S.; Wayne, M.; Carr-Locke, D.L.; et al. Structure and Distribution of an Unrecognized Interstitium in Human Tissues. *Sci. Rep.* **2018**, *8*, 4947. [CrossRef] [PubMed]
72. Kholova, I.; Dragneva, G.; Cermakova, P.; Laidinen, S.; Kaskenpaa, N.; Hazes, T.; Cermakova, E.; Steiner, I.; Yla-Herttuala, S. Lymphatic vasculature is increased in heart valves, ischaemic and inflamed hearts and in cholesterol-rich and calcified atherosclerotic lesions. *Eur. J. Clin. Investig.* **2011**, *41*, 487–497. [CrossRef] [PubMed]
73. Simeone, P.; Trerotola, M.; Franck, J.; Cardon, T.; Marchisio, M.; Fournier, I.; Salzet, M.; Maffia, M.; Vergara, D. The multiverse nature of epithelial to mesenchymal transition. *Semin. Cancer Biol.* **2018**. [CrossRef] [PubMed]
74. Smits, A.M.; Dronkers, E.; Goumans, M.J. The epicardium as a source of multipotent adult cardiac progenitor cells: Their origin, role and fate. *Pharmacol. Res.* **2018**, *127*, 129–140. [CrossRef]
75. Moerkamp, A.T.; Lodder, K.; van Herwaarden, T.; Dronkers, E.; Dingenouts, C.K.; Tengstrom, F.C.; van Brakel, T.J.; Goumans, M.J.; Smits, A.M. Human fetal and adult epicardial-derived cells: A novel model to study their activation. *Stem Cell Res. Ther.* **2016**, *7*, 174. [CrossRef] [PubMed]
76. Van Tuyn, J.; Atsma, D.E.; Winter, E.M.; van der Velde-van Dijke, I.; Pijnappels, D.A.; Bax, N.A.; Knaan-Shanzer, S.; Gittenberger-de Groot, A.C.; Poelmann, R.E.; van der Laarse, A.; et al. Epicardial cells of human adults can undergo an epithelial-to-mesenchymal transition and obtain characteristics of smooth muscle cells in vitro. *Stem Cells* **2007**, *25*, 271–278. [CrossRef] [PubMed]
77. Gittenberger-de Groot, A.C.; Winter, E.M.; Poelmann, R.E. Epicardium-derived cells (EPDCs) in development, cardiac disease and repair of ischemia. *J. Cell. Mol. Med.* **2010**, *14*, 1056–1060. [CrossRef] [PubMed]
78. Bax, N.A.; van Oorschot, A.A.; Maas, S.; Braun, J.; van Tuyn, J.; de Vries, A.A.; Groot, A.C.; Goumans, M.J. In vitro epithelial-to-mesenchymal transformation in human adult epicardial cells is regulated by TGFbeta-signaling and WT1. *Basic Res. Cardiol.* **2011**, *106*, 829–847. [CrossRef]
79. Risebro, C.A.; Vieira, J.M.; Klotz, L.; Riley, P.R. Characterisation of the human embryonic and foetal epicardium during heart development. *Development* **2015**, *142*, 3630–3636. [CrossRef]

80. Viragh, S.; Gittenberger-de Groot, A.C.; Poelmann, R.E.; Kalman, F. Early development of quail heart epicardium and associated vascular and glandular structures. *Anat. Embryol.* **1993**, *188*, 381–393. [CrossRef] [PubMed]
81. Vrancken Peeters, M.P.; Mentink, M.M.; Poelmann, R.E.; Gittenberger-de Groot, A.C. Cytokeratins as a marker for epicardial formation in the quail embryo. *Anat. Embryol.* **1995**, *191*, 503–508. [PubMed]
82. Manta, L.; Rusu, M.C.; Pop, F. What podoplanin tells us about cells with telopodes. *Ann. Anat.* **2018**, *218*, 124–128. [CrossRef] [PubMed]
83. Liu, X.N.; Wang, S.; Yang, Q.; Wang, Y.J.; Chen, D.X.; Zhu, X.X. ESC reverses epithelial mesenchymal transition induced by transforming growth factor-beta via inhibition of Smad signal pathway in HepG2 liver cancer cells. *Cancer Cell Int.* **2015**, *15*, 114. [CrossRef] [PubMed]
84. Tian, H.; Xu, J.Y.; Tian, Y.; Cao, Y.; Lian, C.; Ou, Q.; Wu, B.; Jin, C.; Gao, F.; Wang, J.; et al. A cell culture condition that induces the mesenchymal-epithelial transition of dedifferentiated porcine retinal pigment epithelial cells. *Exp. Eye Res.* **2018**, *177*, 160–172. [CrossRef] [PubMed]
85. Stark, K.; Vainio, S.; Vassileva, G.; McMahon, A.P. Epithelial transformation of metanephric mesenchyme in the developing kidney regulated by Wnt-4. *Nature* **1994**, *372*, 679–683. [CrossRef]
86. Kispert, A.; Vainio, S.; McMahon, A.P. Wnt-4 is a mesenchymal signal for epithelial transformation of metanephric mesenchyme in the developing kidney. *Development* **1998**, *125*, 4225–4234.
87. Gessert, S.; Kuhl, M. The multiple phases and faces of wnt signaling during cardiac differentiation and development. *Circ. Res.* **2010**, *107*, 186–199. [CrossRef]
88. Merki, E.; Zamora, M.; Raya, A.; Kawakami, Y.; Wang, J.; Zhang, X.; Burch, J.; Kubalak, S.W.; Kaliman, P.; Izpisua Belmonte, J.C.; et al. Epicardial retinoid X receptor alpha is required for myocardial growth and coronary artery formation. *Proc. Natl. Acad. Sci. USA* **2005**, *102*, 18455–18460. [CrossRef]
89. Compton, L.A.; Potash, D.A.; Mundell, N.A.; Barnett, J.V. Transforming growth factor-beta induces loss of epithelial character and smooth muscle cell differentiation in epicardial cells. *Dev. Dyn.* **2006**, *235*, 82–93. [CrossRef]

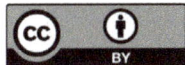

© 2019 by the authors. Licensee MDPI, Basel, Switzerland. This article is an open access article distributed under the terms and conditions of the Creative Commons Attribution (CC BY) license (http://creativecommons.org/licenses/by/4.0/).

MDPI
St. Alban-Anlage 66
4052 Basel
Switzerland
Tel. +41 61 683 77 34
Fax +41 61 302 89 18
www.mdpi.com

Applied Sciences Editorial Office
E-mail: applsci@mdpi.com
www.mdpi.com/journal/applsci

www.ingramcontent.com/pod-product-compliance
Lightning Source LLC
LaVergne TN
LVHW070632100526
838202LV00012B/784